Praise for S.E.X.

"*S.E.X.* is, literally, a lifesaving book: Corinna's vast commonsense wisdom—especially on topics relating to gender roles, queer sexuality, and gender identities—has the potential to improve the physical and emotional health of anyone who reads it, and to help heal our culture's unhealthy, conflicted approaches to sex, sexuality, and gender."

—Lisa Jervis, cofounder, *Bitch*

"Sexpert Heather Corinna is the big sis you wish you'd had when you were a confused, pimply teen. . . . Geared towards 16–22-year-olds of any gender, *S.E.X.* covers the nuts and bolts of anatomy in a tone that's conversational, not cutesy . . . it's her holistic approach and deft handling of other heavy topics, from eating disorders to abuse, that make this book a must-read."

—*BUST*

"If you're a parent looking for an accurate and non-judgmental text for your blossoming adolescent, or a blossoming adolescent or twenty-something yourself, here it is."

—*Toronto Star*

"*S.E.X.* is a positive and informative all-embracing guide to sexuality by a dedicated author. Heather Corinna challenges adolescents and young adults alike to be proactive in owning their sexuality by being true to themselves, all the while laying the foundation of knowledge and acceptance—key factors for the development of a healthy sexuality."

—DR. LYNN PONTON, author of *The Sex Lives of Teenagers* and *The Romance of Risk*

SECOND EDITION

S·E·X

THE ALL-YOU-NEED-TO-KNOW SEXUALITY GUIDE

TO GET YOU THROUGH YOUR TEENS AND TWENTIES

HEATHER CORINNA

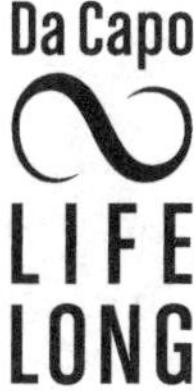

Many of the designations used by manufacturers and sellers to distinguish their products are claimed as trademarks. Where those designations appear in this book and Da Capo Press was aware of a trademark claim, the designations have been printed in initial capital letters.

Illustrations by Isabella Rotman

Designed by Jill Shaffer
Set in 11 point Bembo and 9.5 point Helvetica Neue LT by Eclipse Publishing Services

Cataloging-in-Publication data for this book is available from the Library of Congress.
ISBN: 978-0-7382-1884-7 (paperback)
ISBN: 978-0-7382-1885-4 (ebook)

Second Da Capo Press edition 2016

Published by Da Capo Press, an imprint of Perseus Books, a division PBG Publishing, LLC, a subsidiary of Hachette Book Group, Inc.
www.dacapopress.com

Note: The information in this book is true and complete to the best of our knowledge. This book is intended only as an informative guide for those wishing to know more about health issues. In no way is this book intended to replace, countermand, or conflict with the advice given to you by your own physician. The ultimate decision concerning care should be made between you and your doctor. We strongly recommend you follow his or her advice. Information in this book is general and is offered with no guarantees on the part of the authors or Da Capo Press. The authors and publisher disclaim all liability in connection with the use of this book.

Da Capo Press books are available at special discounts for bulk purchases in the U.S. by corporations, institutions, and other organizations. For more information, please contact the Special Markets Department at 2300 Chestnut Street, Suite 200, Philadelphia, PA, 19103, or call (800) 810-4145, ext. 5000, or e-mail special.markets@perseusbooks.com.

10 9 8 7 6 5 4 3 2

For young people:

At Scarleteen, at the Spruce Street Inn Secure Crisis Residential Center, all the way back to the little preschool I ran in Rogers Park in the mid-1990s, and in many other settings and interactions, I have learned so much about not just this work but about life, love, and living itself from young people. My life has been more rich, meaningful, and unique for all of your places and parts in it than it ever could have been without all of you: **thank you.** I hope this book gives you back at least as much as all you've given me.

For the Liams:

Before you know it, it'll be time in your lives for a book like this one. When it is, I hope you like it and only go "*Eew!*" as many times as it's fun. Know that you can talk with your Aunt Heather about any of this stuff anytime: I promise to only be as silly about any of it as you are.

Contents

Thank You

From idea to bookshelf, the process of riffing, writing, proposing, researching, writing some more, editing, surveying, and then researching again, rewriting, editing again, shopping, shopping again, and then researching yet *again,* and editing once more (with feeling!) took nearly six years. And now, almost a decade since the first edition, there's been yet another big process in revising and updating this book.

There were a lot of people in that many years of work and there isn't anything close to enough paper to thank all of them properly. Those who cannot fit into these few pages still have real estate in my heart. To all of you, my humblest thanks and deepest gratitude. I am incredibly lucky to have a wide, caring, and supportive network of family, friends, colleagues, co-learners, and supporters with so much faith in me. I'm one lucky ducky to have had all of you as part of this endeavor.

To the Grand Pooh-bah and all the staff at Da Capo Lifelong Press for taking this on—the first time, and now again!—and for making the arduous process of publishing so relatively painless.

Boundless thanks to Renée Sedliar: you first found this book a great home when I was sure it would remain ever homeless, fought the good fight, wielded your editorial machete like a peaceable ninja, took my serious stuff seriously, talked me down from the occasional total freakout, laughed at my jokes, and even came back for round two, you silly masochist, you. The prospect of working with you again was literally half my happy at creating a second edition. I could not ask for a better advocate and editor; this is a book made far, far better for your irreplaceable part in it and dedication to it. You're the tops!

To Christopher Schelling: for your tireless attempts to find a home for this book the first time around, your incredible patience with me (and everyone else), and your support.

To the Scarleteam, my incredible staff and volunteers at Scarleteen: for your passionate dedication to sex education, young adults, and sexual health and your constant faith in my unique approach. An additional thanks for your saintly patience with me during the creation of the second edition, when I learned too late that you can't work two full-time jobs anymore when you're middle-aged and do either with any kind of consistent competency. You all had my back, helped cover my butt, and gave even more than you already do of your valuable time and energy to make sure Scarleteen and its users didn't suffer when I was scattered and spread thin. **The Scarleteam RULES.**

To Clare Sainsbury, who has often saved—and keeps on saving—the day.

To the generous people who gave me invaluable aid and information the first time around, especially editorial assistants Laurel Martinez and Kythryne Aisling, and consultants Rebecca Trotzky-Sirr; Janel Hanmer, MD, PhD; Richard Fraser, APNP; Laura Jones; Kerrick Adrian; Erin Seiberlich, MD; Terri Rearick, RN, BS, CIC; Ben Wizner of the ACLU; and Hollie West, RN, BScN.

Great gratitude to a few new additions for round two, all of whom stepped it up for me and this book at the eleventh hour because I lacked the foresight to ask in a more reasonable time frame, including Margaret Hobart, Johanna Schorn, and Amanda Seely. To Dr. Deborah Oyer, who I feel certain is the best abortion and reproductive health provider on the planet, who I'm blessed to call colleague and friend, and whose educated and eagle-eyed comments and corrections were invaluable. To Sam Wall, who not only provided extra coverage at work for me at Scarleteen but also gave me some great feedback on one of the chapters I really needed hers for. To my neighbor and pal Cath Airola, who, lucky for me, was a dedicated public defender for years who cares a lot about people and their rights and supports what I do enough to have leant me some of her time, mind, and patience with my sometimes-cutthroat creative process.

To CJ Turett, soul-brother, beloved friend, and one of the most thoughtful, kind, smart, and also ridiculous people I know: you not only gave me great and generous commentary and correction but also questioned my sanity and intelligence when called for with an impressive amount of grace and love. Plus, I'm always happy for any excuse I can get to work with you, even if it's not the co-writing of songs for *Dangerous, Dangerous Anal* and *Shrimper and the Masturbats* I truly wish it were. (And no tushie tampons for you!)

To my longtime friend and editorial assistant Brandon Sutton, for his fantastic assistance during the maddening first round of edits, his willingness to camp out and work for weeks, and his much-appreciated companionship and good humor throughout. Because you are either just that deeply dedicated to this book, a glutton for punishment, or—and most likely—probably a bit of both, you even let me bring you over here for a *second* time around when I realized, as I entered the final stretches, that it just wasn't the same without you. Thanks for both your insight and your wonderful company, without which this new edition wouldn't be as good as it is and my sanity would have been much more tenuous than usual.

To Isabella Rotman, for lending her formidable talents to the illustrations for this edition, and for her perpetual good cheer even when I'm a stressed-out grumpus, and for being one of the coolest creative collaborators in this work I've had the pleasure of knowing and working with. Shine on, you crazy diamond.

To the Scarleteen users who trusted me with very personal information in surveys for the first edition to ensure everyone got what they really needed, and to the young readers who read faster than they ever had in their lives to participate in the final focus group for the book, especially Celine, Joey, Joanna, Ceylon, Matt, Irmelin, Maggie, Vero, Hannah, Kelly, and Emily.

To Peter Mayle, author of *Where Did I Come From?:* If not for the unbearable cuteness of those wiggly, pink sperms with roses in their teeth and his tale of reproduction for the littlest readers, which was my favorite book at the age of five, I suspect that I and this book might not have wound up where we did.

To the incredible people who have played an integral part in providing initial and ongoing mentorship and support for me in this area of work, most notably: Anne Semans, Cathy Winks, Carol Queen, Robert Morgan, Cory Silverberg, and Hanne Blank. To the women, specifically—especially because in this arena, like so many others, women have been and remain less acknowledged and valued—of my sexual, political, and intellectual ancestry, without whose work mine would not have been possible: Victoria Woodhull, Simone de Beauvoir, Shere Hite, Virginia Johnson, the Boston Women's Health Collective (including two of the amazing founders who wrote the foreword for this book!), the Jane Collective, Sarah Weddington, Natalie Angier, Joani Blank, Judith Levine, Anne Fausto-Sterling, Marge Piercy, Adrienne Rich, Anaïs Nin, Betty Dodson, Annie Sprinkle, Susie Bright, Dorothy Allison, Audre Lorde, Marie Stopes, Margaret Sanger, and others who have fought against the tide to express, champion, and protect equality, balance, and inclusion in human sexuality.

To Brandy, therapist-extraordinaire: there's no way I could have gotten the second edition done and dealt with everything else in my lap without your thoughtful support and guidance, including the occasional f-bombs I so appreciate from you.

To my community and all of the cherished friends who—during the first round of this book, the second, or, for the real masochists of the group, both!—lent me their eyes and ears, shut the computer and dragged me outside, boosted me up when I needed it, supported my endeavors, accepted my utter lack of attention to them for months on end, dealt with my scatterbrain-like champs, and otherwise participated in the care, watering, and feeding of me. For those of you I haven't thanked above already, I'm talking about **you** Becca Nelson, Mark Price, Ben Haley, Audra Williams, Karen Rayne, Megan Anderson, Jacqui Shine, Casey Faber, Elise Matthesen, Sabrina Dent, Kathleen Kennedy, Emily Woods, Jeyoani Wildflower, Justin Hancock, Garrett Coakley, Lauren Bacon, Jane Duvall, Al Potyondi-Smith, MJ Wagener, Lana Crawford, Heather Spear, Jenny Lobasz, Emira Mears, Michelle Demole, Beppie Keane, Stephen Luntz, Trixie Fontaine, Jennifer Andrade-Ward, Molly Bennett, Caroline Dodge, Kaari Busick, Meri Shepard, Emily Burns, Pam Keesey, Jaclyn Friedman, and, my more-cherished-than-I-can-say sister-from-another-mister, Briana Holtorf.

My parents are two of the most wildly different people one can imagine, whose mean average somehow = me. (It's uncanny, really.) I have my mother to thank for my unstoppable work ethic and confidence in my place in my field, my understanding of enough medical mumbo-jumbo so that I can translate it for everyone else, my fierce loyalties, and for being one seriously ass-kicking babe to look up to. Thanks to my father for instilling in me the strong spirit of revolution, empowering my voice in however I have wished to use it; for our amazing and enduring friendship; and for never letting me forget for a minute (even when I wanted to) that, if I think something's broken, I shouldn't give up on trying to fix it.

To Jim: *I* certainly wouldn't want to live with a writer and activist, especially during this kind of process. I will never fully understand why you choose to, but I sure am incredibly glad and grateful for it. Thanks for making such a wonderful home with me and being such a huge, enduring, and important part of my chosen family; for entering into Act Three of our epic trilogy spanning more than two decades; for your support; and for both your care for me when I forgot to do all those nonessential things like eating and sleeping and your forgiveness of the tunnel vision that is unfortunately part and parcel of doing this kind of project. I sure hope that the readers of this book have at least one love as unique, grand, and complex as ours in their lifetimes. All the Xs and all the O's: I love you the mostest.

My dogs can't read, but they would think me very rude if I didn't thank them anyway, so thanks, Trouble Pants and Moo (but not for the barkus-interuptus). I promise to try to make up for all the long walkies you missed during the making of the second edition, and, you're right, I was just the absolute worst for not putting your needs first.

P.S. To the me of my teens and twenties: thanks for being the best kind of big-hearted badass. If I didn't have your high expectations of me to meet, I probably wouldn't have done most of what I have done and am most proud of in my life and work, including this book. You're the best of me, and know I never forget it.

Foreword

JUDY NORSIGIAN AND WENDY SANFORD, COFOUNDERS,
THE BOSTON WOMEN'S HEALTH COLLECTIVE, AND
COAUTHORS OF *OUR BODIES, OURSELVES*

As cofounders of Our Bodies Ourselves, we are huge fans of Heather Corinna—and *S.E.X.*, their wonderful book. Almost forty-five years after the first publication of *Our Bodies, Ourselves*, we admire how this brilliant educator and activist takes up the vital work of providing culturally relevant, up-to-date, and trustworthy resources on sexuality and health. Ever since Heather created Scarleteen.com, for young people of all orientations and gender identities, we have recognized Heather and their team as close colleagues and sisters in the work.

Heather is dedicated to providing utterly useable and highly engaging resources on sexuality and health for young people of all stripes. With a unique voice—accessible, nonjudgmental, humorous, respectful, encouraging, imaginative and clear—Heather is superb at this work, and we are proud to welcome you to this thoroughly updated and expanded edition of *S.E.X.*

Most of us were in our twenties when we first came together to talk openly about our bodies, breaking silences that had for so long kept women in the dark. When we realized how little useful information we had been given about our bodies—from orgasm to menstruation, from contraception to sexually transmitted infections—we decided to learn for ourselves, just like you are in reading this book. We tracked down the factual details. We learned from each other's experiences. And we made a political analysis of the practices and policies that limited women's control over our sexuality and reproduction—from sexist medical school training and laws making abortion a crime to the biases against women of color that were built into the medical care system. To share what we were learning, we created what eventually became *Our Bodies, Ourselves*. Today, so many years later, the book has reached close to five million readers in more than twenty languages around the world.

We were young women educating ourselves and then mobilizing for change. If you're reading this book, you know that young people are as critical a force for change today as they were when we were young, and they have been in all of history. Though Heather asks readers of this book only to enjoy their own lively, self-defined sex and to respect others' right to do the same, their vigorous slant on justice—on the need to counter inequities based on race or class, sexual orientation or gender identity—may just inspire your own activism.

Heather knows the power of information that goes beyond mere facts. Heather knows that people's stories matter and that we must challenge the laws and biases that restrict our freedom to be who we are and to love who we love. This new edition of *S.E.X.* shows a deep commitment to justice and inclusion: gender-neutral pronouns and body part descriptions are used throughout; there's strong support for any person who is stretching or refusing restrictive notions of a male/female gender dichotomy; there is new work on the central importance of consent in sexual relationships, balancing "no means no" with "yes means yes"; young LGBTQ people who counter healthcare discrimination will learn what to do . . . and so much more.

Our work on college campuses convinces us of the ongoing need for clear, accurate, and nonjudgmental information about sex and relationships; we always recommend *S.E.X.* and Scarleteen.com. We hope that many parents, teachers, and others who care about young people will join us in helping this treasured resource reach an ever-wider audience.

We are proud to join Heather in creating an intergenerational conversation that promises to bring us all greater sexual pleasure, acceptance, and respect for who we are. The world will be a better place for that, and we hope you'll join in—for yourself and others.

—Wendy Sanford and Judy Norsigian,
two of the coauthors of
Our Bodies, Ourselves, the classic
about women, health, and sexuality

Who's This Book for, Anyway?

A FOREWORD FOR PARENTS, TEACHERS, MENTORS, AND OTHER PEOPLE WHO CARE ABOUT TEENS AND EMERGING ADULTS

This is a book for adolescents: for teens and emerging adults.

But this book can also be for parents, guardians, teachers, mentors, aunts and uncles, moms' and dads' work friends, grandparents, friends—anyone with an interest and investment in the sexual health and overall well-being of young people.

Anyone who's paid attention to history and current events, basic physiology, psychology, and sociology—and anyone with simple life experience—knows that sexuality is inevitable, important, and integral. Anyone with that knowledge and experience also knows that sexual choices, sexual identity, and sexual health have a huge impact on our world, interpersonally and globally. Sexual choices that just aren't right for everyone involved, sexual dissatisfaction, power inequities, sexual shame, fear or feelings of sexual obligation, manipulation, violence and victimization, sexualization, and some other big bads greatly contribute to or create personal and global problems such as unprepared or unwanted pregnancy or parenting, negative body image and low self-esteem, abusive and unhealthy relationships, sexual abuse and assault, illness, sexism, homophobia, and sexual objectification and exploitation. Some of those things are so normalized, common, and even idealized that it can be challenging to even know or recognize what a healthy, happy sexuality in real life can look like or be like, let alone to create and nurture it.

Accurate, explicit, accessible, and nonjudgmental sexuality information that respects young people and their capabilities offers important and needed protection from the bad stuff and support for the good stuff. When young people know what consensual, enjoyable, and equitable sex is and that it is absolutely within reach, they can understand and feel more confident nixing what is not consensual, what is not enjoyable—physically, emotionally—and what is not.

Learning about preventative care related to sexuality—reproductive health care, safer sex practices, birth control—supports them in caring for their bodies as a whole as well as protecting themselves from sexually transmitted infections and unwanted pregnancy. Learning to love and accept their whole bodies—including, but not limited to, their sexual and repro-

What's in This Book and What Isn't: The Short List

- The term *abstinence* is very rarely used in these pages. However, I *do* discuss celibacy and holding off on partnered sex or a specific kind of sex we can have with partners. Discussion of how this can happen in healthy, responsible ways, and only when it's what everyone involved really wants for themselves, is paramount.
- There's nothing in here that suggests saying no to partnered sex is always better than saying yes. Instead, there's a focus on figuring out what's right for any given individual, uniquely, and recognizing that sometimes no is the right answer for someone, and sometimes yes is.
- Sexuality is not discussed in an essentialist context that only recognizes or champions limited numbers of sexual orientations, genders or gender identities, relationship models, sets of values, religions, or ages. It is discussed as diverse, reflecting the diverse people we are and our diverse sexualities, relationships, and unique circumstances and lives.
- It is presumed and asserted that all living beings are entitled to their sexuality, sexual identity, and right to make fully consensual sexual partnership choices to the degree that they have the agency to make them.
- I use an approach that might be more inclusive or progressive than you're used to or familiar with. Gender-neutral pronouns; a nonbinary approach to bodies, genders, and sexual orientations; and a presentation of sexuality and relationships that aims to represent the highly diverse spectrum of people's lived experiences are employed. This approach is rarely found in older frameworks and understandings of sexuality.
- Because the current pervasive cultural approach to human sexuality and young adult sexuality is often considerably flawed, alternative approaches are often presented.
- I do not claim to have all the answers, nor do I assert that there is one set of sexual choices or behaviors that is best for everyone. My aim here is to give readers information and perspective to help them come up with their own answers and figure out their own best choices. My goal is to be a helper and a guide, not a dictator.

ductive anatomy—promotes their lifelong sexual and general health, well-being, and self-esteem. Learning how to assess and improve the quality of intimate relationships, to figure how they do or don't mesh with another individual's wants and needs—which may differ from cultural standards—and to advocate for themselves within a relationship enables them to be healthy, happy, and whole. Knowing about and accepting the range of positive, realistic, and diverse human sexuality choices protects young adults from others who would—and often do—prey upon and exploit sexual ignorance, fear, or shame. All of these aspects and others open the door to safer sexual lives, sexual lives that are enjoyable, beneficial, satisfying, and empowering.

Chances are good that when it comes to my opinion, my cultural and social analyses, my ethics and values, or my assessments of the sexual lives of young people and sexuality as a whole, you won't always agree with me. That's okay. I probably wouldn't always agree with you either. There's a lot of room in this book for a wide range of opinions, feelings, and beliefs.

Many years ago, I received an unforgettable letter from a parent. He wrote that, although he supported the work I did, he didn't share a lot of my personal views. He told me he was a "once-player," now an avowed "Jesus freak," and that he'd raised his daughter conservatively. He also told me that he was so glad I was around, and that he, quite appreciatively, had directed her to the information I made available. He had explained to her that she'd heard all the things he had to say and that she should go read some different views, too—accurate information—and, thus, be best equipped to make up her own mind, to make her own decisions, wherever they fell along the spectrum.

Ultimately, this book aims to provide information to help lay a solid foundation for clear, usable, informative, and healthy sex education to benefit individual readers and their support networks.

[HOW CAN YOU USE THIS BOOK?]

Read It Yourself, First, and Get Up-to-Date

Many adults didn't get accurate, inclusive sex education and don't keep up with current, sound information unless they've sought it out for themselves and their own sexual issues, interests, or concerns. If you're going to talk to young people in your life about birth control, safer sex, sexual assault, or what makes a relationship healthy and what doesn't, you'll want to make sure that you're not unintentionally endangering them when you want to help protect them. It is challenging to obtain accurate and sound sex information in the first place, plus the information is constantly changing because of new research and new social contexts. I do this work full time and have for almost twenty years now; I am constantly checking new reports, studies, and books and reading new questions, and even *I* have a tough time keeping up.

Read this book yourself before you set it out for young people. Check out information available from other reliable, comprehensive sources such as the

Sexuality Information and Education Council of the United States (SIECUS), the Guttmacher Institute, Planned Parenthood, and the other sound organizations and clearinghouses listed in the Resources section at the end of this book. You can get on mailing lists so that new information and studies are delivered right to your Inbox. Build a small library at home of accurate sexuality and relationships information. Ask a family healthcare provider or counselor to help you learn what you need to know. Check the back of this book, too, for recommended books for parents written by fantastic parent educators that can help you navigate parenting about and with sexuality. More and more low-cost and no-cost classes and workshops are available for parents and guardians that can give you information, ideas about your approaches, as well as a nice support network of other parents who are trying to do this right and who can keep you company in this great, but sometimes quite daunting, adventure.

The information in this book can be useful to you in discussions about sexuality with the young people in your life, and you may even find that the information benefits your own sex life as well. Bonus!

Normalize Sexuality Discussions

To foster comfort, trust, and calm communication, discussions about aspects of

What's Healthy Sexual Development?

Healthy sexual development is much bigger than just avoiding disease, unwanted pregnancy, or sexual abuse or about having—or not having—any kind of sex with partners at a certain age.

The fifteen key domains of healthy sexual development identified in the *International Journal of Sexual Health* are as follows:

i. Freedom from unwanted activity
ii. An understanding of consent and ethical conduct more generally
iii. Education about biological aspects of sexual practice
iv. An understanding of safety (This is meant in the widest possible sense, including physical safety, safety from sexually transmitted diseases, and safety to experiment.)
v. Relationship skills
vi. Agency (In this context, agency includes young people learning that they are in control of their own sexuality and of who can take sexual pleasure from their bodies.)
vii. Lifelong learning
viii. Resilience
ix. Open communication (This includes communication about sex and sexuality within families.)
x. Awareness that sexual development should not be "aggressive, coercive, or joyless"
xi. Self-acceptance
xii. Awareness and acceptance that sex can be pleasurable
xiii. Understanding of parental and societal values
xiv. Awareness of public/private boundaries
xv. Competence in mediated sexuality (This refers to skills in accessing, understanding, critiquing, and creating mediated representations of sexuality in verbal, visual, and performance media.)

sex and sexuality should be relaxed, ongoing, and commonplace from the get-go rather than taking place when the issue is fever-pitch or personal. There's no need to wait for a time, year, or event to have that One Big Talk.

"The Talk" is not only never going to cut it—sexuality is much too diverse, ever shifting, and complex for any one talk to cover everything a teen needs to know—and when parents or guardians try to come at this that way, The Talk often never even happens or happens much, much too late. It's pretty easy to put something off that's so intimidating. And, your comfort (or lack thereof) with the topic aside, trying to construct one perfect talk that covers all of sex is intimidating because it's also impossible.

Instead, do your best to cultivate and nurture regular, less formal, and more relaxed discussions about general health, body issues, development, relationships, and sexuality. Talks about sex that concern cultural or world events or rules and policies at school can take place over dinner, for instance, and are excellent ways to take a lot of steam out of the overheated engine of parent/teen sex talk. By the time your children are developing sexually, physically and otherwise, and they have started thinking about or are having sexual partners, talking with you about sex should feel pretty comfortable, even if there are still some (inevitable) rough spots.

It can be trickier if you're feeling that only *now* is the time to start these discussions and the young person or people in your life are already in their late teens or even heading off to college or to live independently. A whole lot of sexual information and personal sexual ethics and values are ingrained before puberty even gets going, so if your child is already in their teens or twenties, I'm afraid you're running late. But just as any birth control is always better than no birth control, any time you choose to foster open, honest, and sensitive sexual discussion with a child or teenager is far better than never doing it at all.

If you're picking this book up to start talking for the first time about sexuality to the emerging adult in your life:

- ▶ You might want to open the discussion by explaining why the subject hasn't been discussed before (for instance, because you were worried about bringing it up at the wrong time or in the wrong way and lousing it all up, or because you lacked modeling from your own parents, so just didn't know how to do this).
- ▶ Ask more questions at first rather than doling out answers: **listen more than you talk, and try to be responsive, not reactive.**
- ▶ If you've avoided talking about sex until now or you tried before and gave up because of embarrassment, know that you're not alone. Talking about something so intimate is difficult for a lot of people. It may have been tricky for you to figure out how to talk about it without feeling that you're crossing boundaries or grossing your teen out. Let them know that. If you feel embarrassed, say so. If you're worried about boundaries, tell them. That sort of humility and realness can be a good icebreaker because often they feel exactly the same way.

▶ You can let your child or children know you'd be open to and interested in discussing the book or other sexuality information with them and ask whether they'd like to initiate those discussions or have you do it. You could even organize an informal family or group book club about it if that's your usual dynamic. As with anything else, the best approach depends a lot on your family and your unique child: what's comfortable for one may be embarrassing for another.

[THE SILENT TREATMENT]

One of the toughest things many adults face when it comes to talking to teens or emerging adults about sex is that many aren't always going to—or just plain don't want to—talk to them. That can happen to even the most open, honest parent, to the parents who have great relationships with their children and who have had good talks about aspects of sex throughout their lives. It can happen to the parent whose child truly thinks of them as their

"I" Statements Are Your Bestie

Voicing what your subjective viewpoints and ethics are and explaining that they are *yours*—not theirs, not universals—are very big deals. One of the easiest ways to isolate a young person who is in the process of forming a personal identity is to give the impression that your choices and experiences must or should be theirs. It's also one of the best ways to shut down communication and openness rather than to support and encourage them.

Remarks like "casual sex is disrespecting yourself" or "you'd be better off focusing on your homework than boys/girls right now" are not "I" statements and probably won't be welcomed. Statements like "sex before marriage is wrong" or "you just think you're bisexual, you can't know that" are dogmatic and subjective. Young people aren't stupid; they usually know these sorts of statements are based on your opinion and in your own unresolved issues. Strident presentations often leave them feeling resentful, controlled, and disrespected. If you've made the same choices you're telling them they shouldn't make, they may feel (validly) that you're being hypocritical and they may tune you out completely. Judgmental statements like these often do an excellent job of telling a young person that you're the last person they should talk to about any of this.

Try this on for size: "Starting to have sex at fifteen was too early for *me* because I didn't understand the risks or consequences of sex, and I think it kept me from achieving my goals." Or this: "I just don't understand how you can know you're bisexual now, because I'm forty-one and even I'm still not sure about *my* orientation." Or, "I'm concerned that if you start dating now, other things I know are important to you might get lost in the shuffle," or "I feel sex before marriage is wrong because we're Catholic, and in our religion, premarital sex isn't okay." Then follow any statement like that with: "What do *you* think? Why do you feel that way? How do you think I can support and help you while respecting our differences?"

best friend. And that can be heartbreaking for that adult, obviously.

Most of our sex lives are private; for a young person, there's no exception. (One teen in the surveys for this book said, *"My parents don't talk to me about their sex life, why should I talk to them about mine?"*) Healthy boundaries and positive separation between parents and teens or emerging adults also mean allowing for privacy about or around sex and sexuality. Beyond that, for many young people, talking to parents about their sex lives is just a little too intimidating. They may not be toddlers anymore, and they may say they don't care, but to many, parents are still the sun, moon, and stars. That can make it difficult even for a teen who is behaving very responsibly or who isn't even sexually active yet. Even voicing doubts about whether they want to be active in the future, and how, can be uncomfortable if they're worried about parental judgments, as the vast majority are. You thinking well of them means so much, risking your disapproval is a big and seriously scary deal.

Many teens or emerging adults are more likely to talk to almost everyone else besides their parents: friends, partners, other relatives, teachers, you name it. That's not necessarily a bad thing, even though it might make you feel like you're out of a loop you should be in or that you've erred in your parenting somehow.

Allowing them the freedom to talk to someone else can help open the doors of communication between you and your child so they can know you're available and you *can* have productive discussions with them. Giving them room to get a range of perspectives, information, and avenues of support can make them feel more inclined to *also* talk with you.

And if you're waiting for them to initiate discussion, stop waiting! One of you has got to take the leap, after all, and it's harder for them to do so than for you.

[GIVING THIS BOOK TO TEENS AND EMERGING ADULTS]

This book is intended for an adolescent readership, those roughly between the ages of fifteen and twenty-five. Some readers could utilize and absorb it at younger ages, and plenty of readers will still find a good deal of this information new at older ages. If you're an attentive and involved parent, guardian, or mentor, you probably have a pretty good idea of when a book like this is appropriate for the young adults in your life. Trust your instincts.

I suggest you make this book and others like it readily but casually available: don't hide it or pass it over as if it were the Dead Sea Scrolls. Dedicate an area of your bookshelf to books that concern shared family issues—or, heck, books about sex, period. And when they're curious and interested, they'll seek out the information. Young minds do a great job of knowing when, how, and what they're curious about and can absorb. If your child asks a question about sex that you don't know how to answer, pull out this book, or another like it, and find the answer together. This shows them where and how to find accurate information and has the added benefit of showing them that you are invested in providing them with this information. Further, this approach illustrates the fact that sex is a very big and complex topic about which none of us has all the answers: not them or their peers, not the media, not you.

I have never—not in years of reading hundreds of thousands of young people's postings online about these issues, not in thousands of e-mails—seen even one young person express that a parent who was down-to-earth, honest, compassionate, respectful of boundaries, and primarily concerned with their well-being, in other words, a parent who just really tried to do their best with all this, had seriously screwed things up in addressing sex with them. **Never.**

IS IT EVER TOO EARLY?

Giving a book like this to a ten- or eleven-year-old—maybe with the idea of being as supportive and proactive as possible—is unlikely to be in any way damaging but probably won't be very helpful either. For instance, even very intelligent ten-year-olds are unlikely to read information about birth control, sexually transmitted infections, or communication with sexual partners and somehow store it in their minds for later. Likely, it just isn't applicable to them now; what information we retain has a lot to do with how relevant it is to us at the time we encounter it. This book also isn't written in a style that's very accessible for younger readers, and the size and scope of it alone may freak them out. For some preteens and even plenty of teenagers, making a big presentation of a book like this too early may actually feel like pressure or a statement that they *should* be ready for or interested in these issues. If they're not interested yet, this can make them worry about what stage of development and sexual interest they should be in. For a list of recommended sexuality books for young children, younger teens, and young people with developmental or learning disabilities who might find the depth or volume of this book overwhelming, see the Resources section.

Of course, I certainly have heard more than a few express how they felt embarrassed or insulted when parents brought up sex in any number of ways or gave them sexuality books or items. But that "Ugh! My super-uncool mom/dad/aunt!" stuff has never struck me as overriding the positives these kids gleaned from caring parents or guardians who were doing their best to ensure that their teens were comfortable with their sexuality and had all the information possible to make the best choices about a healthy, happy sex life.

And even if you do stumble—maybe you freak out at a teen coming out, becoming sexually active, taking up with a partner you don't like or feel is unsuitable, or even starting puberty—most of the time, brushing yourself off and plopping a Band-Aid on the wounds heals them up in no time. All you can do, all anyone can do, is their best, and your best is awesome, even in places where you might struggle.

Ultimately, if you care about young people, accept they're becoming adults, and love and seek to support the people they're becoming—maybe not who you want them to be, I'm talking about who *they* are—you're going to do just fine, and so are they.

Every young person is different. Some of the "facts" in this book might surprise you. You may have thought, for instance, that the average age when people become sexually active these days was younger or older than it is. Some of the issues addressed in this book may be pertinent to the young people in your life, some may not. Some parts of this book may make you feel much more comfortable about young adult sexuality; some may make you more uncomfortable. You may have various levels of comfort with your child even reading parts of this book at all.

But they do need this information. Every day, between twenty thousand and thirty thousand readers worldwide visit Scarleteen.com, and they often come to us only after finding loads of inaccurate information or after already forming very busted frameworks or false beliefs about their bodies, minds, hearts, sex, sexuality, or sexual health. The information at the website and in this book is informed by all the questions we've been asked over the nearly two decades Scarleteen has been in existence, by candid and open discussions young people themselves initiate and sustain.

We field as many pregnancy scares, rape crises, and anal sex questions in a day as we do questions about breast development, weight gain, gender inequity, bisexuality, orgasm, and how to ask someone out or break up. What young people want to know about sexuality at any specific moment is incredibly varied and individual. Given the annual number of unplanned and unwanted pregnancies in young people, given that for decades older teens and emerging adults have had the highest rates of new sexually transmitted infections, given the body image and self-esteem issues so many young people grapple with, given the rates of sexual assault and abuse, given the dangerous social isolation of many queer and gender-nonconforming youth, given the endless mixed messages from the media and the inaccuracy and politicization of so much school-based sex ed, as well as the misinformation peers and partners disseminate, they don't just want this, they **need** this.

At this point in their lives, they are already establishing ideas about and patterns in their sexual identities and behavior that form the foundation of their sexual lives and intimate relationships for their whole lives. If they feel unable to say no or yes now; if they feel ashamed, afraid, or confused now; if they don't learn how to practice contraception or safer sex now; if they don't learn what they do or don't want sexually now, they may well never learn it.

They need this information.

And they need *you*. They need you most of all.

This book, and others like it, paired with proactive, informed, and relaxed (as relaxed as it gets, anyway, when it comes to sex) parenting and modeling in loving, supportive environments will nurture a much different world than we have now—a much better world.

In other words, this book is valuable, but it increases in value substantially when you—parents, extended family, mentors, teachers, role models, and other caring adults—are just as big an influence as it is.

So, who's this book for?

Everyone.

I Pledge Allegiance . . . to Myself and the United State of My Sexuality

AN INTRODUCTION FOR READERS

As you start to read this book, I invite you to make a bold choice: to envision, create, and stand up for a healthy, happy, and satisfying sexual life that you make and live exactly to fit and benefit the unique person *you* are and anyone else you decide to share it with. I'm talking about a sexuality and sexual life that are all yours and that come from who you are and what you want, not one based on scripts, standards, or ideals that someone else—often someone who's never even met you—came up with.

We all *have* the power to do that, no matter our age or gender, whether we're currently choosing to be sexually active with partners, or whether it even feels too soon to do *anything* in terms of our sexuality. You have the power to shape every choice you make about sexuality into a choice that supports your happiness, health, and well-being, one based on your unique criteria, and, if and when you add anyone else to the mix, one based on how both of your sexualities, wants, and needs can work together.

For sure, spelling out sexuality isn't simple: sexuality is a big, bubbling stew of sociology and chemistry, physical and emotional development, and individuality, nature, and nurture. Each person's sexual self not only is always shifting and evolving in a whole bunch of ways throughout life but also is a very personal and individual combination of desires, identity, and self-image; relationship wants and needs; interpersonal patterns, ideals, and previous experiences; and emotional, chemical, and physical ways of being and experiencing all of life, including sexuality. Add to that simmering pot life and cultural contexts and circumstances like personal and public health issues, reproductive issues and choices (or a lack thereof), laws, cultural and community values, attitudes and expectations, personal ethics, and sexual fantasy and reality. **You really *are* a special snowflake.**

That's a lot to sort out, process, and learn to juggle and fit into the rest of your life. Take it all on the road with other people in relationships, add all of *their* stuff to yours, and it's pretty easy to see why so many people can feel overwhelmed.

But when you make smart, healthy, and informed choices that really do feel right for you, at a pace that really works for you—including when you have enough accurate information even to know how to figure that out—it's not that hard to stay safe and sound and to *enjoy* your sexuality and your sexual life, which is what they're for in the first place.

You've got more freedom to create and claim what is best for you sexually than your grandparents or even your parents did. Now more than ever before complete and accurate information is within reach: about sexuality as a whole, about infection and disease, about reproduction and birth control. That information is also a lot less biased than it was even just a few decades ago. We have greater access to information and to sexual health services and support. Even though media, public health, politics, and the ever-changing values of our world add extra complications and confusion—especially given the mixed messages we tend to get about sex and sexuality—you can choose a lot of what you make part of your life and your frameworks of sexuality and all of what you sign on to for yourself (or don't). When it comes to sex and sexuality, you even have the ability to positively influence the media and public health policies, both with your personal choices and with your collective actions as a generation.

You have a unique opportunity to create, explore, nurture, and enjoy an authentic, personal sexuality that is beneficial for you and others, that's healthy and feels balanced, that is informed and empowering, and that can allow you to find and express intimacy, joy, fun, and pleasure in your life.

So, I hope you make a choice to do just that, and I hope this book helps you do that. This choice alone nearly guarantees that every other sexual choice you make will be a good one.

Maybe you picked up this book because you felt like you wanted to begin exploring your sexuality or because you felt like you couldn't get away with ignoring your sexuality any longer. Maybe someone gave you this book because you asked about sex, because you're at a time in life when you're likely to be curious about sex, or just because they're a cool person who loves you to bits and wants you to have all the sexuality information you need when you want and need it.

No one person, group, or book can—or should—tell everyone which choices are right for them, because there is no *one* right set of sexual choices for everyone. Not even close. What is absolutely right for one person can be absolutely wrong for someone else. Only you can figure out what your sexuality should be like, what you want from it, and how to define and design it accordingly.

What this book *can* do is to give you a solid foundation of information so that you can make those choices more soundly for yourself. I may be something of an expert when it comes to sexuality, but the only person who is an expert when it comes to *your* sexuality is **you.**

There's no one right way to use this book. You might find that some parts of the book are more useful to you than others, that you're already past some of the material, or that some of it isn't information you need yet. (You might feel ambivalent about certain parts or even feel a little scared, weirded out, or overwhelmed by the book now, and that's okay, too.) Some parts may be more useful to a sibling, friend, or partner than they are to you. Some of what's addressed may be within your personal experience; some may be outside it. The information in here might be something you want to digest and process alone, or you might want to use it to initiate or further discussions with friends, partners, or family.

You can read this book cover to cover if you like, but you'll more likely use it as the reference book it is, reading whatever section or topic you need or are curious about. What you do and don't need from this book at any time will have to do with what sex education you've got under your belt so far and your unique life circumstances. It should give you a whole lot of answers, and it should also present you with some new questions. However you use it to help you make choices that are best for you at any given time is the right way.

I want this book to be something that can help you enter into or continue your sexual life confidently, gladly, and comfortably—and with as much information and support for what's best for **you.** It's intended to help *you* spell out what *your* sexuality is and how *you* want it to be.

I don't aim to be the expert on you, your relationships, your sexuality, or your sexual life: I'm not, I shouldn't be, and I can't be. No one else can be the expert on us, whether we're talking about an educator like me or a sexual partner. You are the expert on you, and you can become more and more of one throughout your life. My aim is to do what I can to help you uniquely create and enjoy exploring and expressing a healthy, happy, and fulfilling sexual life that's good for you and for everyone else in it and to help you feel confident being your own expert.

2

Your Sexuality and Your Body: An Owner's Manual

[WHAT IS "SEXUALITY"?]

Sexuality isn't technically "adult" or something that pops out of the blue when anyone reaches a certain age: it's been with all of us from day one; it just hasn't always been—and won't always be—the same for every phase of our lives. When as infants we comforted ourselves by sucking our thumbs, by nursing, by touching our own bodies, even our genitals, part of what we were experiencing was sexuality. When as children we enjoyed the smell, the feel, or the sounds of things, when we learned about the world by putting everything we could grab into our mouths, when we wanted to peek into underpants other than our own, and when we asked about our parents' adult bodies, we were experiencing some of our sensual and sexual nature and curiosity. If we played doctor, experienced our interest in being physical with others, masturbated or examined our own bodies, began getting crushes on peers or adults, started to become more and more curious about sexuality, our sexual selves were further developing, just as they'll continue to grow, change, and develop for the whole of our lives.

Sexuality isn't just about your genitals, though, or about having sex. It's a mix of many different things—of physical, chemical, emotional, intellectual, social, and cultural aspects—and that mix is different for, and unique to, everyone.

Our physical and emotional development from children into adults shifts our sexual wants, needs, and identity. Infant sexuality and adult or adolescent sexuality are very different. By the time we're well into or finished with puberty, our sexuality usually becomes or has already become something that can feel new to us even though it really isn't and that usually feels like a much, much bigger thing than it ever did before.

What Can Be Part of Sexuality?

The Physical

The physical part of sexuality includes the development, health, and function of our whole body—including our brain, central nervous system, and reproductive organs, the three biggest players in our physical experience of sexuality—and our experience of being in our body. It also includes our very unique and personal experience of our senses and sensuality.

Physical sexuality encompasses our experience of our sexual responses and something called "skin hunger," which is the physical experience of desiring touch. As teens and emerging adults, we tend to experience less and less touch from family members as we get older. People often don't recognize how big a part just plain wanting to be touched can play in a young person's developing sexuality.

The Chemical

I'm talking neurochemicals—hormones—here, not recreational substances or medications but the chemicals our body makes and distributes all by itself. All too often hormones take the blame for hasty or poor sexual choices, choices no other way of accounting for seems to exist, as in "Those dirty hormones made me do it!" Hormones are not at all close to what

Sexuality Is Epic

You might say sexuality is about our minds, bodies, and neurochemicals (aka: hormones); about our feelings and our relationships; or about touching and being touched. You might think it's about doing and engaging in one kind of sex or any kind of sex or about wanting, seeking, or experiencing certain kinds of pleasure. You might say it's about parts of our identity, like our gender identity or sexual orientation. You might say it's about reproduction: about making babies (or not). You might say it's about our desires to be close to—or far away from—other people in ways we define or experience as sexual or about feeling horny, lusty, tingly, mingly, hungry, itchy, twitchy, or whatever words you use to express a strong feeling of "I can haz sex NOW, plz."

There's no one exactly right model when it comes to defining sexuality. I'm going to talk about it a couple of ways here, based on our current definitions and frameworks in sex education and sexology, the scientific study of sex and sexuality. But if they don't feel like a perfect fit for you, adjust as you like. These things get adapted and adjusted all the time, including by those of us who work in this field. Even in just the last fifty years, the way we talk about sexuality and the models of it we create have changed a lot. In the next fifty years, this may change, too.

our total sexuality is—nor are they some kind of Evil Overlord that can make people do sexual things against their will. They are not a sound scapegoat for poor sexual decision making, though they can certainly play a part in it. *Sex* hormones—testosterone, estrogen, and progesterone—usually get most of this blame, but there are others—such as GABA, adrenaline, serotonin, vasopressin, oxytocin, dopamine, and endorphins—that influence sexuality, often in a much bigger way than the previous three mentioned.

The Emotional and Intellectual

Emotional and intellectual parts of sexuality include our feelings, values, and ideas about everything that informs our sexuality, such as body image, gender identity, and sexual orientation; sexual desires and fantasies; sexual activity with ourselves and with partners; relationships and sexual self-image; and the way we feel about sexuality and sex as a whole, not just our own.

Feelings *are* part of our sexuality in every and any sexual interaction or desire, though what kind of feelings they are varies. Sometimes we hear people say they've had or want to have sex "without feelings," but the only way we could do that, seriously, would be to cut off our heads. Although we may not have, be open to, or experience the same kinds of feelings in every sexual interaction, because we're alive and conscious emotions are always part of the picture—it's just that *how* we feel is very varied and diverse. We can't magically turn our emotions off in any part of life, including sex and sexuality.

The Social and Interpersonal

Social and interpersonal facets of sexuality include all our relationships with sexual partners and potential partners, friends, and family. The myriad other kinds of relationships and interactions we have with others is also involved, as is the influence our relationships and interactions have on our feelings about and our experiences with our sexuality.

What we want and need sexually from and with others are part of the social and interpersonal aspects of our sexuality. So is how we experience the ways others express their wants and needs and how we might assume those wants and needs play into this part of their sexuality.

The Cultural

Because we are all individuals and members of larger groups, our sexuality is influenced by how the rest of our world—including peers, local and larger communities, government and other larger cultural systems, media—views sexuality as a whole and our sexuality (including sexualities assigned to us, even when they're so not ours).

Cultural influences on our sexuality include what messages, overt and covert, about sexuality we get from our cultures and what we feel or experience as allowed or disallowed, "good" or "bad," idealized or admonished. These influences affect us, whether we're aware of it or not.

Circles of Sexuality

Things in each of these groups overlap a lot. That's because we just can't completely compartmentalize them: we can't really put them each in tiny little boxes where everything always stays neatly in its own container without touching or influencing anything else. The Circles of Sexuality model, designed by Dr. Dennis M. Dailey, does a great job of defining and explaining sexuality and illustrates this overlapping nicely.

Sensuality: Sensuality is about physical senses, our awareness and experience of them. Sensuality also involves our awareness and experience of our body as a whole, including our body image and our experiences of physically exploring or sharing the bodies of others, and not just with sex. Sensuality is about our experience of all kinds of pleasure: seeking, exploring, and experiencing it, alone or with others.

Intimacy: Intimacy is the ability and desire for closeness with other people. It can include sharing, caring, emotional risk taking, and vulnerability. Sex can be a

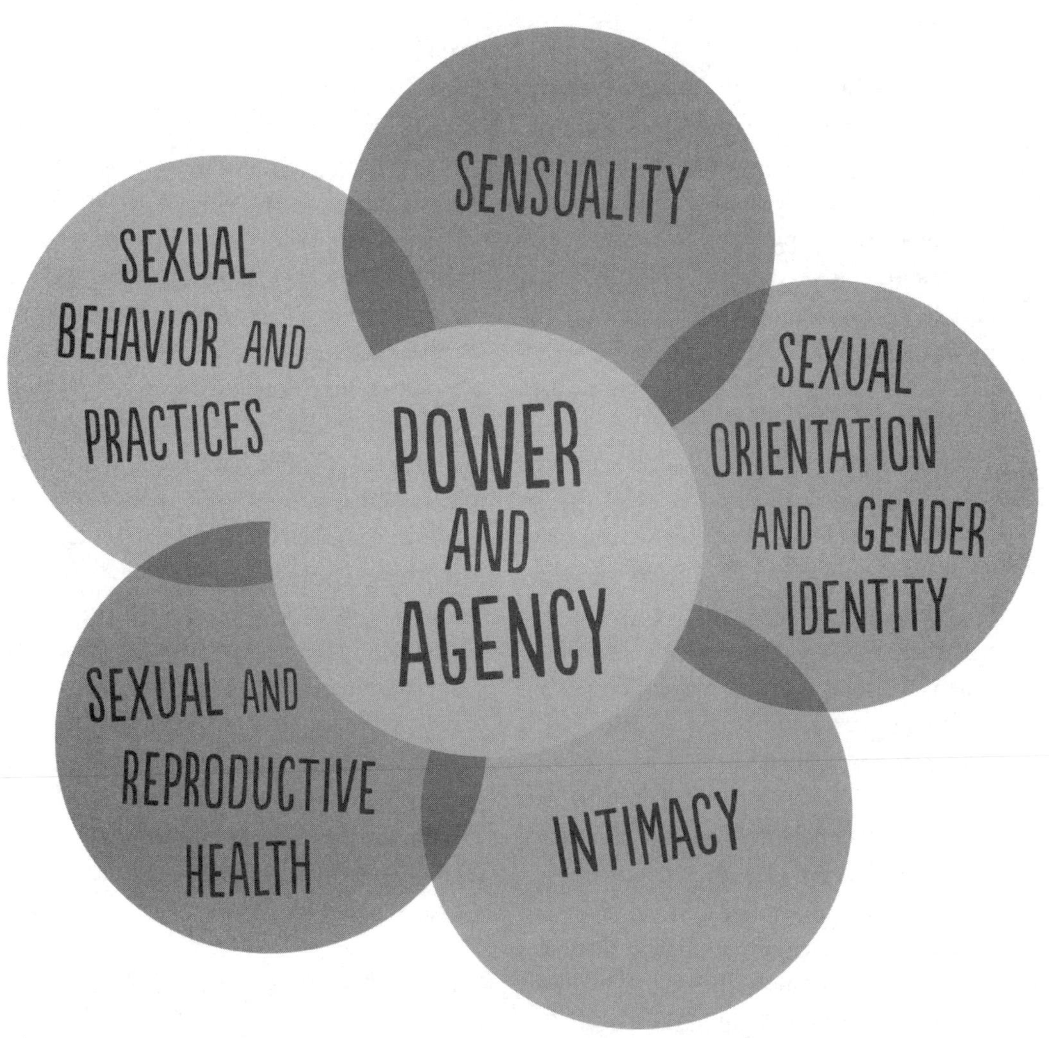

way to explore and experience intimacy, but sometimes sex isn't about intimacy at all—it depends on the experience. Intimacy also doesn't always look or feel the same way for everyone—including for people sharing an experience together—or with every experience. When and if we seek sex with others, we're usually seeking intimacy. Such encounters might not deliver the same kind of intimacy every time or the kind of intimacy someone else is seeking. Usually, we are just looking to share an experience in which we're close to someone else in some way.

Sexual Orientation and Gender Identity: Gender identity is a person's feeling, sense, or understanding of who they are related to their gender. Sexual orientation, one part of most people's larger sexual identity, includes the ways they express that part of themselves and what parts gender plays in sexual feelings and desires they experience, want, or are part of with other people.

Our biases, stereotypes, and fears can play roles here, too, just like they can in all the other circles. In other words, ways we think about other people or ourselves regarding gender or sexual orientation—just like ways we may think of others when it comes to physical ability or disability, race or ethnicity—can also play a part in our sexuality.

Sexual and Reproductive Health: Our capacity or ability (or lack thereof) to reproduce, feelings about and experiences with reproduction, and behaviors and attitudes about sex and reproduction all play a part in our sexuality. This includes the information we have about sexual anatomy, sexual activities, reproduction, contraception, sexually transmitted infection (STI) prevention, and self-care, among other topics, and the messages that information gives us about all of those things. This circle is also about our experiences of sexual wellness and illness, including ability and disability, and how these experiences influence our sexuality and sexual desires and experiences. Having emotionally healthy sexual relationships is also a part of sexual and reproductive health.

Sexual Behaviors and Practices: Sexual behaviors and practices are what we or others actively do sexually to explore, enact, or express our sexuality. They include who is doing what when it comes to their own body parts and those of a sexual partner or partners and, for example, whether sex toys and other objects are involved. This part of sexuality isn't always a "do" or "have done" for everyone: some people may want or desire certain behaviors or practices but have not yet engaged in them for any number of reasons, including lack of opportunity or ability, fear, or something else. Even if someone doesn't or hasn't yet actively done a particular sexual act, the behaviors and practices that person is interested in or wants often play a big part in their sexuality. Sexual behaviors and practices aren't just about sex with partners; masturbation is part of this circle, too. What we do *not* want to do sexually can also be part of our sexuality and how we experience it.

Power and Agency: Power is the ability or capacity to do something and can be about strength or force or the ability or capacity to exercise control over ourselves or others. *Agency* is a sociological and philosophical term that addresses a person's capacity to act: what a person has the right, ability, or power to do. How much power or agency each of us has in general and in specific situations varies a whole lot, in really big ways—based on what power and agency we may or may not have in the world because of how rich or poor we are, what color we are, what our gender is, how our bodies do or don't work—and then in smaller, more situational ways, such as in one given relationship.

Power and agency play a huge part in all aspects of sexuality, which is why this version of the circles model puts it smack in the middle connected to everything. Power and agency influence our sexuality from our sense of self-worth and our understanding of our sexual preferences and values, which can enable us to realize sexual well-being and health, or, when we lack or don't feel our own power and agency, can be a barrier to all the good things. We may or may not have or feel varying amounts of power and agency to influence, negotiate, decide, consent, or decline when it comes to sexual experiences. We or others may use power or agency to manipulate, control, or harm others in our sexual experiences, too.

Not everyone's sexuality or the way they express it is healthy, and what's emotionally healthy or isn't tends to have a whole lot to do with power and agency. If we feel and use whatever power and agency we have when it comes to sex to care for ourselves and others, to seek out mutual pleasure and well-being, and we act from a secure emotional place where we give ourselves and others high value and worth, then chances are good we're using or enacting our power and agency sexually in emotionally healthy ways.

Power and agency are also in the middle of all the other circles because how much power and agency people have, what they do with power and agency, as well as how they are affected by others' power and agency connect power and agency to all the other issues.

Let's Talk About Sex

In common language, *sex* is often used to mean genital intercourse or other kinds of sexual activities with someone else. But what the word *sex really* refers to is how we divide a species into two categories based on the appearance of the external genitals, which often corresponds to an individual's chromosomal structure. *Sex* as used in this way is usually understood and most often presented as binary, with only two categories: male and female.

Some basic aspects of human sexual development and reproductive anatomy and function differ on the basis of sex. So, before we get started talking about the stages of puberty, it's helpful to know where we stand when it comes to our gonads.

Most of us were assigned a sex at birth as a result of a visual examination of our genitals, or we were assigned a sex while still in utero based on genital appearance as seen with an ultrasound.

How our genitals look, in utero and at birth, usually has a lot to do with our sex chromosomes, which are in the nucleus of every cell of our body and which guide

Intersex

The Intersex Society of North America defines *intersex* as "a general term used for a variety of conditions in which a person is born with a reproductive or sexual anatomy that doesn't seem to fit the typical definitions of female or male." Intersex is a socially constructed category that reflects real biological variation; this means *intersex* is a word people have come up with to describe sex diversity.

Some names for ways of being intersex are Klinefelter's syndrome, androgen insensitivity syndrome, adrenal hyperplasia, Sawyer's syndrome, and Turner's syndrome. As many as one in every one thousand to twenty thousand people born are born intersex. That's a big spread, I know—it's that murky because so few people ever have anyone looking at their chromosomes or ask a healthcare provider to evaluate conditions that can be related to being intersex, such as later puberty, variations in body shape, and fertility issues.

The bodies of many, if not most, intersex people look just the same and just as different and diverse as anyone else's.

If you think you might be intersex—because of your sexual development, general appearance, or fertility; because you're experiencing what seems like a serious delay in the onset of puberty; or because you have a profound feeling that your sex doesn't "fit" you—talk to your doctor. Intersex conditions usually don't need any sort of medical treatment, unless you can and want to treat them, but knowing you are intersex can be important when it comes to managing health issues and in terms of forming and claiming your identity.

the endocrine system in how it generates hormones that influence the development of our brains and other body parts, including our genitals and reproductive systems. Sex chromosomes, and the hormones they generate, aren't the only things that influence the development of our body, though, and they don't influence every body in the same way. In fact, a far greater amount of sex diversity exists than most people realize, and that diversity isn't limited to the appearance of genitals or other body parts.

The classic sex chromosome pattern for people who are classified on the basis of their chromosomes as male is called XY (because that's what the chromosomes look like under a microscope), and for those classified as female, XX. But other chromosomal combinations besides XY and XX exist (and other factors and processes contribute to physical sexual development, including the ways the body interprets and responds to hormonal signals). Some people think these are the only two sexes, but that isn't true. It's just that XY and XX are the most common.

Sex chromosomes matter because they guide the development of gonads, and gonads matter because they produce sex hormones, and sex hormones matter because they strongly influence the process of sexual and general physical and psychological transition—puberty—that we're about to discuss.

[MEGA-METAMORPHOSIS: PUBERTY]

During puberty, the entire body experiences growth spurts until a person's bone mass, overall body size and shape, sexual

Throughout this book, I may use language or an approach to gender and people's bodies that's new to you. As I just discussed, the whole idea of sex as a simple binary category is just plain old wrong, because there are more than two sexes. And *gender*—a person's sense of how masculine or feminine, both, or neither they feel; characteristics that our world links to sex; ideas that are cultural and, for many people, that feel like a thing that exists inside of them or that has to do with certain body parts (see Chapter 5 for more)—is even *more* varied than sex. For some people whose body has a vagina or a uterus, talking about their body as the body of a woman is right because they conceptualize themselves as a woman. But for others, that doesn't feel right at all, either because they identify as a female or a woman and don't (or no longer) have a vagina or a uterus or because they have a vagina or a uterus but don't feel like or identify themselves as a woman, or even as a man *or* a woman.

The way we assign a sex to people is iffy at best, but our way of assigning people a gender is *really* busted: gender, like our sense of faith (if we have one), ethnicity, or relationship status, is about who we feel we are and how we ideally want to identify ourselves—not who someone else decides we are based on our body parts or anything else besides how we tell them we want to be identified. I don't want to misassign gender to anyone reading this book; I want to do my best to respect what feels right for you in terms of your identity and how your body parts may or may not relate to that identity.

In most cases when I need a pronoun, I use a third-person gender-neutral pronoun—that is, *they* and *them*—for everyone. And when I talk about certain kinds of bodies, I won't assign gender to them—because it's not my place or anyone else's to assign gender to anyone!—so I talk about people who have a penis or testes, rather than boys, and people who have a uterus or a vagina, rather than girls. So, you'll see I use "people who have a penis" or "someone with a vulva" like you might say "people with freckles" or "someone with brown eyes" to describe other physical characteristics. If and when I say *cisgender,* I'm talking about someone whose gender identity feels like it matches their assigned sex; when I say *gender nonconforming* or *transgender,* I'm talking about someone who feels that their assigned sex, or the cultural roles or ideas associated with it, does not feel like it fits with the gender they identify with.

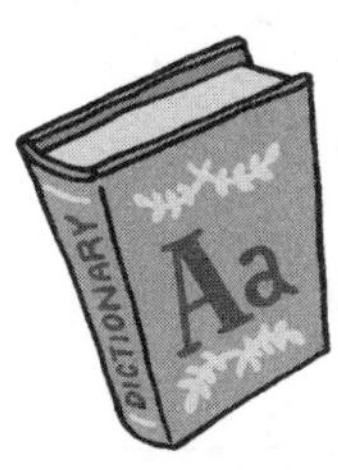

If any of this is new to you, it might feel a little *Huh?!?* at first, but you should get used to it in no time.

organs, and secondary sexual characteristics have finished their basic development. A ton of brain development and change, including neurochemical change, also happens throughout puberty. The human body—including our brain—never, ever stops changing, but puberty is a stage in which some of the most rapid and whole-body changes occur. Puberty often feels intense because **it is**.

On average, puberty begins for most people between the ages of eight and fourteen years. It usually starts earlier for someone with a uterus and later for someone with testes. Currently, puberty is considered to be "precocious," or early, if it begins before the age of eight; it's considered late if no development related to puberty has occurred by the age of fourteen. No matter when puberty starts, most people are finished with it by their mid-twenties. Puberty ends much later than most people realize.

It's common to feel awkward, overwhelmed, and self-conscious during puberty. A lot of people struggle with body image issues. Bodies gain weight as a necessary part of puberty, and they can become proportioned in ways that don't match cultural beauty ideals. Parts of our bodies during puberty can be in places for a while where they won't eventually land, and that can make a lot of people feel worried. Acne, voice changes, body hair, breast development (or slow development), unwanted erections, and the arrival

BASIC STAGES OF PUBERTY

If You've Got a Uterus

- **Breast development:** Most often, the first part of puberty is initial breast growth, called "breast budding" because growth starts with small lumps just under the nipples. These lumps do not always appear at the same time; sometimes one forms before the other. Breast development includes changes in the size and shape of the areolas, or nipple areas, as well as the rest of the breasts.

- **Vaginal discharges:** At or around the same time as breast budding, vaginal discharges become apparent. As a person gets further into puberty, or after they become sexually active, it's common to become far more aware of what's going on down there. So, if you've just noticed discharges because you weren't paying attention until now, it's likely nothing new.

- **Body hair and pubic hair growth:** After breast budding, pubic hair and other body hair usually begin growing. For some, pubic hair may appear before breast growth occurs.

- **Menarche:** Usually about two years after breast budding, the menstrual cycle begins, starting with first ovulation and then with the first period, called menarche. Menstruation may be delayed or super sporadic if someone is underweight or malnourished, overexercises, diets excessively, or has or develops an eating disorder.

- **Body size and shape changes:** The body both grows taller and changes shape. By the time a person has their first period, their peak growth—the most growth they'll have in life—in terms of height and bone mass is almost complete. It's normal during puberty to be gaining weight and to be eating more than before and probably more than you'll eat after puberty. It's also normal for the shape of the body to feel a bit disproportionate sometimes, which is one reason why adolescent body ideals should not be based on adult bodies (or vice versa).

If You've Got Testes

- **Penis and testicles:** Puberty most commonly starts with testicular growth. During the whole of puberty, the penis and testes will eventually grow to their adult size. It's common for the length of the penis to grow faster than the width of the penis and for testicle growth to start before penis growth. Growth of the penis and

of menstrual periods can be sources of body image woes. Adults and peers—often without even realizing it—may call unwanted attention to your changing body. A parent may feel their child needs a brassiere before the child wants one (if they ever want one) or may make a public joke about their child's wet dreams without thinking. Things like that often seriously increase the very common social shudder of puberty.

Our bodies feel simpler during childhood (mostly because they are). We don't have to navigate the challenges puberty brings. Developing more complex sexual feelings, the visible maturation of our reproductive and sexual organs, and the attention from others that comes with these developments can be big-time

testicles often is not complete until the end of puberty.

■ **Growth spurts:** Through puberty, people become taller and their muscle mass increases. It's normal to be gaining weight and to feel out of proportion at times. It is also common to experience nipple swelling, and some breast development is normal for larger people.

■ **Erections:** Whereas even infants can get erections, during puberty, erections occur frequently and involuntarily—something that is a source of embarrassment for many young people but that is completely normal. Many people get erections several times a day or more. Often, an erection isn't about sex or arousal; it can happen as a result of friction, temperature changes, and hormone fluctuations. An erection does not mean someone wants or needs sex right at that moment, and sex or masturbation isn't required to make an erection go away. Erections can be waited out and pass in a relatively short amount of time.

■ **Ejaculation:** When the ability to ejaculate develops—well after the ability to achieve an erection—it's typical for people to have "wet dreams," ejaculation that occurs while sleeping, as a result of sexual dreams, high levels of semen accumulation, stimulation from the touch of sheets and blankets, or having a full bladder. First ejaculation is sometimes called "spermarche," just like a first period is called menarche.

■ **Body and pubic hair:** Pubic hair—around the base of the penis as well as on the thighs and around and between the buttocks—is usually the first adult body hair to crop up and continues growing around the anus, buttocks, and legs. Growth of underarm hair usually follows, and chest and facial hair often develop last, sometimes even after the end of puberty.

■ **Voice changes:** During puberty, the voice deepens and may go through stages of being all over the place. At times, someone may experience voice cracking or croaking.

For Every Body

■ **Skin changes:** During puberty, it's normal for the skin to become oilier and for perspiration and body odor to become stronger because certain hormones are shuttling through the body at higher levels than in childhood, working their way up to levels where they'll stay when puberty is over. Pimples and zits, suck as they may, are as common as the sun in the sky. ■■

uncomfortable. Plenty of folks going through puberty have times when they truly hate or don't feel at home in their bodies; some people experience certain developing parts—such as breasts, pubic hair, or an erect penis—as gross and feel ashamed of them. For anyone who doesn't feel a harmony between their gender and assigned sex, puberty can even be traumatic.

Wishing you could avoid some or all of these changes is hardly uncommon. The ideas people have about young adult bodies as they're developing can be hard to deal with sometimes, like the insistence that you should be excited about development that doesn't thrill you at all or that you should hide things you really can't or don't want to hide.

Preteens or teens who start developing earlier or later than most of their peers can experience added stresses. Late bloomers may feel like babies—or be treated like them—compared to their friends or siblings and may feel left out. Those who start puberty early can find themselves the center of unwanted or inappropriate sexual attention or teasing and may feel weird compared to most of their peers who haven't started yet. People assigned male sex usually start puberty later than people assigned female sex, so the former group can encounter expectations of sexual development or desire from their peers that they don't feel ready for yet or just don't want at all.

Alas, just like other times in life when we experience a lot of physical or emotional changes that are outside our control, puberty is unavoidable, and there's no healthy way to curb the strain of certain parts of it. Excessive dieting, for example, to try to stop developmental weight gain, breast growth, or menses is only going to make you sick. You also can't make puberty hurry up by using herbal supplements or hormones, by weight training, or by behaving in certain ways. Puberty has its own timetable, and no matter what you do, it's going to stick to the schedule for you as an individual, which is mostly determined by your genetics and influenced by environmental factors such as nutrition and stress. But puberty is also temporary: it does end, and you only have to go through it once.

Braaaaaaaaiiiinnns

Before I move on to discuss what most people think of and what's most commonly called sexual and reproductive anatomy, I have something very, very important to tell you: when it comes to sexual response and pleasure (not just reproduction), **sex is mostly between your ears, not your legs.**

The largest, most important, and most active sexual organ in the body isn't genital, or "down there," but up much higher. It's the brain and its structures.

The brain is responsible for our emotions, our perceptions (including of pain and of pleasure), and our memories and for regulating and controlling our central nervous system, our cardiovascular system, our endocrine system, and our senses. The hypothalamus of the brain is responsible for the secretion of hormones that influence sexual feelings and response. The brain receives and processes messages from your sensory organs, giving you and other parts of your body information about how something (or someone, including yourself) looks, sounds, tastes, smells, and feels. It's also the brain that sends and receives signals regarding blood pressure, heart rate, body temperature, and respiratory rate—all huge parts of sexual function, experience, and response.

The pleasure center of your brain processes signals that indicate what's happening feels good (or doesn't), and your brain and nervous system transmit the feelings and sensations of orgasm. Not only is sex about communication between people but also it's about the systems of your brain and the rest of your body communicating. The beauty of bodies and brains is that they don't all communicate the same way. It may take time to figure out how your personal communication system works—it's definitely worth the effort.

Without your brain, you wouldn't be able to feel pleasure or pain, even if you were touched in a way or in a place many people find pleasurable or painful. The brain is primarily responsible for orgasm and what people feel during orgasm: during sexual pleasure, all the nerve endings of your body (including those of your genitals, which are all linked to your nervous system) work in concert and are in communication with your brain, and vice versa. Without all that goes on in our brains, we wouldn't have any interest in sex at all; nor would we find sex anything of interest.

The ways that sexuality is chemical, emotional (yes, even for those who say sex isn't at all emotional for them), psychological, intellectual, social, cultural, and multisensory, as well as physical, is all brain stuff. No matter what other parts of our body are involved in what's going on with us sexually, our brain is our biggest, most important, and most active sexual organ.

Once you understand this—how the brain functions and all the systems it controls and responds to—it's a lot easier to see why we, as a people, can be so sexually diverse and experience sex so differently from one another and from experience to experience. After all, if sex was only or mostly about our genitals, even considering the genital diversity I discussed earlier, we could expect that those of us with the same basic parts would all have the same basic experiences and the same sexualities. But we don't—not by a serious long shot—and that's primarily because of our brains. Once you understand how the brain is our largest and most significant sex organ, you can begin to see how thinking differently isn't necessarily a negative when it comes to sexual pleasure.

Tingly Bits

You might (or might not) have heard the term *erogenous zones*. It was popularized in the field of sexology in the 1960s and 1970s and describes areas of the body with high sensitivity. People often (but not always) find stimulation of these zones particularly sexually exciting.

High sensitivity in this context means that some areas of the body more than other areas have higher numbers of sensory nerve receptors (nerve endings that react to stimuli and pass impulses from sensory nerves to the central nervous system in a continual hey-how's-it-going/good-how-about-you running conversation between specific body parts and your brain). These are places where we're generally more sensitive to both pain and pleasure than in other areas of the body. When it comes to sensory nerves, see, not all parts of the body are created equal. That's why, for instance, we can find a lot of people who feel highly stimulated by someone rubbing their nipples (an area of high sensitivity) and fewer people who feel as highly stimulated by someone rubbing their elbows (an area of lower sensitivity).

Lists of erogenous zones can sometimes seem arbitrary—like someone is just listing what they personally like best—but for many people, typical erogenous zones are the lips, tongue, palms and fingers, soles of the feet, inner thighs, nipples, neck, ears, armpits, and genitals. Our skin, as a whole, really is an erogenous zone. Mucocutaneous regions of the body (those made of both mucous membrane and cutaneous skin) are also usually particularly sensitive; these are parts like the foreskin, penis, external clitoris, inner labia, perineum, mouth, and nipples.

Bear in mind, not only is individual sensitivity different—what feels great to one person may feel ticklish or like too much to someone else—but also what we carry in our brains about a given part of our body and what's happening there influences our sexual response.

If we have had violent or negative experiences or have ideas about a given part, even if that part is packed densely with sensory nerve receptors, stimulation there can feel unpleasant instead of pleasant. If someone we aren't into touches one of those areas without invitation, it tends to feel a lot different from when those parts are touched by someone we very much want to have touching us. When a relationship is really great, a partner touching us in such a place, in a certain way, might feel amazing. But if that relationship later goes straight to hell, that same person touching us in the same place in the exact same manner can feel lousy or even like nothing at all. One day, a given kind of stimulation might result in orgasm, whereas the very next day, it won't.

There goes the brain at work yet again, demonstrating how we can't segregate physical sensations from the overall experience and how what's going on with us up between our ears has a whole lot to do with what goes on down between our legs.

REPRODUCTIVE AND SEXUAL ANATOMY: WHAT'S UP DOWN THERE?

Although way more than our genitals and reproductive systems is involved with sex and sexuality, some body parts are pretty universally or scientifically classified as sexual anatomy.

Every Body's Got One: The Anus, Rectum, and Perianal Region

The anus—the external opening of the rectum, visible between your butt cheeks—is surrounded by two concentric rings of muscle: the internal and external sphincters. We can voluntarily control the external sphincter (in other words, you can think about opening it or squeezing it closed and make that happen); we can't control the internal. The anus is rich with sensory nerve endings: it has half the nerve endings of the whole pelvic region, and they are interconnected with other pelvic muscles. Same as for the vagina, most of those nerve endings are concentrated around the opening and just inside the opening (rectum). The anus is unlike the vagina in that it does not self-lubricate.

The nerves and muscles within and around the perianal area play a huge part in the genital sensations of sex and sexual response even when those parts might not be directly stimulated. In other words, not just anal sex involves this region: any kind of genital sex or genital sexual response does, no matter what you are (or aren't) doing.

You've Got Some Nerve!

The pudendal nerve is located in the perianal region at the bottom of the spinal cord, and for folks whose nerve pathways aren't being disrupted in some way, it's quite the powerhouse. It supplies nerves to the bladder, anus, perineum, penis, areas around the scrotum, and clitoris. It divides into two terminal branches: the perineal nerve, and the dorsal nerve of the penis or the dorsal nerve of the clitoris. A lot of the sensations people experience in their genitals and pelvis during orgasm—including the spasms people often feel with orgasm or ejaculation—are because of the pudendal nerve as well as the pelvic nerve.

The Vulva, Vagina, and Uterus: From the Outside In

What people usually call a vagina isn't actually the vagina at all. The external part of the genital system I'm about to talk about

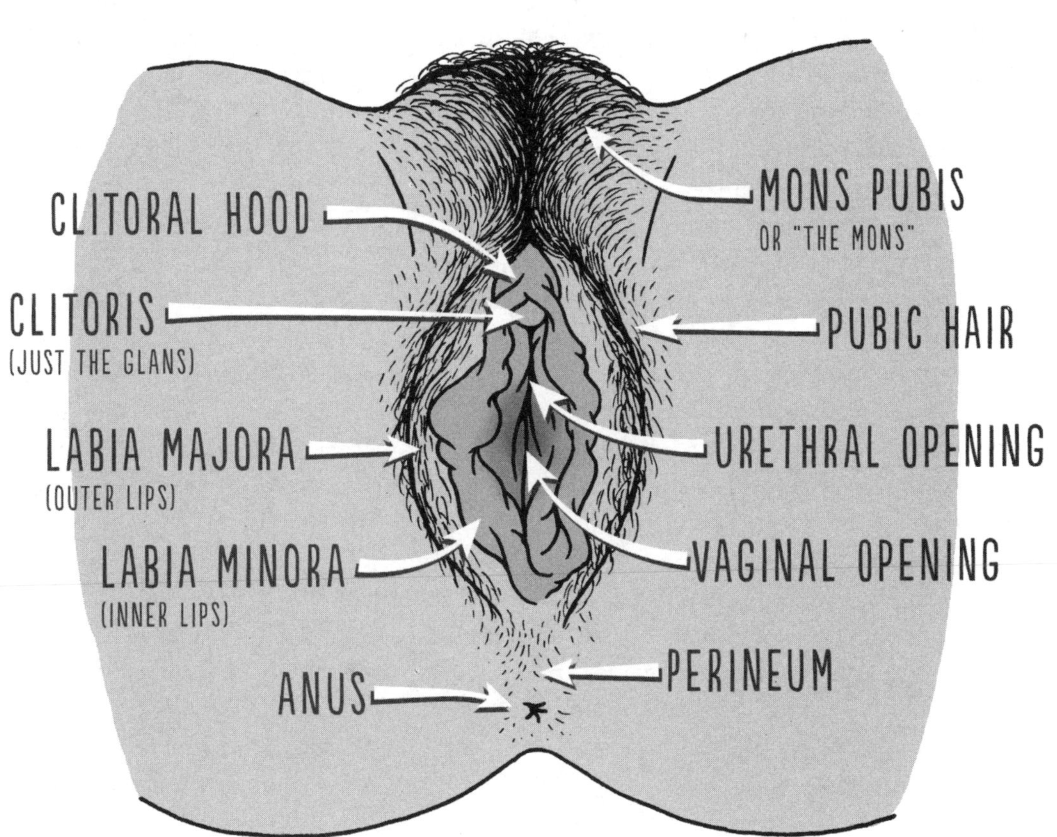

is, instead, called the vulva. Cunt, pussy, fanny, twat, coochie, muff, and snatch are some common slang names for the vulva.

The vulva begins with the *mons,* a fatty area of skin below the lower abdomen, where most of the pubic hair is. The mons continues downward to form the *labia majora,* or outer labia (*labia* is Latin for *lips*). The mons and outer labia are skin like that on our arms and legs rather than mucous membrane like that of other parts of the genitals. The size of the labia majora varies a good deal among people, as does the flatness or puffiness of the mons, depending on body size and shape and bone structure (the pubic bone is just beneath the mons). (If you've ever been horseback or bicycle riding for a long time, you know *exactly* where your pubic bone is because that's what usually feels mighty sore afterward.) And it's normal for the mons to be a bit puffier in teens than it is for people who are done with puberty.

Between the labia majora, you may see the *labia minora,* or inner labia, peeking out. Because the length of the inner labia varies a lot—not just among people, but even between one person's own pair—some inner labia peek out even when someone's legs are closed, and others aren't visible unless the legs or even the outer labia are spread open. Even then it might be tricky to differentiate the labia minora from the tissue of the vaginal opening for people with very small labia. The inner labia are made of mucous membrane, contain sebaceous glands and sensory nerve endings, and tend to look a lot like flower petals or two little tongues. They can vary a lot in color, from pink to red, brown to violet. More people than not have asymmetrical labia minora, with one labium longer than the other. The labia minora also aren't very uniform in shape—many have ragged-looking edges, and that's normal.

The inner labia are important: not only do they help to keep bacteria and other ickies from getting into the *vestibule*—the area between the inner labia, which houses the clitoris, urethra, and vaginal opening—they're also connected to the clitoral hood, so they often play a part in genital stimulation and sexual arousal.

Clit Lit

Just inside the vestibule—beneath the *fourchette,* where the inner labia connect—is nestled the visible part of the infamous *clitoris* (sometimes called the *clit*). Beneath the clitoral hood (a little skinfold) is the *glans,* or the tip of the clitoris, often mistaken for the whole of the clitoris. If you explore your own clitoris with your fingers, you may feel an intense tingle or a tickle, especially if you're turned on at the time. Pressing down on it, you may be able to feel a firm portion that is the *shaft* of the clitoris. The clitoris also has little "legs" inside the body, called the *crura,* which run down the sides of the vulva, inside the labia majora. There is one more portion of the clitoris, the *vestibular,* or *clitoral, bulbs.* They are also internal, beneath the inner labia, and they surround the vaginal opening. The bulbs—which are erectile tissue, much like what the penis is made of—and the crura can provide some clitoral stimulation during vaginal sex. You can see, then, that the clitoris is a

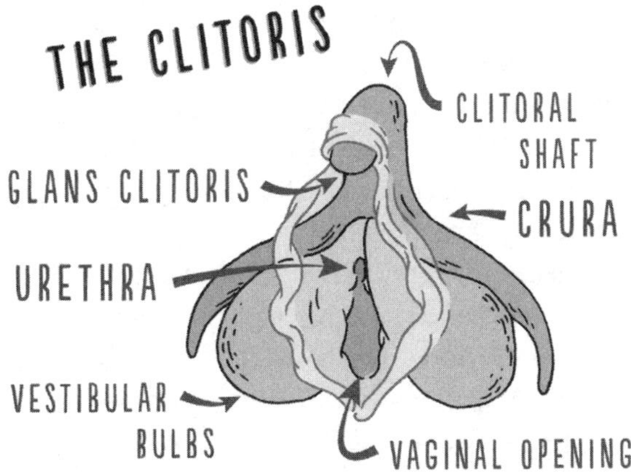

whole lot bigger than it looks. If you had X-ray eyes, you could see that the entire clitoris is similar in size to the penis.

The clitoris is usually the most sensitive spot of the whole vulva, and much more so than the vagina. In fact, the tiny glans of the clitoris alone has more sensory nerve endings than the penis or any other part of the human body—and the clitoris is the only organ in the human body whose *only* known purpose is to provide sexual pleasure. It's attached to ligaments, muscles, and veins that become filled with blood during sexual arousal and that contract during orgasm.

The clitoris is the part of the genitals most people with one usually give the most airplay during masturbation, and they tend to find it the most stimulating with any kind of genital sex with partners, just like most people with a penis often enjoy a lot of focus on the penis with both solo and partnered sex. Because of differences in sensitivity, preference, and tolerance, people differ in how and where they like the clitoris touched, just like people differ in how they like any part of their body touched.

Right below the clitoris is a little dot or slit, which is the *urethral opening,* the door from the *urethra,* where a person urinates (pees) from. You may or may not be able to see it easily, because it's so tiny. Just inside the urinary opening and on the upper wall of the vagina inside are glands called the *Skene's glands,* or *paraurethral glands,* which drain into the urethra. The equivalent of the Skene's glands for someone with a penis is the prostate gland.

Below the urethral opening is the *vaginal opening,* the opening to the *vagina,* a canal that has this opening on the outside of the genitals but that is actually an organ inside the body.

Just inside the vaginal opening, there may or may not be a visible *hymen* or *corona,* but there always are some traces of one, whatever your age or sexual experiences.

It's a pretty safe bet that everyone with a vagina is born with a hymen, and before puberty, barring injury, it is just inside the vaginal opening, mostly covering the canal behind it. It isn't any kind of seal: it contains small holes and perforations called *hymenal orifices,* the size and shape of which vary widely. After puberty starts, estrogen, menstruation, and physical and sexual activity start to wear the corona away. For the rest of someone's life, usually very gradually, it wears away more and more. But it's not like the hymen is a "Now you see it, now you don't!" situation: the hymen isn't there one day and—*poof!*—gone the next. When someone talks about "popping a cherry," they are referring to the hymen. But really, hymens are rarely "popped" or "broken."

Some hymens look like . . .

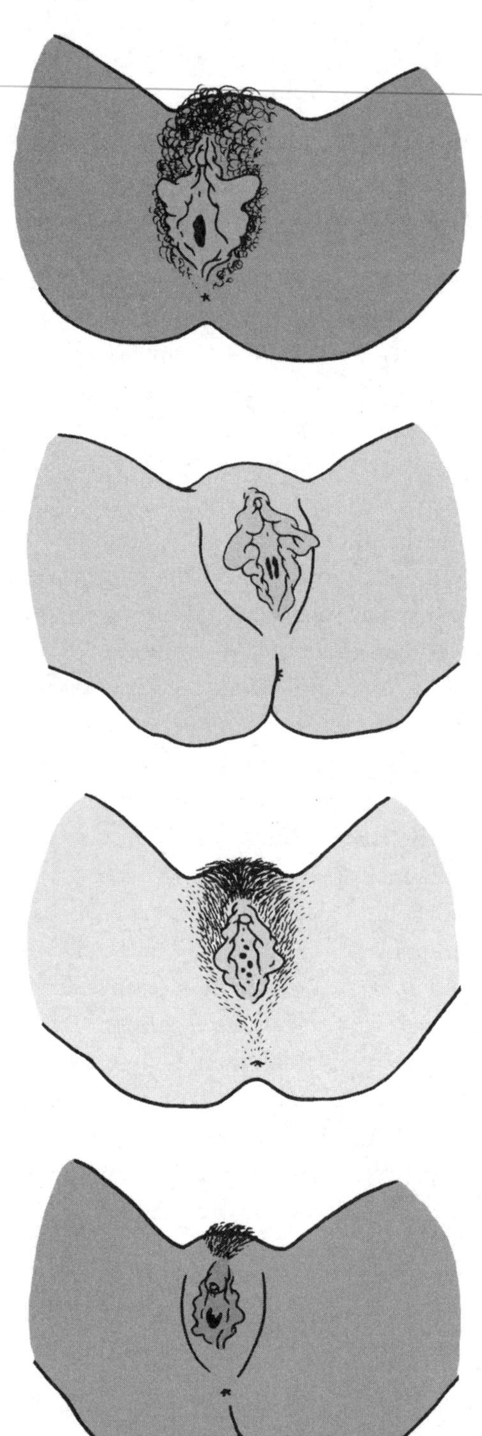

The corona itself doesn't have sensory nerve endings in it. Some people who experience pain or discomfort during initial vaginal entry or intercourse may feel some hymenal microtearing or stretching, which *can* put pressure on the parts of the vaginal opening the hymen is attached to, and these parts *do* have plenty of nerve endings. That's normal, and it's just as normal *not* to feel pain or discomfort—or for the hymen to be stretchy enough or worn away enough so that it's not in the way of intercourse. (Pain and discomfort can happen for different reasons altogether; for more on pain or discomfort during vaginal intercourse, see page 234.)

Even after the hymen has been worn away, little folds of its tissue often remain just inside the vaginal opening. Hymens are forever!

Below the vaginal opening, there is an area of skin called the *perineum.* It leads to the *anus,* the external opening to your *rectum,* through which bowel movements pass.

Life on the Inside

If you slide your finger inside the vaginal opening (yours or someone else's), you're in the *vagina. This* is where and what the vagina is: it's a muscular tube between the external genitals and the internal reproductive system: the cervix, uterus, and fallopian tubes. It's where the action happens during kinds of sex involving vaginal entry, and it's also where an infant passes through during a vaginal childbirth.

Just inside the vaginal opening are glands called the *Bartholin's glands.* During sexual arousal, these glands often provide some lubrication.

The vagina isn't a passive body part. In other words, it *does* things and isn't simply an empty place that just sits around like a slacker playing video games and eating chips. When nothing is inside it, the walls of the vagina lie together, pretty much closed. When something is inserted into it—be it a tampon, a finger, a penis, or a dildo—it can hold whatever it is pretty intensely: it's flexible and muscular! When whatever was inside it is removed, the vagina goes right back to its collapsed "resting" state. You or a sexual partner can feel that, with your fingers, and you can feel some of the muscles that surround the vagina, including the PC—*pubococcygeus* (and if you want to sound like a smarty-pants, it's pronounced pew-bo-cock-eh-GEE-us)—muscles, too. If, while urinating, someone squeezes to stop the flow of urine, those are the PC muscles at work.

The vaginal canal is curved, not straight—if you could see it inside in profile, you'd see an arc from vaginal opening to cervix—and there are a lot of different textures within it. On the front wall of the vagina, you may be able to feel a small spongy or textured area, kind of like what's on the roof of your mouth. That is the infamous *G-spot*, or *Gräfenberg spot*, another potential contributor to sexual pleasure and response.

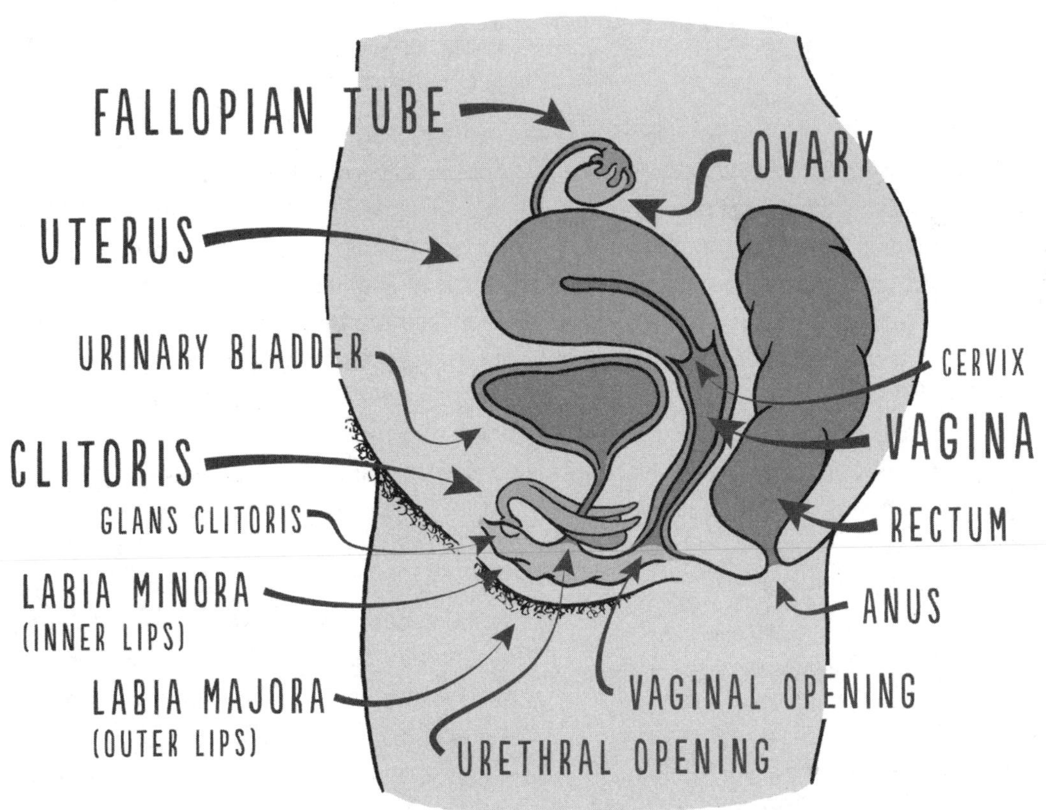

Even farther back into the vagina, you might feel something deep inside, sticking out a bit, the edge of which has a little dimple. This is the *cervix* (Latin for *neck*), and the dimple is the opening of the cervix, the *os* (Latin for *mouth*). The cervix is the passage from the uterus to the vagina. There's no reason to ever worry about losing a tampon, a toy, or anything else in the vagina: the os is very, very small. The very back of the vagina, slightly above and around the base of the cervix, is called the *fornix*. During sexual arousal, the fornix gets larger, or "tents," to make extra room for whatever might be inside the vagina.

Inside the body, the cervix leads into the *uterus* (also called the *womb*), a pear-shaped and muscular internal organ that's about four centimeters thick and about eight centimeters long. The uterus is the area of sexual anatomy where a fetus can develop and grow. The lining of the

HONORABLY DISCHARGED

Vaginal discharge and secretions are a normal, healthy part of the reproductive system and fertility or menstrual cycle.

The vagina is a passageway between the outside of the body and the internal reproductive system. The pH balance of the vagina is acidic, with "good" bacteria that help keep infections away. The vagina is a self-cleaning organ. Secretions are its way of cleansing and regulating itself, in the same sort of way that secreting saliva helps keep our mouths clean and healthy. So, although we need to wash the external genitals, there's no need to try to clean inside the vagina with soap or douching. It does it best all by itself!

Normal vaginal discharge:

- Can be clear and thin. This sort of discharge usually occurs around ovulation, and vaginal secretions during sexual arousal also tend to have a similar appearance and consistency.

- Can be white or slightly yellowish and thick. This sort of discharge tends to occur during less fertile times in the monthly cycle.

- Often has a mild, but not a strong or unpleasant, odor. Vaginas and vulvas, as it turns out, smell like vaginas and vulvas, not like flower gardens, cookies, or air freshener (which would be mighty weird).

- May have a brown or reddish tint. This kind of discharge often occurs usually just before or just after menses.

- Will appear on underpants, around the vaginal opening, and on the inner labia a lot of the time.

Normal discharge is just that: *normal.* It's nothing to be worried or embarrassed about, there's nothing wrong with it, and it's an important part of reproductive health and function. During times when vaginal secretions are especially profuse, or more "wet" than at other times, some people feel more comfortable using a washable or disposable panty liner, but there's no need to do that if you don't want to: underpants are more than absorbent enough to handle most vaginal secretions.

Bacterial, yeast/fungal, or sexually transmitted infections (STIs) can create changes in the amount, consistency, color, or scent of vaginal discharges, so if in doubt about whether your discharge is normal, ask your healthcare professional. For more information on general vaginal infections, see page 284, and for information on STIs, see Chapter 10 and Appendix A. ■■

uterus, called the *endometrium,* builds up every menstrual cycle to prepare for a fertilized egg, and this is what a person sheds each cycle when they have their period.

On either side of the uterus is a *fallopian tube.* Eggs travel through the fallopian tubes, also called the *oviducts,* to get to the uterus. Finger-like structures called *fimbriae* at the end of the fallopian tubes sweep the eggs from the ovary into the tubes. At the end of each fallopian tube is an ovary, which both stores and releases eggs, or *ova,* one at a time during each menstrual cycle (though some people may ovulate more than once in a cycle, and a person may also sometimes release more than one egg at a time). The ovaries produce the hormones estrogen and progesterone, which are responsible for the development of sex characteristics but which also keep the genitals flexible, elastic, and lubricated and help keep the vaginal lining healthy. Some estrogen is also produced by fat tissue. The ovaries also produce the hormone testosterone (and the adrenal glands elsewhere in the body produce this hormone, too).

The Menstrual Cycle. Period.

The menstrual cycle isn't just something that happens when someone has their period. Periods are only one part of a complex hormonal, physiological, and emotional fertility cycle that takes place approximately every month, some parts of which have effects on a person every single day.

The menstrual cycle is divided into three phases: the menstrual phase, the proliferative phase, and the secretory, or luteal, phase.

Oocytes

Oocytes—the name of ova, or eggs, before they are released—aren't created every month but are all lying in wait, around a half million of them, at the time puberty begins. They then mature randomly in one of the two ovaries and are released one at a time (usually) until menopause, which typically happens for people sometime in middle age. If you do the math—one ovum (usually, but occasionally two) released around once a month for about forty years—you'll see that most oocytes never see the light of day; that's because, during each cycle, about a thousand of them naturally degenerate, and the cells are just absorbed by your body. Some ova remain at menopause, so no one runs out of ova before then.

Every menstrual, or fertility, cycle begins on the first day of each menstrual period, starting the **menstrual phase**. A menstrual period is the uterus shedding the lining it built up in the previous cycle because a pregnancy didn't occur. The idea that menstrual flow is all blood, blood like the kind you see from a cut, is in error. On average, menstrual flow is only about 35 percent blood. The rest of its contents are endometrial tissue and other vaginal and cervical secretions, so it's perfectly normal to sometimes see globs rather than simply liquid, and those globs aren't clots; menstrual flow doesn't clot because even the blood in it isn't like other blood. Instead, those globs or clumps are either tissue coming out in more solid form or menstrual flow mixed with the thick vaginal discharge that's

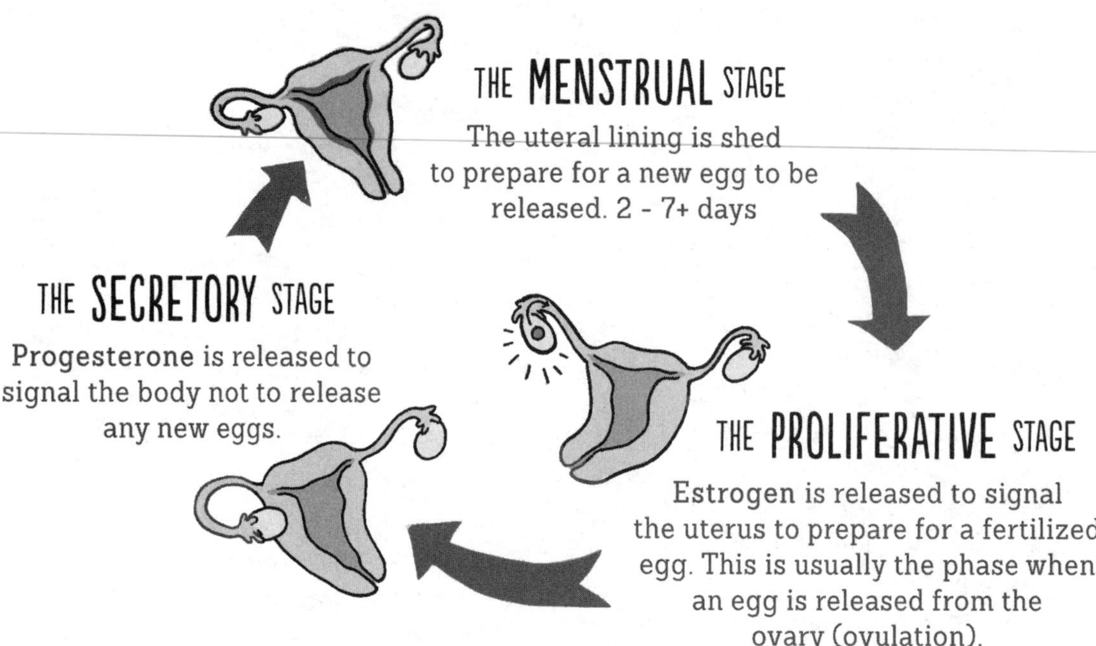

often present during a period. They aren't anything to worry about.

THE MENSTRUAL STAGE
The uteral lining is shed to prepare for a new egg to be released. 2 - 7+ days
THE SECRETORY STAGE
Progesterone is released to signal the body not to release any new eggs.
THE PROLIFERATIVE STAGE
Estrogen is released to signal the uterus to prepare for a fertilized egg. This is usually the phase when an egg is released from the ovary (ovulation).

The menstrual phase usually lasts anywhere from just a couple of days to around eight days, with flow varying from light to heavy. There may be hours or even a day when there doesn't seem to be flow at all, and then it starts up again. Vaginal discharge often has a brownish hue a couple of days after the end of a period because it is carrying slight residue from the previous days.

The next phase is the **proliferative phase**. In a section of the brain called the hypothalamus, substances are produced and released that travel down to the pituitary gland and stimulate it, kind of like jumping a car battery. The pituitary gland then releases two hormones: the follicle-stimulating hormone (FSH) and the luteinizing hormone (LH). These chemicals create changes that cause an ovum to mature and be released. This occurs at the end of the proliferative phase and is when a person ovulates: when the egg is released from the ovary and begins moving through the fallopian tubes.

When someone is most fertile—when they're most likely to become pregnant—varies, but the majority of people are most fertile during the end of the proliferative phase and the start of the secretory phase. Sometimes the time just before and during ovulation is called the **ovulatory phase.**

Right at ovulation the **luteal,** or **secretory, phase** begins. At this time, the hormone *progesterone* is produced by the ovary, and this hormone prepares the lining of the uterus, the endometrium, to nourish and house an egg should an ovum be fertilized. During this phase, vaginal secretions become thinner and more fluid, with a stretchy, egg-white consistency. This happens because that type of mucus provides the right environment for sperm cells. If an egg is fertilized and implants in the lining of the uterine wall—this is what *conception* means and signals the creation of a pregnancy—even more progesterone is released. If conception doesn't happen, then the level of progesterone drops; it's that hormonal drop, and the shedding of the endometrium—a period—that starts the cycle all over again.

Where Can Aunt Flo Go? Menses Management

Menstrual flow—about three or four ounces over the course of each period—has gotta go somewhere. There are several options for managing that flow, and which you choose is mostly about what you have access to, what you can use, and personal preference. When used properly, all of the following methods are safe, healthy, and valid choices. And you don't have to pick just one—you can combine or alternate methods.

Pads: Pads are usually the best choice for first starting menstruation, for heavy flow, and while sleeping. Disposable pads come in various levels of absorbency and have an adhesive backing that attaches to underwear. If you use disposable pads, avoid any with added perfumes because these can irritate the vulva. Most pads are a blend of natural and synthetic fibers with plastic backing. Some people experience vulval irritation from the synthetic fibers, bleaching, plastic backing, or casing of some commercial pads. Organic, unbleached cotton pads are also available.

Washable, reusable pads are a better choice for the environment and the body than disposable pads. In the long run they're also much less expensive, even though they cost more at the outset. They are made of natural fibers and come in different levels of absorbency. Some brands have a heavier "filler" you can add or remove as needed. Most have snaps on little wings that just wrap around the crotch of underwear (they won't work with boxers though; you need to use them with close-fitting underpants that stop at or around the bottom of your butt). There are also washable menstrual underpants with a pad sewn right in. They can be washed just like any other piece of clothing. When you wash your underwear, it's clean enough for wearing again—same with washable pads. Menstrual flow is no different from daily vaginal discharge when it comes to bacteria. You can find washable pads at most natural foods markets or health stores, and some standard pharmacies have started to carry them as well. You can often find the best selection online, or you can even make them yourself.

Tampons: Tampons are handy while swimming or participating in other sports, for special occasions, during outercourse (sexual activities such as manual or oral sex), or if you just like them. As with pads, tampons without fragrance or perfumes are healthiest. Although menstrual flow, like other vaginal fluids, does have its own scent, the idea that it is a "bad" or foul scent is nothing but a marketing ploy—at the expense of vaginal health. A person menstruating smells just fine so long as they're good with basic hygiene and changing menstrual supplies often enough. Perfumes aren't meant to be inside the vaginal canal and can incline a person to infections that truly *are* stinky. Because tampons are absorbent, pulling fluid from the vagina, they can increase vaginal or menstrual scent as well as cramping.

Some tampons come with plastic or paper applicators, and some come without; which to use is a personal preference, though those without the applicator usually are easier to learn with. Nearly all commercial brands of tampons do contain some manmade fibers, like rayon, and bleaches. Those aren't the best for a body, and they suck for the environment. Unbleached tampons made with all natural fibers are the best way to go.

Sometimes, tampons—especially those left in for too long—may separate or shred when removed, and extra fibers may be found coming from the vagina even a week later. Although that's nothing necessarily major, if you discover you've got other symptoms, such as itching, redness, soreness, extra spotting, headaches, dizziness, or a foul scent, you should see your doctor or gynecologist pronto.

TSS

Tampon use can pose a risk of toxic shock syndrome (TSS). TSS is rare, but it can cause severe medical problems and even death. TSS is caused by a staph organism that produces toxins that colonize the fibers of the tampon. Staph in and of itself is a nasty infection, but the added toxin production of TSS is serious bad news.

Symptoms of TSS appear nearly immediately and are pretty obvious: during tampon use, should you suddenly feel dizzy, nauseated, weak, or faint or develop a sudden high fever or body rash, you need to seek medical attention immediately. If you use tampons only during the day, change them often—every four to eight hours—and use the lowest absorbency you need, you don't have to worry much about TSS. If you use pads or a menstrual cup, you don't have to worry about TSS at all.

Natural sea sponges: Sea sponges are multicellular living organisms that have been harvested from the ocean and then processed for human use. Like washable pads, they're reusable. To use them as a menstrual product, you just soften them with a little water, bunch them up, and insert them inside the vagina. To change them, just pull the sponge out gently, rinse it with warm water, and put in a fresh one. At the end of each cycle, sponges can be sanitized by soaking them for a few hours in a cup of warm water with a teaspoon of baking soda, a half cup of hydrogen peroxide, or a few drops of tea tree oil. Sponges are a good alternative for someone who feels "poked" by tampons, has trouble inserting tampons, feels uncomfortable with tampons as a result of dryness, or wants an environmentally sound product. Natural sponges can be found at most natural foods stores and should be replaced every few months.

Menstrual cups: Reusable cups have the adaptability and ease of a tampon but without the waste and the downside of fibers and the endless costs. A menstrual cup (such as The Keeper or the Divacup;

see Resources) can save you serious cash. A menstrual cup you use for just five years (and you can often use one for longer than that) will cost you around $30 to $35; five years' worth of tampons or pads costs around ten times that amount.

Made of gum rubber or silicone, reusable menstrual cups collect and hold menstrual flow within the cup until you remove it, empty the cup, and reinsert. At the end of a period, you can clean your menstrual cup by boiling it or using a cleaning agent designed for use with it.

Disposable menstrual cups are also available but tend to work less well—they leak far more often for most people—and are far less cost-effective.

Because they collect flow rather than absorb it, cups don't disrupt the moisture balance of the vagina, and some users report less cramping than when they use tampons. Menstrual cups can often be in place in the vagina safely for longer periods of time than tampons.

To date, cups have not been associated with TSS. Menstrual cups might be harder to obtain in some areas, but as with washable pads, natural foods stores carry them, and you can order them online. Some drugstores and big-box stores carry them now, too.

For very light flow, for the end of your period, or for someone who just doesn't want to use anything at all—you don't *have* to. Some people keep undergarments to use just for menses or sheets that they're cool staining with flow at night so they can go productless. Using nothing generally doesn't work very well for work or school, but there isn't a thing wrong with just letting flow go if that suits you.

When the Rag's a Drag

Cramps: It's normal to experience cramping before or during a period, mostly as a result of chemical and hormonal changes that happen around and with menstruation (namely, increased prostaglandin, which decreases blood flow to the uterus and causes it to contract, which is what causes flow to come out). It's also common for periods to be more painful or heavy when you're younger.

There are many ways to relieve cramps. Over-the-counter anti-inflammatories, such as sodium naproxen or ibuprofen, or another analgesic, are often very effective. Warm baths, beverages, or compresses can be very helpful with cramps. Deep stretching, yoga, other exercise, activity, or self-massage are helpful, and acupuncture can also save the day. Calcium, magnesium, and vitamins E and K, which are usually in a regular daily multivitamin, can help with cramping and other menstrual discomforts. Some foods that tend to make cramping and other menstrual unpleasantness worse are caffeine, processed foods, sugar, salt, alcohol, and dairy products. It's best to go for light, healthy meals while menstruating and to try to avoid or limit the foods or drinks that tend to increase cramping, bloating, and digestive distress, even though they're the things—silly bodies!—many people tend to crave most before or with periods.

Irregularity: It tends to take several years for the menstrual cycle to become regular, for the cycle to start to be around the same length each time. Twenty-eight-day cycles are an average length—from day one of one period to the start of the next—but like all averages, there's a lot of variation on both sides: some people's regular cycles may occur every twenty-three days; others' may be around forty days. Just because someone doesn't have perfect twenty-eight-day cycles does not mean their cycle isn't regular. The standard deviation for regular cycles is between two and three days, so someone whose period doesn't come on exactly the day they expect it each time doesn't necessarily have irregular cycles. A regular cycle really just means that a person is having periods with a similar number of days between one cycle and the next. So, someone whose cycles over a few months were 26 days, 29 days, and 27 days would, in fact, be considered to have a very regular cycle. An irregular cycle would look more like 26 days, 42 days, and then 30 days. Many people have irregular cycles during some times of their life, and some always do.

It's also typical during the first few years of menstruating to have longer or shorter cycles than you will when you're older.

If periods go missing outright for more than a couple of months, or if after a few years of menstruation they're still often very late or missing, diet and exercise are common reasons why. Not eating enough, having disordered eating, being very inactive, or overexercising can throw a body out of whack and cause missed or irregular periods. Experiencing unmanaged stress, including stress from a pregnancy scare, can also make cycles go wonky. Obviously, if there has been a pregnancy risk and a missed period, a pregnancy test is in order, because pregnancy is one reason for a missed period. If you're concerned about your cycles for any reason, it's always smart to check in with a healthcare provider.

PMS: Common symptoms of PMS, or premenstrual syndrome, include acne, bloating, feeling very tired, backaches or general body soreness, tender breasts, headaches, constipation or diarrhea, food cravings, mood swings, serious crabbiness or depression, and troubles with concentrating or managing stress. Some degree of PMS is normal and it can usually be easily managed, however annoying it may be. Getting enough rest and activity, reducing the amount of sugar and caffeine you consume, and taking extra-good care of yourself before periods can reduce PMS. Some people also find that a blood-thinning medication, such as aspirin, helps with PMS symptoms and may reduce cramps at the onset of a period. Recent studies have also found that a combination of calcium and vitamin B supplements can reduce PMS symptoms.

Severe effects: If your period produces more severe side effects, such as highly painful and constant heavy cramping (dysmenorrhea), deep abdominal pain, very heavy flow (menorrhagia), irregular vaginal bleeding during other times in your cycle, heavy-duty acne, strong loss of appetite, very intense mood swings or depression, extensive PMS symptoms—or if you have stopped getting your periods altogether (amenorrhea)—talk to your healthcare provider. Many menstrual maladies can be remedied with the proper treatment or medication, and some may be a result of other conditions, such as pelvic inflammatory disease (PID) or endometriosis, which require diagnosis and treatment. Hormonal methods of birth control or some intrauterine devices (IUDs) can alleviate some of these symptoms for some people. To find out what kind of treatment is most likely to help you, work with your healthcare provider and make sure to tell them about these symptoms. Some people have learned to believe that people are supposed to suffer with menstrual periods, like it's some kind of cross to bear just for having a uterus. That's sexist hogwash: as with any other kind of physical pain, there is usually a cause that can be addressed with medical interventions so you can feel better.

Breast Basics

Breasts are composed of connective tissue and fat. For someone with a uterus, breasts also contain mammary (milk-producing) glands known as *lobules* and lactiferous (milk-carrying) ducts. The breasts sit on the rib cage, over the chest or pectoral muscles, and are connected to the body by ligaments.

There's no muscle in the breast. The parts of the breasts that create their size and shape are fat and glands, though how much or how little muscle someone has beneath the breast influences how the breasts look on the body. Between the ligaments of the breast are pockets of fat that contain the mammary glands (lobules), and those lead to the lactiferous ducts.

The area of the breast that is darker and that surrounds the nipple is called

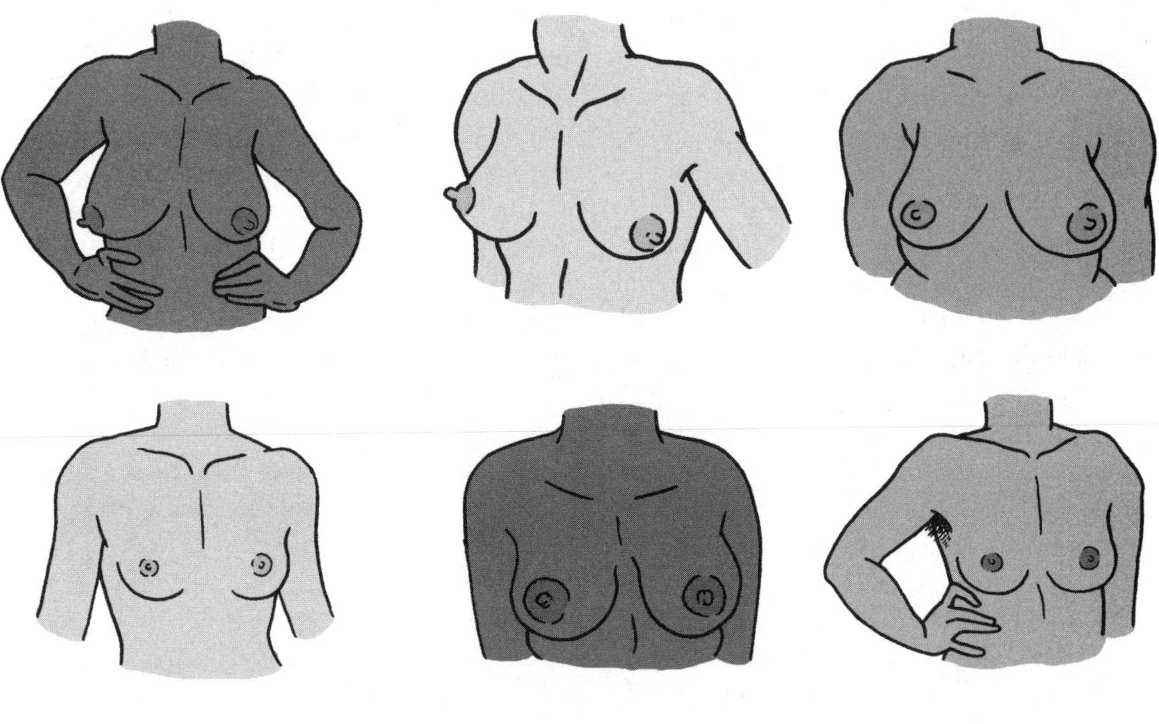

Bogus Boob Stuff

- Bras aren't needed for good health, and there has yet to be any viable data that show that brassieres prevent breasts from sagging over time. Wearing a bra is an individual preference based on comfort.
- No supplements or creams on the market can increase breast size. Using some of them may cause the skin to swell, but not only are those results temporary but also some of the supplements contain compounds that can be dangerous to long-term health.
- Breast implants, although safer now than they used to be, still pose risks such as inability to nurse a baby properly, rippling (wrinkling), scarring, sensory loss, and serious and even life-threatening infections—cosmetic surgery comes with health risks just like any surgery does. Food and Drug Administration (FDA) scientists have found a significant link between silicone gel implants and fibromyalgia, a disorder that causes pain and fatigue in the muscles, tendons, and ligaments. According to the FDA, 43 percent of all implant patients have complications within just three years of surgery. Considering that breast implants cost the very big bucks, are not one-time surgeries but require upkeep every few years and even removal or replacement, and pose all sorts of risks, if they're something you're considering, do your homework and make this choice very carefully.

the *areola*. For those who have them, milk ducts behind the areola—about fifteen to twenty of them in each breast—lead to the nipples from the mammary glands; during a pregnancy and after a delivery, those glands produce milk, which comes through the ducts to nourish an infant. There are also glands called *Montgomery glands* within the areola, which can sometimes be seen and look like little bumps. Most nipples protrude slightly (and noticeably when someone is sexually excited or just cold), but some people have what are called inverted nipples, which turn inward into the breast—a totally normal variation.

Breasts come in a lot of different shapes: some look round or globe-like; other breasts may appear more triangular. For people with very small breasts, only the areola and nipple may protrude or have visible shape. Some people have what are called tubular breasts, which have less glandular tissue than other breasts and look long and cylindrical. No one breast shape is necessarily more functional, beautiful, or otherwise better than another, just like no one color or texture of hair is.

Areola size doesn't necessarily correspond to breast size. People with large breasts can and do have small areolas; people with smaller breasts can and do have larger areolas. It's normal for breast size and shape to differ slightly in one set of breasts. Areola and nipple size, however, tend to be pretty symmetrical.

The size and shape of breasts vary so widely because each person's breasts are made up of different amounts of various sorts of fatty, mammary, and fibrous tissues.

Also, an individual's skin, fat, and muscle composition and structure as well as their hormone levels (of estrogen, progesterone, and prolactin) vary widely. That's one reason why even for one person, in a given month, breast size can vary slightly as can the tenderness of the breast. Most of breast size and shape is determined by genetics, but because genetic combinations are so unique, it's still possible for a given person's breasts to look nothing like the breasts of their close relatives.

The Penis and Testes: From the Outside In

Let's start from the top, or rather, from the tip.

At the end of the penis—the name for the external genitalia, not including the testicles and anus, which you might call the dick, cock, willie, johnson, schlong, or little Elvis if you're feeling retro—you'll see the *urethral meatus,* or the opening of the *urethra.* All fluids from the penis, including urine, come through the urethra; the urethra has both a urinary function *and* a reproductive one: semen and pre-ejaculate come out through the urethra, too.

The urethral meatus is at top and center of the *glans,* or the head of the penis. The glans is mushroom-shaped, and the ridge along the edge at the bottom of the glans is called the *corona,* or coronal ridge (oddly enough, the hymen has been recently renamed the corona, too). On the underside of that ridge, on the side of the penis facing away from the stomach when erect, is the *frenum,* or *frenulum.* Many people experience this and the glans as the most sensitive areas of the penis.

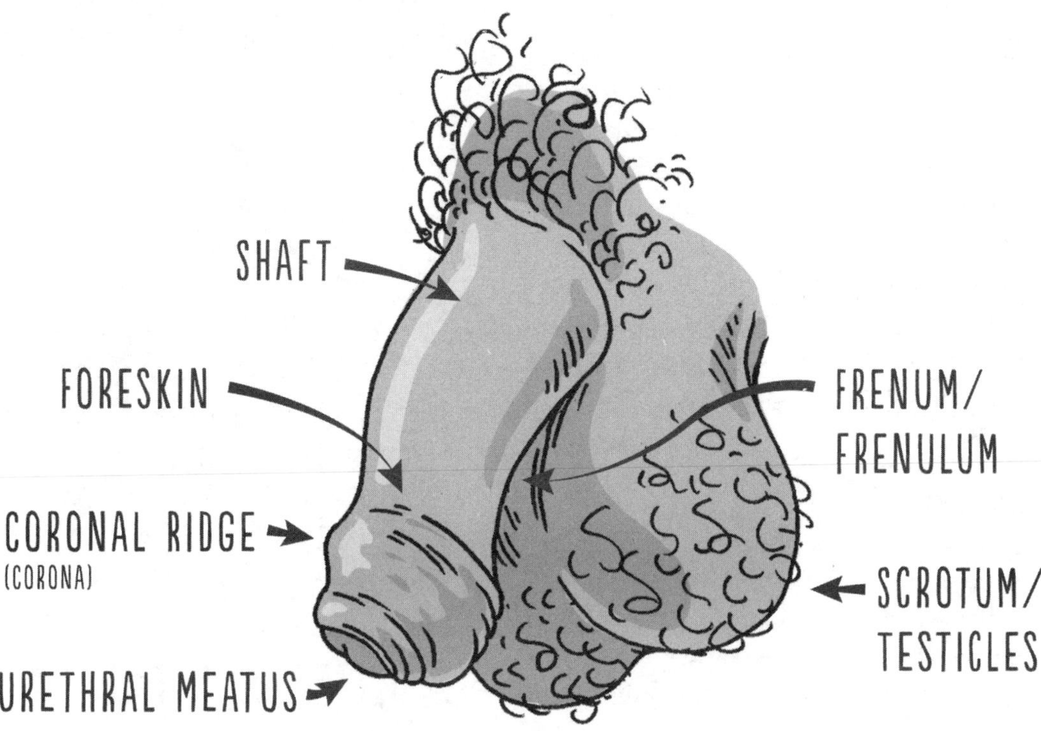

At birth, the *shaft,* or area of the penis from beneath the coronal ridge to the base, is covered by a loose tube of skin, called the *foreskin.* This is attached to the penis in two ways: at the base, and along the length by the *frenar band,* which extends from the frenulum and runs in a long loop within the foreskin.

The Foreskin (or Not)

The foreskin is full of sensory nerve endings and looks a lot like a turtleneck sweater for the penis. When a penis is flaccid—not erect—the whole of the shaft and the glans are covered by the foreskin. When erection occurs, the foreskin retracts: it slides backward down the shaft of the penis so that the glans and some of the shaft are visible outside the foreskin. When an intact (uncircumcised) penis is erect, the foreskin essentially blends in with the shaft, so it is generally easier to see the difference between circumcised and uncircumcised penises when they're flaccid. The foreskin should slide and retract at least past the head of the penis comfortably, by itself, with the hands, and during sexual activity; if you've got a foreskin and yours doesn't do this, check in with your doctor because most infections and conditions that cause foreskin problems are easily treatable.

Intact penises are self-lubricating to allow the foreskin to move comfortably along the shaft (though people with foreskins may still find they or their partners want or need additional lubrication, especially when using condoms). It's normal for *smegma,* a white and waxy substance, to be found beneath and around the foreskin. It's made up of shed skin cells and secretions from glands within the foreskin, called the *Tyson's glands,* and glands of the testes. Basic, gentle hygiene takes care of most of the smegma, but it's likely

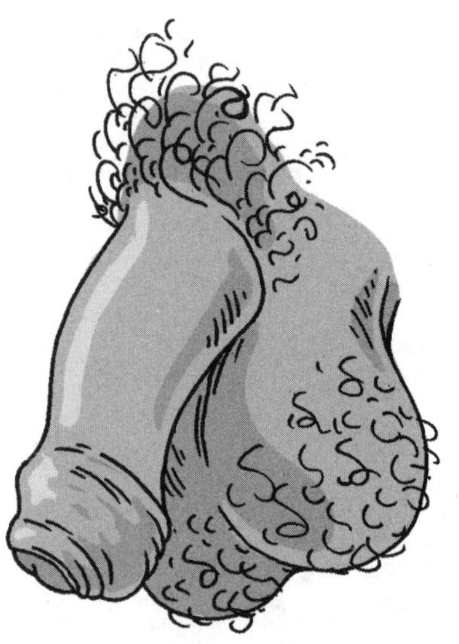

UNCIRCUMCISED PENIS

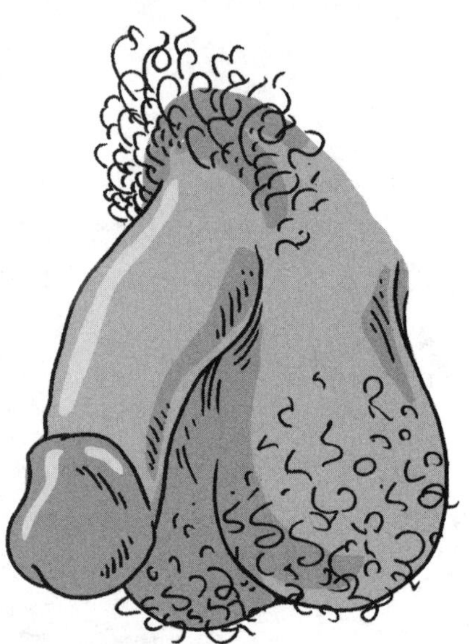

CIRCUMCISED PENIS

to be present in some amounts at all times, and that's both normal and healthy (it also can often be found around the clitoris or labia).

People born with a penis are also born with a foreskin. But about 20 percent of people with a penis worldwide, and about 80 percent in the United States, have been circumcised: their foreskin was surgically removed, usually in early infancy, because of either cultural traditions or the belief that an uncircumcised penis poses health concerns. (For the record, where we're currently at on the topic of foreskins is that circumcising and not circumcising both present health issues and risks, just not the same ones.

Penises with and without foreskins are healthy and hygienic. It's normal—common—to have a foreskin or not to have one.

In people who have been circumcised, the frenulum isn't attached to the foreskin or frenar band, so it may look like a small V-shaped area. Because circumcisions vary, different degrees of the frenulum, and sometimes the frenar band, may remain. On both circumcised and uncircumcised people, a line, called the *raphe,* can be seen on the side of the penis that faces downward. The raphe continues down through the testicles to the anus.

It's normal for the skin and shaft of the penis to be several shades darker or deeper than the skin of the rest of the body, either all the time or just when the penis is hard. It's also normal for the penis to change color slightly when it gets hard. The coloration should return to normal once the erection goes down. The shaft, when erect, can also look veiny and bulgy in places; that's normal, too.

How Big Is It Supposed to Be?

Penises vary in size pretty widely when they're not erect, but the average is a little over three inches in length. The size of a flaccid penis doesn't dictate the size it may be when erect. According to most studies, the average erect penis of a fully grown person—someone *all* the way done with puberty—is about five to six inches long and four to five inches in circumference. The way averages work, that means an awful lot of people have penises both smaller and larger than that size, and people who are not yet finished with puberty have size ranges smaller than the range for adults.

How big or small someone's penis is, is a lot like how big or small someone's breasts are. In other words, weight or height doesn't dictate size, but genetics do.

Try not to get too focused on or worried about the size of your penis. If you're convinced you've got a serious health issue or abnormality that is creating any kind of problem with how your penis functions or feels, talk to your doctor. Otherwise, you've got bigger fish to fry and much better ways to spend your time—like finding out what's really going on in there.

Life on the Inside

Despite being called a boner, the penis has no bones. In fact, there isn't even any muscle, except the *bulbospongiosus,* a

small muscle used to squeeze out urine and ejaculatory fluids, and some muscles and ligaments at the base of the penis that attach it to the body. Most of the penis is composed of three long cylinders of tissue: two *corpora cavernosa* (singular: *corpus cavernosum*) and the *corpus spongiosum,* through which the urethra runs.

Erection occurs because of blood; during arousal, blood flows into the penis and fills up the cylinders of tissue in the penis. The corpora cavernosa run along the top of the penis, and the corpus spongiosum runs around the urethra. When the corpora cavernosa and the corpus spongiosum are filled with blood, they get stiff and the penis becomes both hard and erect, leveraged up by the extension of those structures a little into the body.

The urethra is a small tube about eight inches long that runs the length of the penis and connects to several internal organs: the bladder (where urine is stored), the testes, and the ejaculatory ducts. The urethra ends at the urethral opening.

Get the Ball Rolling

The *testicles, testes,* or "balls" hang below the penis in a sac of skin and muscle called the *scrotum*. There are two testes but just one scrotum, which is divided in half by a wall of tissue. You can usually see where that division is from the outside via the raphe, which runs down the center of the scrotum. The testes produce sperm cells, the hormone testosterone (which is produced in almost everyone's body, but people with testes usually have more of it), and other androgens.

The testes are outside the body because the ideal temperature for the sperm cells inside them is slightly lower than body temperature. The size of the testicles varies: some are the size of olives; others as

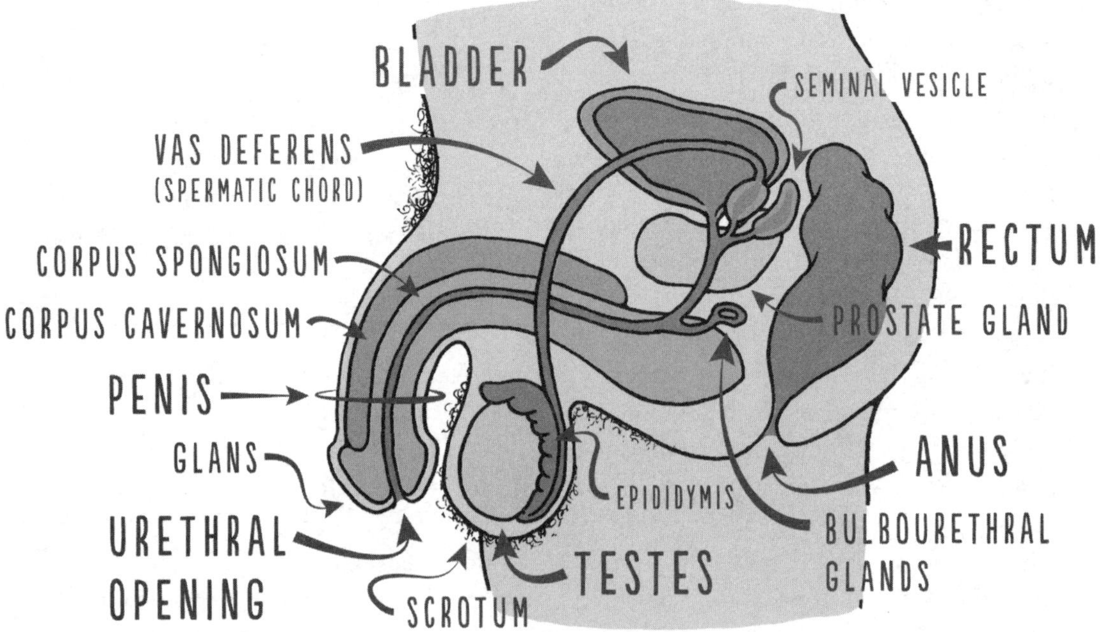

THE EJACULATION SITUATION

What's the Difference Between Sperm, Semen, and Ejaculate?

Ejaculate is just another word for semen. Semen—the fluid that comes from the penis during ejaculation—contains sperm. Semen and sperm are not one and the same, though. Sperm cells, between 50 million and 130 million in a given ejaculation, are only a small part of what is in ejaculate. Sperm compose only about 2 to 5 percent of the volume of the semen ejaculated; the rest of semen is composed of fluids produced by the prostate gland and the bulbourethral or Cowper's glands as well as fluids produced by the vas deferens and the seminal vesicles. The prostate produces fluids that are about 30 percent of the total volume of semen. Each fluid is added to the semen mixture at various points along the route the semen takes to be ejaculated. Most ejaculations are about one teaspoon of fluid, but volume can vary a lot from person to person, or from day to day.

When Does Ejaculation Happen?

Ejaculation and orgasm aren't the same thing, but they are usually related. Whereas ejaculation usually happens after orgasm, orgasm can occur without ejaculation (for more on ejaculation, see pages 75–76). Although people get erections from infancy on, ejaculation doesn't occur until *after* puberty has begun, and some people may not even begin to ejaculate until they're in their late teens.

It's okay for someone not to ejaculate during masturbation or partnered sex activities, either because they haven't begun ejaculating yet or because, for whatever reason, it just doesn't happen. Not ejaculating doesn't mean anything is wrong. As well, no volume of ejaculate is better than another, nor is "dribbling" rather than "shooting" anything to be embarrassed about—how much and with what force someone ejaculates vary based on levels of semen from day to day. To date, there have yet to be any Olympic competitions or cash prizes for ejaculating, so as long as somebody is physically comfortable and everything feels fine, chances are everything *is* fine.

What's Healthy and What's Not?

Semen/ejaculate tends to be whitish, milky, or somewhat translucent. It may sometimes also have a slightly yellowish tint (because it can contain some urine, by virtue of using the same pipe, the urethra, to travel through). Urination or ejaculation should not cause a person with a penis any discomfort.

Don't worry if you have stains on your underwear or sheets; that's perfectly normal. Just wash them.

If urination or ejaculation causes pain or discomfort, if other discharges are coming from the penis, or if urine or ejaculate is discolored or contains any blood, however, it's time to see the doctor.

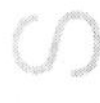

big as plums. They're *incredibly* sensitive to touch and pressure.

The scrotum's muscles are used to pull the testes closer to the body in order to protect or warm them (this is why when it's cold the scrotum can shrivel up); when the muscles relax, the testes hang a good deal lower, and the scrotum often looks longer.

Sperm cells are formed in the testes and then move into the *epididymis* to mature. Composed of a bundle of squiggly tubes, the epididymis is a small organ that lies against the top of the testicle. When someone is going to ejaculate, sperm are moved from the epididymis into the *vas deferens,* the continuation of the epididymis that takes sperm up and out of the scrotum area and into other ducts so they can be ejaculated. New sperm cells are constantly created and moved to the epididymis. Sperm that don't get ejaculated stay there for around four to six weeks before they die and are reabsorbed into the body. This is why it's impossible—even if you never ejaculated in your whole life—to have "excess" sperm build up in your body with nowhere to go.

The epididymis and testicles are anchored to the body by what is called the *spermatic cord.* The spermatic cord is a bundle of nerves and blood vessels that serve the testicle and epididymis, plus the vas deferens.

The vas deferens leads into the body, through a canal toward the bladder—which is also connected to the urethra—and into the seminal vesicles, where sperm get mixed up with some of the other ingredients of semen.

The bulbourethral glands, or Cowper's glands, are two pea-sized glands connected to the side of the urethra. They produce a liquid sort of mucus called *pre-ejaculate,* or *precum,* that is excreted when someone becomes sexually aroused, usually with an erection. Pre-ejaculate may be emitted more than once during arousal, and many people won't feel it or be aware of its presence, especially during intercourse or other partnered sex activities when the tip of the penis can't be seen or when other body fluids are already in the mix. It's a fluid intended to neutralize any acid (from urine) that might be inside the urethra. Since sperm cells do not thrive under acidic conditions, pre-ejaculate helps to make the conditions in the urethra favorable for sperm to survive. The same fluid is also a component of semen itself.

Just above the bulbourethral glands is the prostate gland. A chestnut-shaped gland about one and a half inches around that surrounds a small part of the urethra, it's below the bladder and toward the rectum, the canal between the bowel and the anus. The seminal vesicles empty into the urethra at this location, mixing sperm cells with other fluids from the glands to make ejaculate and provide lubrication.

The prostate, like the G-spot, clitoral glans, or the glans of the penis, is sensitive to touch, so plenty of people enjoy prostate stimulation during sexual activity. Some people call it the "P-spot." Because of its location, it is stimulated by receptive anal sex or stimulation or deep massage of the anus or perineum.

Once fluids from the prostate have been added to the mix of fluids and

WE ALL GET—AND ARE—HORMONAL.

What are called and thought of as sex hormones—testosterone, estrogen, and progesterone—aren't the only hormones out there or that influence how we feel emotionally or sexually. In fact, they're not even the biggest players in the area of sexuality; neurochemicals such as dopamine, GABA, serotonin, and endorphins are the real MVPs with sexual stuff. The hormones that cause the hormonal changes that happen for people with a uterus aren't the only hormones that influence how people are feeling; neither are people with a uterus and a menstruation-related fertility cycle the only people who experience hormonal changes wrought by their reproductive systems.

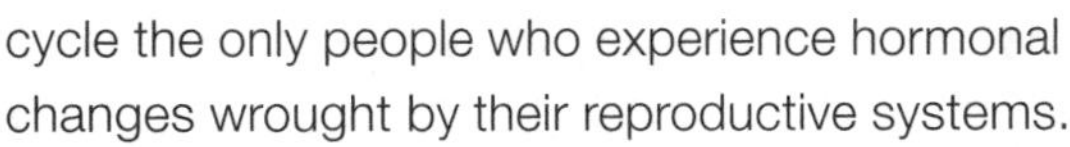

The cyclical fertility changes that happen for someone with a penis happen differently, but they happen. There are two different arenas of constant hormonal changes in that kind of reproductive system. There are daily hormonal changes—testosterone levels are usually highest in the morning and decrease through the day—that occur in cycles of around twenty-four hours. And then there are additional cycles every seventy-two days in which the hormones FSH and LH are at work, just as they are in the menstrual cycle. These regulate the production of sperm. So, if you have the idea that only one group of people can be "hormonal" or only one sex goes through mood changes because of their reproductive systems, think again!

sperm cells that has traveled to this point, semen is ready to be ejaculated. Ejaculation occurs through the urethra, usually as a result of sexual arousal and stimulation, with the aid of contractions that continue all along the path that the sperm and fluid take in order to leave the body.

During ejaculation, a muscular gate called the urinary sphincter, which is located at the opening of the bladder, closes so that urine, if it's present in the bladder, isn't released during ejaculation. During urination, that gate is voluntarily opened.

Vasocongestion (aka Blue Balls)

Blue balls . . . aren't about balls at all. Nor are "blue balls," correctly termed vasocongestion, exclusive to people who have testicles. Every body can, and probably will, at least once, experience a similar sensation.

During sexual arousal (as explained on page 44), the genitals fill with blood. When we orgasm or ejaculate, the swelling from vasocongestion usually subsides and quickly goes away. If we do not orgasm or ejaculate after sexual stimulation and arousal—and sometimes even when we do—vasocongestion can stick around for a bit and can cause pain or discomfort, which we feel in the genitals.

Discomfort when arousal is not followed by ejaculation is vasocongestive pressure often felt in the penis, testicles, or general pelvic area. In many ways, vasocongestion is like having a tension headache in your genitals: blood pressure is increased, but the blood vessels that the blood must flow through are constricted.

DID YOU KNOW? . . .

As different as the genitals of people who have testes and a penis are from those of people who have a vulva and uterus, when we were all embryos, our genitals were identical for a while. Only after the tenth week of development, based on levels of hormones dictated mostly by our chromosomal structure, do fetal genitals usually turn into either the head of a penis or clitoris, do the genital folds turn into either testes or inner labia, and do the genital swellings become the scrotum or outer labia.

When high blood pressure and high blood volume meet narrowed blood vessels—like trying to force the flow of a kitchen faucet through a soda straw—it's uncomfortable and can be downright painful. The reason someone may feel vasocongestion most profoundly in the testes is that the testes are so sensitive.

Taking care of vasocongestion is pretty simple. You can masturbate to orgasm, take a pain reliever, use a cold or warm compress, get a little rest, or engage in some simple physical activity to redirect your blood flow.

If you've got a sexual partner, your vasocongestion is not their responsibility, just like the headache you got or the muscle you pulled trying to get to their house quickly because you wanted to see them so bad isn't. No one can "give" anyone a "case of blue balls," and no one should be manipulated or pushed into doing something to relieve this condition or be made to feel like this response is their fault or doing when it's really all about your own body, and not a big deal to boot. *Just no.*

Too Loose/Too Tight! Too Long/Too Short! Too Large/Too Small! Or, What Goldilocks and the Three Bears Have to Do with Your Genitals

Too Loose!/Too Tight!

There's no one standard resting "size" or width of any given vaginal opening or canal, because when nothing is inside the vagina, any vagina, it's a loosely closed tube that doesn't have an open space of any width to measure. How "loose" or "tight" it feels when something is inside of it depends mostly on how relaxed or aroused someone is (or isn't) at a given time. The vagina is very elastic, and how it feels is mostly about the muscles around it and how the person with the vagina feels. Someone who is very nervous or anxious or who doesn't want what's trying to go inside their vagina will generally feel "tight" in a way that feels uncomfortable. When someone is relaxed, comfortable, and wanting what's inside the vagina to be there, they won't feel an uncomfortable tightness, and in some ways that area will feel looser because the muscles of and around the vagina are more relaxed instead of tense. If someone is very sexually excited on top of that, they'll often feel the comfort from that lack of muscle tension and a feel-good kind of muscle tension.

Ideas some people have that the vaginal canal or opening is "loose" or "tight" when nothing is inside the vagina or that how the vagina feels to the person with the vagina or to someone else is about anything besides what I just talked about are fictions based on a lack of education about anatomy as well as some crummy

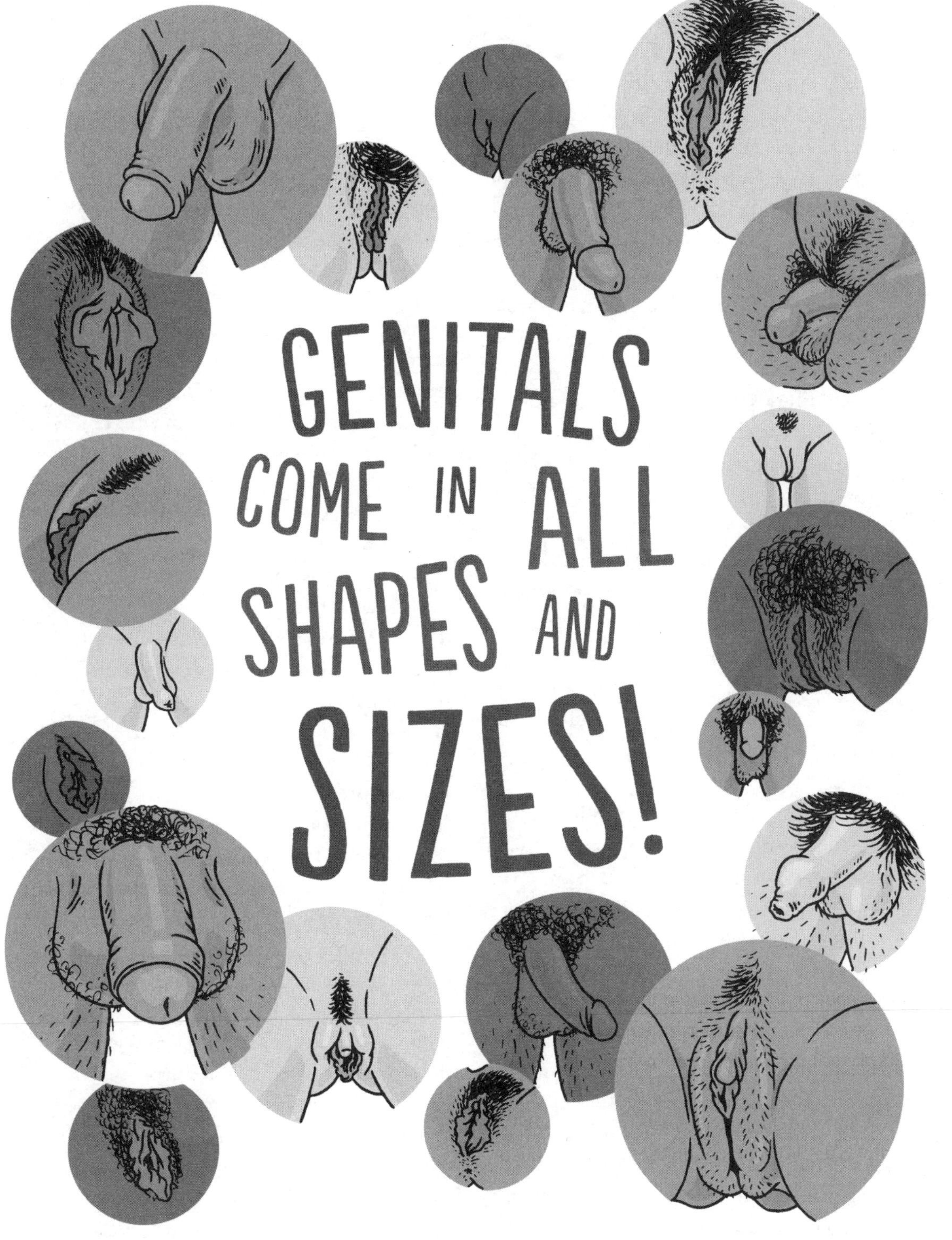
GENITALS
COME IN ALL
SHAPES AND
SIZES!

cultural constructs and history about people with vaginas and sexuality and about other people wanting to control both.

If, during masturbation or partnered sex, you or a partner feel you are "too tight," relax (and ask them to relax as well, for crying out loud). Stressing out is only going to make it worse. Take the time you need to chill out, to become aroused by activities that don't involve the vaginal opening and canal (like snuggling, massage, kissing, or stimulating the clitoris) before you attempt vaginal entry with a penis, fingers, or sex toys. You can always opt out entirely of any kind of vaginal sex when it's just not feeling good. Usually, sex of any sort really and truly should not be painful.

Someone saying you're "too loose"? Maybe that person's previous experiences have been with people who felt "tighter" because they weren't aroused or who were feeling nervous (which, in the case of young adults, isn't unusual). How many friends do you know who are *expecting* sex with vaginal entry to be painful? Expecting pain often prevents full arousal: it's pretty difficult to feel excited when we're just waiting for pain. Because many people think that sex with vaginal entry is supposed to be painful at first, a lot of them don't know how to do it only if and when they're truly aroused or how to make any of this comfortable (for more on that, see Chapter 8). So, if a partner is saying you're "too loose," either they're simply experiencing a relaxed, aroused partner for the first time or they're blowing smoke—because they think it's the thing to say or they were expecting to feel trapped in a vise, which is not how this should feel for either partner.

In the first place, it's very unlikely for those in their teens or twenties to have vaginal or pelvic muscle tone issues unless there have been complications from a childbirth. But, if you like, you can do Kegel exercises to strengthen the muscles of the pelvic floor, which can be felt within the vaginal canal. You've likely done Kegels already: when you're finished urinating, you know how you squeeze your muscles a bit to force out those last few drops of urine? That's a Kegel. Often, people are advised to do them after childbirth because pregnancy can weaken the pelvic floor, and some people find that Kegel exercises heighten their orgasmic and sexual response as well as increase bladder control. Some folks—including people who have a penis, not a vagina—just enjoy doing them because they feel good. So, squeeze away, rhythmically, whenever and wherever you like—no one else can see you doing them.

Too Long!/Too Short!

A lot of folks have the idea that there are "ideal" inner labia and that what's ideal is any length or size that is diminutive and hidden; in other words, that inner labia are only okay if someone can barely tell they're there at all. Some people make lewd jokes or comments about various types of labia or insult labia of a certain size or shape. This is not surprising: we live in a culture that often acts ashamed about genitals and sexuality, especially genitals also associated with women, so it's no big shocker that the "ideal" is genitals that are as hidden from view as possible.

People who are raised as men often want their penises to be larger than life; people raised as women often wish their genitals were small, shy, and nearly invisible. But the reality is that fully functional, operative, and "pretty" genitals, whatever someone's sex or gender, are diverse and come in a range of sizes, just like everything else.

Like people's mouths or noses, labia minora come in a wide variety of shapes, sizes, textures, and colors. All of these variations are okay, with no one "kind" somehow better or worse than the rest. Some people with longer or larger labia worry that they've altered them by pulling at them or by masturbating, but that's very unlikely.

Gynecologists have seen a whole lot of vulvas and labia, of every imaginable shape, size, and hue. So, if you're seriously concerned or convinced that yours are abnormal or problematic, ask a gynecologist or another kind of healthcare provider who provides sexual or reproductive health care to take a look and give you an honest assessment. Chances are good that what you think is totally abnormal is completely normal. It's so easy to feel insecure about parts we hardly ever get a chance to see. (For others who look at our parts, especially those who don't have these parts themselves or haven't seen many of them on others, it's easy to think something looks "weird" when it's just unfamiliar.) There are a few good books available that do show the real diversity of the vulva, such as Joani Blank's *Femalia* or Wrenna Robertson's *I'll Show You Mine.*

Pornography is often a poor place to look for "normal" genitals. Not only are actors and models in porn chosen to meet whatever "fashion" or size of genitalia fits fantasy fodder (which is usually exaggerated in one way or another) but also shaving, waxing, tucking, primping, photo editing, retouching, and lighting, and sometimes surgical adaptations, have been employed to alter genital appearance. If your own genitals were given that kind of treatment, you might not even recognize them yourself!

In the same vein, what peers have to say about what's "normal" in genital appearance often comes from their own very limited viewing of other genitals (if they've even seen any at all), from seeing genitals in photographs or porn, or from what they've heard from someone else. Too, a lot of times when someone proclaims another person's genitals are abnormal, it stems from a place of insecurity about their own.

When you attempt to figure out what's normal in terms of genitals, remember that appearance and function aren't the same thing. What's most worthy of concern is the latter, not the former, and if your genitals are functional, chances are pretty darn good that they're normal as far as appearance goes, too.

Too Big!/Too Small!

Let's be honest: How often do we hear complaints from people with penises about their penises being too big or earnest brags about being smaller? Not often. Most of the worries we hear are about penises being too small, and often, those concerns are about vaginal intercourse or about partners with penises who compare sizes. Here's a tip: it may seem like a pretty remarkable coincidence, but the average vaginal canal is about the same length as the average penis. (The average rectum is shorter.)

Moreover, the vaginal canal (as do the rectum, mouth, and hands) contracts to hold the size of whatever is inside of it, the first inch or so of the vagina is where most of the sensory nerve endings are (thus, where people are really feeling a lot of sensation), *and* the most sensitive, sensory-nerve-ending-rich part of sexual anatomy isn't the vagina at all but the internal and external clitoris.

TECH TIP

If you're looking online at images of penises, know that you're probably not seeing very realistic representations. In pornography, actors who have larger-than-average penises are almost always chosen. And even on user-generated sites or tools where people are posting their own penis pics, the people posting are often just as worried about size as anyone else, so they probably pick angles that exaggerate the size or shape of their penis (including showing it erect) or they are not even posting pics of their own penises at all.

Concerns that *you'll* get less sexual sensation or satisfaction because of the size or shape of your penis are also misplaced: sensation and arousal have nothing to do with size (unless you let anxiety about size get the better of you or get excited about the idea of having a given size or shape). Shorter penises can experience and create just as many pleasurable sensations as do those that are longer. A bigger penis isn't "better" any more than a taller person is "better." We're all just different—no big whoop.

So, being worried that a particular penis size won't satisfy a partner, of any gender, is generally pointless, because *no* specific size or shape of penis is likely to produce instant satisfaction or orgasm via intercourse. If we're talking about anal sex (see page 239) or oral sex (see page 231), more times than not, less is more when it comes to what's most comfortable in the mouth or anus. In studies about sexual satisfaction, penis size is not something reported as a major player.

If you have an e-mail account, you probably get daunting amounts of spam telling you about this device or that one, these pills or those, all of which can increase your penis size—the whole lot of it is rubbish. And most of what you hear about people preferring a larger penis size is the same sort of parroting you hear about people only liking larger breasts or blond hair. What people publicly state as their preferences often has a lot more to do with what they *think* they should be saying than with what they actually feel, know, or prefer.

The truth is, with partners of any gender, sometimes a person wants greater or lesser depth of entry into their genitals. If someone with a vagina has a partner with a larger penis, at times they may prefer vaginal play with just a finger or two instead of a penis. If they have a partner with a smaller penis, sometimes they may want greater vaginal stimulation with a sex toy (see page 247) or manual sex (see page 229) with a few fingers—and that shouldn't be a big deal. One of the cool things about sex and bodies is that the experience doesn't have to be about just one or two parts: most often we have our whole bodies to work with, and approaching sex in a whole-body way tends to result in people having a really good time.

Sometimes, oral or manual sex may feel better to you than vaginal or anal intercourse. It's the same sort of thing: when we drop the false idea that our genitals are supposed to be some sort of one-size-fits-all tool for satisfaction, rather than just one of many body parts that we can feel and give pleasure with in numerous ways, it's easy to get a lot more comfortable with normal size and shape variations.

(Not) On the Straight and Narrow

It's most common for a penis to have *some* curvature when erect; perfectly straight, symmetrical penises aren't at all common. If you discover that you have any pain or discomfort when you become erect, or that the curvature of your penis is profound (basically, if you're looking at something like a 90 degree angle), then speak to your doctor. But, otherwise, some penises curve up, some down, some to the left or to the right, and some don't seem to curve at all. Each of those variations is normal. In terms of partnered sex, mouths, vaginas, and rectums are all flexible and have curves of their own. So, whereas two particular people may find they're an exceptional fit in some ways or positions than others, curvature is in no way a problem.

When it comes to partnered sex, if any of these vast and normal variations were all that problematic, we'd have a lot less sex going on, and a lot fewer people on the planet. Don't sweat it.

Circumcised/Uncircumcised

There is nothing wrong, dirty, or gross about having an intact foreskin (see page 42); at birth, all penises have one (just like the clitoris has a hood), and the majority of people worldwide are uncircumcised. Intact folks just have to make a few adaptations: you do need to pull back your foreskin and clean it gently when you bathe, and you need to use a condom a little differently (for more on that, see Chapter 10 on safer sex). You may also need to be on the lookout a little more cautiously for yeast or fungal infections. But none of that is any big deal, just some basic habits to pick up if you haven't already.

A circumcised penis, if that's what you've got, is also fine and functional, and *it's* not wrong, dirty, or gross, either. Circumcised people can have slightly less sensitivity in their penises than uncircumcised folks do, but that needn't be a trauma or a problem: the whole body, not just our genitals, is involved in sexual activity and sensation, and we experience *most* sexual arousal and satisfaction in our brains and nervous systems.

Also, there isn't one sort of penis that is more prone to STIs (Sexually Transmitted Infections; see page 265). Some data on uncircumcised penises have shown that uncircumcised people may be at greater risk for some infections, but other data on circumcised penises show that those who are circumcised may be at greater risk for different infections, particularly with or after circumcision. And research shows that, if you're going to have genital sex with partners, the only thing that *really* does the job preventing STIs isn't whether you are circumcised or not but whether you practice safer sex, including the consistent and correct use of condoms.

In a few countries and areas, the look of an uncircumcised penis may be unfamiliar to some, but uncircumcised penises are the most common around the world.

Ultimately, you have whichever you have. Although some doctors will perform elective adult male circumcision, that procedure carries risks and downsides, and it's not recommended save for a few very specific health conditions.

Sometimes, just like partners who find the first few times being up close and personal with vulvas unusual or daunting, some sexual partners may feel or act awkward or intimidated around a certain type of penis. Although it's hard not to take someone's fascination, curiosity, or even amazement about something so personal personally, it's helpful to recognize that it's just how humans react sometimes.

A Few Short Words on the Short and Curlies

Because we're mammals, all of our bodies, male and female, are naturally covered with hair—and that includes our genital areas. Hair grows naturally around the genitals, down to and around the anus and thighs, and over the pubic mound. Lately, whereas pubic hair on men is generally accepted, popular culture, mass media, and fashion have been dictating that women should or must remove or modify their pubic hair—even to the point that certain patterns and shapes are considered preferable or fashionable.

If You're Going to Remove Your Pubic Hair

- Shaving or waxing just before sexual activity can increase STI risks because of small cuts or scrapes, so best to shave or wax a day or two before you have sex with a partner rather than just prior.
- Be careful: you really don't want to cut, burn, or tear the inner labia or scrotum. *YEEEOOWCH!* When pubic hair is removed in any way, it's also normal to get ingrown hairs, red bumps, and itching. You can exfoliate daily with a loofah or the like, and keep the area moisturized, to help reduce irritation.
- Same goes with waxing or sugaring—genital tissue is delicate. So, if you're waxing yourself, be sure not to apply the wax to genital tissue but only to the *external* genitals: thighs, mons, outer labia, and area around the base of the penis, not the penis itself or testes. Because waxing and sugaring the genitals can be tricky, it's probably best to have a professional do your waxing, at least at first.
- Shaving doesn't permanently darken body hair. Body hair that grows back after shaving does appear darker and more coarse because it's been cut and hasn't been exposed to sun, water, salt, and air for years like body hair you don't mess with has. So, before you shave any body part, just consider that the hair you may have there afterward will likely not be as fine or light-colored again once you start shaving it.

As with the hair on your head, you can do whatever you want with your pubic hair. Plenty of people—more, worldwide, rather than less—leave it be, and plenty of people do something to it. Just like the hair on your head, pubic hair is totally acceptable in any length, thickness, or color, and just like the hair on your head, what you do or don't do with it is hopefully about what you like, your style and comfort, and what works with your life. If you don't want to mess with it at all, you don't have to. If you want to try shaving or waxing it, you can; like any hair, it grows right back, so it's fine to experiment to find out what you prefer and what works for you.

TECH TIP

On a few great sites or feeds out there right now, people are doing their best to post realistic pictures of their own bodies, including their genitals, with the aim of showing our true diversity and more real representations of bodies than we often see in any media, including online media. To find these sites, try searching using the keywords *body positive* plus the name of the part you're looking for, such as *penis, breasts,* or *vulva.*

What's "Normal" Down There?

Most teens and emerging adults (and most people, period, really) haven't seen a lot of genitals up close and personal in real life. At best, maybe you and your best friends have looked at one another's, perhaps you've spied a few brief glimpses in the locker room, maybe you've seen your parents' genitals, and possibly you've seen the genitals of a few sexual partners. Plenty of books out there include illustrations of genitalia, but sometimes it's hard to compare what pen and ink have created to what's there in the flesh.

Ultimately, when we say that genitals come in a seriously diverse array of shapes, sizes, colors, and textures for all genders, it's not a bunch of malarkey meant to comfort and quiet you. It's a fact.

We often confuse the word *normal* with the word *ideal.* Normal doesn't mean perfect; it simply means what is most common. And what's normal is diversity!

3

The Problem with Perfect: Body Image

OR, WHY APPEARANCE ISN'T ALL IT APPEARS

Start a revolution: Be kind to your body!

When you've got a healthy, holistic, and realistic body image, you're more likely to take good care of your body and all of who you are. You're more likely to be aware of when you're sick and when you're in good health. You're more likely to truly use your body as a vehicle for really living and experiencing your life—however it looks.

When we've got positive body image brewin', we feel more positive, powerful, confident, and capable. Positive body image allows us to have greater self-esteem, because we're better able to see that our bodies and what they look like are just parts of who we are, not all, and that our bodies are about way more than just what they look like. Positive body image can also help us make smarter choices when it comes to sex, to feel more able to set and maintain our limits and boundaries and to fully enjoy the sex we're having.

Too often, we and everyone around us place more value on how we look than on who we *are* and what we can *do;* appearances are often given more weight and attention than character, ideas, and accomplishments.

We don't have to ignore appearances or how others look at them and there's nothing wrong with noticing or appreciating them. In our teens and twenties, when there's often so much added focus from peers and parents on how we look, ignoring our appearance is nearly impossible to do, even if we wanted to. People

Body image

Body image describes your view of your own body, in function, health, experience, and appearance. *Self-esteem* describes what level of regard, respect, and value you have for yourself—not just your body but the whole person who lives in it. Body image and self-esteem are often linked, especially in young adults, and all the more in a culture that fixates on physical appearance. *Lookism* or *looksism* describes discrimination based on physical appearance, or the fixation of a person, group, or culture on physical appearance.

are amazing critters, bodies are pretty fascinating things to look at, and visual sexual attraction and attention to appearance are parts of our nature—but only *part, and we want to be sure to strike a balance.* Our bodies also enable us to do everything we do each day: to go to work or school, build cities, make art, and create cultural movements; to enjoy a stack of steaming pancakes or a swim in the sea; to nurture families and friends; to live out our whole lives, enjoying and accomplishing all the things we can do.

Your body can seek out, nurture, and enjoy pleasure, alone and with partners. Your body is your partner in emotional intimacy. Your body can even potentially create new life, new bodies. You'll also inevitably experience pain, discomfort, or illness in your body during your lifetime. At some point, you may be dissatisfied with your body for far more pressing and challenging reasons than because your thighs aren't thin enough or your muscles big enough. You may be unhappy because you've experienced a serious injury or illness, because you have developed a disability or increased challenges over time because of a disability, or because you can't feel or experience pleasure in the ways that you're used to.

Maybe you've already managed the fantastic accomplishment of having a strongly positive body image; maybe you're not there yet. Maybe you feel as if you're drowning in insecurity, can't see how you'll ever get out of it, and think that if you hear the phrase "positive body image" one more time, you'll scream. Wherever you are on the spectrum—even you screamers—listen up.

[TEN BODACIOUS WAYS TO BOOST BODY IMAGE]

1. Make the real the ideal. Less than 5 percent of the entire population looks like celebrities, models, and other uncommon people who meet most cultural beauty standards. Especially without all the lighting, makeup, retouching, and everything else involved in producing the media they are in, celebrities or models often don't even look like their famous personas. To make the real the ideal, collect photos of people you admire for all sorts of reasons, not just for the way they look; make your collection realistic and well rounded. For every photo of one mostly-because-they-look-so-awesome, add photos of at least ten other people whose external appearance isn't the most notable or valued thing about them—friends and family, writers, musicians, teachers, scientists, activists, folks whose smiles or wrinkles are as interesting as their backsides—because **that's** a more realistic and inspiring collection. Creating a realistic collage is an easy, visual way to get a better idea of what an actual range of whole-person beauty is rather than the very limited, often unattainable, and on-the-surface-only beauty the media sell us.

2. Exercise your enjoyment. Engage in physical activity or movement that offers you something more than thinner thighs or six-pack abs. Moving our bodies is not just about trying to get them to look certain ways or reaching the "right" number on a scale. It's about health and enjoying the physical and emotional feelings movement can provide; about becoming stronger, more flexible, more resilient; about learning new skills and exploring personal goals. It's about getting our ya-ya's out. It should be fun and should feel *good, in all ways.* Don't try to force yourself to do exercise that feels like drudgery or training for a beauty contest. Consider self-defense or martial arts classes. Try yoga, hula-hooping, or paddleboarding. Pick a team sport. Indulge in a nice, long stretch each day. Get outside and go hiking, biking, swimming, or horseback riding in places where your exercise also lets you enjoy some extra oxygen, a beautiful day, or a new place to hang out.

3. See every body. *Spend time in places with real-deal body diversity.* Shoe stores don't have just one shoe that's universally better than all the rest; there are different kinds of shoes for all sorts of activities, aesthetics, and preferences, and they come in a dizzying array of materials, styles, sizes, shapes, and colors. Human bodies are the same way.

Community centers, grocery stores, airports or bus stops, public parks, and swimming pools are all good places to see diversity. When we're regularly exposed to only one town, one age group, one social class, or one locker room, it can be too easy to forget how incredibly different we all are. Just as it's not sage to assume that the whole world is like your hometown, it's smart to keep in mind that our idea about how bodies look, and how people choose to present them, is often pretty limited.

4. Be a positive body image warrior! If you pick up magazines with articles or images that make you feel bad about yourself, or that support negative body image, use your voice. Almost every magazine includes inserts for subscriptions that require no postage to send. Get out a pen and write what you're feeling on those cards, and then toss them in the mail. Write an article for a school or college paper about media lies and myths about bodies, health, dieting, or beauty. How about starting a no-makeup or comfy-clothes-only day once a month with your friends, in your dorm or at a workplace?

Start at home by changing what you expose yourself to and how you process it. Recycle your fashion, fitness, or beauty mags or catalogs, or use them for kindling in a fireplace. Reduce the number of hours you spend immersed in mainstream media. For just one day, count how many times you look in mirrors, fuss with your hair or clothes, or think or talk about appearance-related things; just becoming aware of how much time and energy these things take can deliver a pretty loud wake-up call. Sit down and figure out how much money you spend each month on makeup, hair products or styling, clothing, weight-loss products, and work to cut that amount at least in half—save the money you don't spend on that stuff for something you really want to do for your *whole* self.

5. Ditch the dissing. Most of us aren't even aware of how often we judge other people based on how they look. In our heads, or even worse, out loud, we may call others fat, ugly, cheap, skinny, skanky, gross, what have you, so much that we no longer think anything of it or recognize it as big-time bad juju. Start paying attention. Think about *why* you judge people the way you do. When you call someone fat, even out of their earshot, is it because you're concerned about their health or because it makes you feel less insecure about *your* body? Does dissing them give you a break from insulting yourself? If you talk about someone having a small penis or a "loose" vagina—likely without any idea of what their bodies are like or without accurate ideas about sexual anatomy in the first place—how does that really benefit you? Who is that helping (probably no one) and who is it hurting or keeping down (probably everyone, including you)?

The same goes for tuning out and turning off any of *your* body image bullies. Often, other people who diss your body or get in a snit about it are doing it for the same lousy reasons you do: out of fear and insecurity. It's not always easy to be direct about an insult, but it can sure feel better than sucking it up or pretending it doesn't hurt. So, if Mom says you look a little chubby or teases you about your size, remind her that what she says is hurtful and that there are better ways she could express any concern she might have. If a friend or peer dogs your appearance, let them know that you're not interested in being a target for their own insecurities. If you're getting harassed or teased at school, fight back productively by filing a report with the faculty or participating in or starting up grassroots actions against school harassment.

6. Look deeper: looks aren't everything. A poll from the Eating Disorders Awareness and Prevention Center in Seattle found that teen girls were more scared of being fat than they were of a nuclear war or of losing their parents. **Yipes.** That's how big and bad things can get and feel when we—or others—focus on appearance that's way out of whack and when we or others not only create or perpetuate narrow beauty standards that fit almost no one but also assign a greater or lesser *value* to people based only on what they look like. That all really *is* scary.

It's hard to have a positive self-image and solid self-esteem when you don't feel important or valued, even if you feel fantastic about the way you look. Put yourself in environments where you can *do* something and be someone you're seriously proud of. Volunteer to help build low-income housing (bonus: it's also a great workout). Help with a community garden or with landscaping at a community center, school, or domestic abuse shelter. Escort at an abortion clinic. Be a Big Sister or Big Brother, or tutor a kid in your apartment building who's struggling. Help coach a Little League team. Join a letter-writing campaign for women and men in other countries who are fighting for their right to education, jobs, or freedom.

Remember, too, that you have many relationships of value in your life, not just sexual or romantic ones—friends, family, teachers, and mentors, and those to whom you are the mentor or role model. All the different feelings people can have for you are important, not just feelings of sexual attraction or aesthetic appeal. And becoming someone you are truly proud of will also help you achieve more fulfilling, richer, and healthier sexual and intimate relationships.

7. #iwokeuplikethis (for real). According to a study done by facial cleanser company Albolene, 73 percent of American women wear makeup, and 42 percent report that they never leave home without it. Makeup and grooming aren't bad things, but feeling that hairstyling, shaving, or clothes that accentuate this or hide that are required is an express bus on the road to poor body image and self-esteem. Ditch the stuff sometimes. Go places—not just hang out at home—without makeup, without straightening or styling your hair. Wear clothes that are comfortable, without spending time worrying about what statement they make or if they're in style right now. If you are in a sexual partnership, get comfortable being together now and then without a metric buttload of preparation first: the shaving or waxing, the makeup, the clothing. You don't have to look like you've been living on a deserted island for a year, and I'm not advocating that you shouldn't shower, wash your face, brush your teeth and hair, or clean your clothes.

But sometimes, let the basics be all you do. You'll be amazed at how many people don't see a profound difference, and it's a cool thing to get comfortable really looking like you, turning off the messages that say you have to look like anyone else—and saving all that cash, too!

8. Self-validate. Remember that neither partners nor friends can magically deliver positive, lasting self-esteem. When someone you find attractive or are in love with tells you you're beautiful, sexy, or hot, of course you get a boost—but it can't usually make you feel those things about yourself by yourself. By basing your body image and self-image on what others think, you put other people in charge of your own self-worth. That can be particularly easy to do in your teens and twenties, when you're still in the process of some heavy-duty personal development and when the pressures on you to conform and fit in are so intense. But, if you base your self-image on what a partner says, what are you going to do when that partner's gone, when their opinions change, or even when they're having a hard day and are focused on things besides what you look like?

Self-validation can look like positive self-talk or simply doing something that makes you feel good about yourself and your abilities. Bonus points if the activity you choose helps with stress management because many body image issues become more pronounced during stressful times or when people experience a loss or lack of control. Instead of taking out frustration on your body, do things that make you feel powerful.

DID YOU KNOW? . . .

Bad Self-Talk: Talking to ourselves very negatively and destructively is probably Public Enemy Number One when it comes to body image. Unfortunately, loads of us do it, because it's been so normalized for us, and fewer of us make our self-talk positive and supportive in large part because that hasn't been normal. In most cultures, feeling bad about ourselves, in general, is a lot more supported than feeling good about ourselves. But it really is all self-fulfilling prophecy of the worst kind. If we tell ourselves we're ugly, too thick or too thin, worthless, stupid or terrible, we're going to feel that way. And the more we say it, the more we're going to believe all those things to be true, even when confronted with clear evidence to the contrary. The opposite of that is, however, also true: when we make our self-talk the kind of talk that comforts and supports us, that aims to make us feel better instead of worse, we'll tend to feel better and we'll be much more likely to feel and believe the things we say. If it's not something you'd ever dream of saying to the person or other creature you love most of all in the world, you shouldn't be saying it to yourself, someone who deserves that big love and care, too.

9. Do unto others. Imagine how you might feel if, a couple of times during the day, someone walked up to you and said, "Your tooth gap is the coolest," or "That was a *great* presentation you just gave," or "That skirt you made is awesome. How did you do it?" or "I love your laugh." Start the chain. And that doesn't just mean compliments about appearance, either; give others credit for their *accomplishments,* too. Not only can that be a serious day-maker for someone else, you'll find that doing it makes you feel more positive about yourself, too.

10. Make friends with a healthcare provider. If you have body concerns; if you feel you need to diet, be at the gym twice a day, or go ballistic with weight training and protein powder; if you wonder whether your body parts are normal; or if you just feel like crap about your body—a doctor or nurse is a great person to talk to. They can let you know what you really *do* need to be doing for your body as well as what's realistic for your body and your age. Healthcare providers see a vast array of bodies every single day, up close and personal, so they tend to have a good bead on what bodies really look like and how diverse they are. They're also concerned with health rather than appearance, which often makes them excellent people to talk to about body image and body concerns.

DISORDERED EATING AND EATING DISORDERS

A majority of young people have been or are on diets, and *diets* usually means fad diets, skipping meals, vomiting after eating, or using diet pills or weight-gain supplements. Over 50 percent of teen girls and 30 percent of teen boys use unhealthy weight control behaviors such as skipping meals, fasting, smoking cigarettes, vomiting, and taking laxatives. Polls from sources like *People* magazine have shown that well over 80 percent of young women are unhappy or dissatisfied with their looks or bodies, and studies have also found that the more mainstream media someone consumes, the more likely they are to struggle with body image. (For more about the impacts of media and other external influences, see Chapter 6.)

In 2003, the Centers for Disease Control and Prevention surveyed fifteen thousand high school students in the United States about eating habits. They found that over 44 percent of them (59.3 percent of people classified as female and 29.1 percent of those classified as male) were trying to lose weight. Many young people start dieting as early as the age of eight or nine. Obesity rates have been increasing for young and grown adults, even though the majority of them are also dieting. This

DON'T MAKE A MATE A MIRROR

When we have sex partners, poor body image or self-image can make it harder to talk honestly about sex, to insist on things that keep us safe: limits and boundaries, safer sex practices, birth control. When we're insecure about our appearance or our worth, we may feel we owe favors to someone who finds us beautiful or interesting. We may find it hard to say no or ask for things we need, because we feel the other person is giving so much just by accepting us when we can't accept ourselves. We may tolerate or agree to sexual activity or partnership we don't want because we think we can't do better and we believe that something will always feel better than nothing. Our character judgment of partners may be skewed by virtue of our messed-up self-judgment.

If you're going to enter into sexual partnership, do yourself a solid and make it a real partnership, not just a performance or form of self-validation. When you seek a partner, ask yourself: is it because you want a mutually beneficial relationship or is it because you need someone around to make you feel better about yourself, to prove to you that you have value and worth? Are you willing to have relationships that are less beneficial and enjoyable to all partners because so much effort needs to go into securing your self-esteem? Some people seek out sexual partnership to try to fill a void in terms of self-esteem or positive body image, and then they discover—alas—that the sex or boyfriend/girlfriend doesn't fill that void. They then get even more depressed and self-loathing, thinking something must be wrong with them, screwing up their relationships in the process.

Whoever you're with, whether they're a friend, a casual hookup, or the Juliet to your Romeo (or the Romeo to your Mercutio, for that matter), you should be able to feel like yourself, act like yourself, look like yourself, and have sex like yourself: Be yourself *for* yourself. It shouldn't feel like an audition—you already got the part.

Most of us are going to spend decent parts of our lives single, without sexual partners or spouses, living by ourselves, being by ourselves. It's important to learn that we can stand alone; that we can love and accept our bodies, whether or not anyone else shows attraction to them at any given time; that we can love and accept ourselves, even during the days, weeks, or months when no one says anything good about us and even when we get negative feedback. We need to value ourselves when we're not in relationships or sexual partnerships; we need things we enjoy doing, be they work or hobbies, and we need a sense of body love that isn't just about how our bodies look but about how they feel and what they enable us to do each day.

That would be that *self* part of self-esteem, self-love, and self-worth.

isn't a surprise: dieting is well known and has been clearly shown, through a lot of study, to make more people *less* healthy, physically and emotionally, rather than healthier, especially in the long term or when it starts at a young age.

Many young people believe that if they could only be the "right" size or shape, they'd feel better about themselves, even though there's plenty of evidence to support that, realistically, even people who lose weight when it is medically advised often find that doesn't do much for poor self-esteem or body image by itself.

Disordered eating can range from mild to severe. Skipping meals now and then, trying a diet, or binging on ice cream post-breakup would be considered mild. For some, occasional disordered eating becomes a serious eating disorder (ED)—such as anorexia (starvation), bulimia (binging and purging), or binge eating—which can jeopardize their health and well-being, even their life.

All types of disordered eating have side effects, long and short term, benign and severe. EDs carry serious risks such as malnutrition, heart failure, bowel problems, permanent damage to the throat, permanent gallbladder or reproductive damage, and diabetes, to name just a few, as well as serious emotional and psychological effects.

Fad diets, starvation, binging, or purging can mean permanently, irreversibly screwing up your body and your health. And if you permanently screw up your metabolism, all the dieting and starving in the world aren't going to fix it; you will usually end up less healthy and *less* able to influence your size and shape than you are now.

DID YOU KNOW? . . .

During adolescence, to be as healthy as we can and to develop properly, physically and intellectually, we need to eat more calories than we do in any other phase of life. The average teen needs about 2,200 to 2,500 calories each day. And if you're consuming most of those via fresh, whole, healthy foods, while keeping moderately active within your abilities and managing your stresses, you are setting yourself up with the best foundation possible for sound short- and long-term health and good looks.

Who's at Risk of Disordered Eating, Body Image, or Self-Image Problems?

More than five million people in the United States—some still in elementary school—are currently affected by eating disorders. Although the onset of most eating disorders has typically been around the age of thirteen or fourteen, now disordered eating starts in some young people before puberty even hits. At least 10 to 15 percent of people with eating disorders will literally die because of them.

Some issues can increase risks of developing an ED. Low self-esteem is a biggie, as is depression or anxiety. During adolescence, it's easy to feel out of control and also easy to feel controlled. Teens can be at an increased risk when their parents, friends, or communities exert a lot of control over appearances, such as how someone dresses; do not allow for healthy and normal social opportunities, freedoms, and responsibilities; or push for particular goals, such as college, marriage, or certain professions. Research has found that young women whose mothers or sisters have eating disorders or are obsessed with diets are at a greater risk for developing EDs (a finding that would probably be similar for children and parents of any gender). Plenty of parents don't realize how much their own eating is disordered and how those behaviors affect their kids. Many teens and emerging adults are under extreme social, academic, and familial stress that is dismissed or that goes unrecognized, and those stresses can increase ED risks. The highly, and narrowly, gendered socialization processes that overemphasize appearance as part of ideal femininity or masculinity that most of us grow up with are often another player in disordered eating.

Although disordered eating is primarily associated with women, men aren't immune to EDs. Some coaches or trainers support or enforce disordered eating. Plenty of men—especially gay men, men who participate in certain sports, and young men who are "late bloomers"—deal with an overemphasis on appearance and body perfection just as many women do. Young men may binge eat, overdo protein supplements or other weight-gain formulas, or engage in steroid use. And some young men are also anorexic or bulimic; both disorders are currently on the rise among young men.

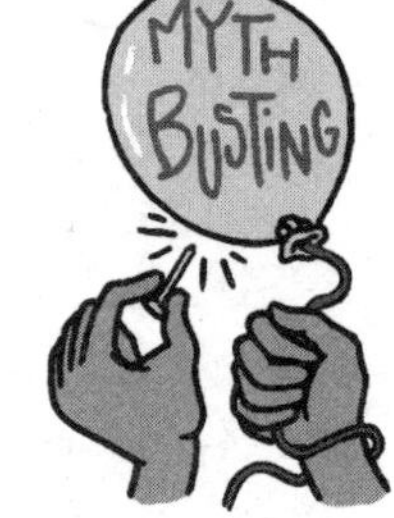

The bottom line is that EDs are serious illnesses caused by a complex mix of factors. EDs are much more than "a diet gone too far" and often have very severe physical and psychological repercussions.

If you think you might have an ED or be on the road to one, talk to a physical or mental healthcare provider. It's always okay to err on the side of caution, so even if you're not sure, ask. It's a whole lot easier to prevent an ED than to get past it once you've gotten into those patterns.

If you have a friend you suspect may have an eating disorder, seek out capable help. It's often impossible to help someone else through an ED alone, and time isn't on your side: the longer someone with an ED goes without getting effective help, the more sick they become, and the tougher recovery is. Even the well-intentioned ways people try to help often feed the problem. For instance, saying, "You're so skinny!" to an anorexic only validates the illness. Most people with eating disorders work very hard to hide their behaviors, so it may not be possible to get them to admit that they even have an ED. The better road to take—for yourself and your friend—is to talk to a trusted counselor, doctor, or parent and let them know what you suspect. For more information on dealing with an eating disorder, your own or someone else's, see the Resources section.

[THE IDEAL SPIEL]

We're constantly bombarded by messages about sexual appeal and performance that promote often unattainable and unrealistic

TECH TIP

Selfies for Yourself-y!

In common practice selfies are something about you (well, kind of), but not *for* you. Often, they are for other people or to get the opinion of or validation from other people. There's nothing inherently wrong with that: as people, we generally seek outside validation to some degree; it's just a thing we do. No big. There's also nothing inherently wrong with—I sure don't think so, anyway—selfies as a thing. People like to look at themselves and at each other; it's also just a thing.

But selfies that we don't share with or make for other people or use to find out how they view us can offer us some things that the other common kind can't. You can take selfies just to discover a different way of seeing yourself, by yourself, and something about that one step removed that the camera provides can offer you new ways of viewing yourself, including ways you really like, and self-affirmation. You can use selfies to present yourself however you feel like you really want to be when no one else is looking and the only person you have to think about pleasing and making choices for is you. This process of self-discovery can be a big deal for anyone, but it's a superbig deal for people who don't yet feel safe or comfortable expressing their gender identity the way they really want to and for people hit hardest by the restrictive and narrow cultural beauty standards, such as young women and people with physical disability.

So long as you don't share these photos—make sure that you don't accidentally save them to the cloud and that you delete them when you're done—you can rest assured no one but you will ever see them. You can even take pictures of your own naked body or your genitals. If you're a minor, this is often not lawful (for more on the law, see page 212, and for more on making or sharing sexual selfies with or for others, see page 240), but when the pictures are *only* for you and stay with *only* you, you're all good when it comes to the law.

You can use your camera to see your own parts—or angles of parts you can't get with your eyes. This can make your body feel more familiar to you. Anyone else who might see your body now or later is going to know your body in ways you can't. Seeing your own naked body with that kind of one-step-removed view can also be a good half-step toward being sexual with other people when you still feel too self-conscious about your body to let anyone see you naked just yet.

Typical selfies are anything but candid and authentic; they're more often carefully posed and edited and very much intended to be all about how you want other people to see you. Showing yourself the way you are and the way you want to see yourself—without it having anything to do with what you think others will like, approve of, or applaud and without worrying about what others might insult or treat callously—*to* yourself, in any way you feel safe and free to do so, can provide some big-time positive self-image mojo.

ideals. These messages often center on heteronormativity—a way of defining what's "normal" based on what is heterosexual—or gendernormativity—a way of defining what's "right" for a given gender based on the most pervasive or socially accepted gender roles and identities, which often come from and best represent people with the most power and privilege. These messages also make a lot of people a whole lot of money: playing into people's insecurities is a surefire sales technique because when someone becomes convinced that whatever you're selling will "fix" whatever they think is flawed, wrong, or broken, they buy, buy, buy it.

But you're no dummy. The littlest bit of self-awareness clues you in as to what is realistic for you and what isn't, what's authentic and what's hype, what's real and what's ideal. Even if some folks can't figure it out—or choose to misrepresent reality for their own purposes—you've got a little voice in there (and maybe even a nice, big loud one) telling you what the real deal is. Trust it.

We're all bound to have moments of insecurity about sexuality, about how others perceive us sexually, about our performance in bed, about our sexual normality. It is okay to enter into solo or partnered sex without being the most confident person in the universe, and moreover, most people go through a lot of insecurity, especially at first, feeling nervous and having doubts about themselves. But the better we feel about ourselves and our bodies, the better the sex and the sexual relationships will be.

If you're having issues with sexual self-esteem with a partner, take a look at your overall self-esteem. If you're worried about your body or your sexual performance with a partner, talk it out with them, with friends, with family or other people you trust and value. Getting those feelings out into the open and hearing about other people's perspectives and experiences can be a big help. Pace yourself however you need to—you might find that, in general, or sometimes, you're just not in the right frame of mind about yourself to be with a partner. If your insecurities are about partnered sex, go as slowly as you need to. If you don't feel right about showing your body to someone else, give yourself the privacy you require, whether that means dressing modestly or waiting to let a partner see all or any of you in your birthday suit. If you feel that you just can't measure up to some ideal—yours or a partner's—give yourself time for whatever reality check you need.

[WHOLE BODY/WHOLE SEXY]

What's "sexy"? Potentially *anything* that elicits sexual feelings in a person can be called or considered sexy. So, when you experience something or someone, or some part of something or someone, that makes you feel what you know to be sexual, or sexually curious, that's what people usually mean when they say "sexy."

Take a partner or potential partner out of the equation for a minute, and then take what you or others *see* out of the picture as well. Your sexuality, your body, and your mind aren't just visual; you've got other senses to work with that are just as much a part of you and your sexuality as your eyes and your appearance. And pleasure isn't just about sex, but it is most often very sensory. The word *sensuality* describes the way our senses bring us pleasure.

For instance, when you're eating, what foods make you feel sensual, sexual, or both? How does letting chocolate melt on your tongue make you feel? How about eating a ripe, sticky, messy mango? What smells make your head spin? Spicy cinnamon, rich vanilla, a fresh-squeezed orange, salty sea air, fresh-mowed grass, peonies or roses, sweat, just-washed hair? Your sense of smell not only can connect you with remembered scents from times you felt sexual, sensual, sexy, or had a sensual or sexual experience but also can allow you to enjoy scents that are evocative and heady. How about how things feel under your fingers or on any other tactile part of your body—warm sand, the soft down of hair on the back of your neck, cool paper, slippery silk or soft cotton, coarse brick, a squishy pillow, the inside of the lips, the warmth of thighs? When you've just worked your muscles during exercise, when you've had a great massage, when you're in a hot bath or waking from a nap, how do those things feel to you? How are tastes different then? So much of what really turns us on is about multisensory experience, and engaging as many of those senses as possible not only enhances the sex we may be having but also allows us to savor our bodies completely, not just how they look.

And when you *are* looking, open your eyes! On both your body and that of a partner there are so many parts to explore and appreciate, beyond the parts our culture sexualizes. What parts of your own body, when you touch them, expose them, or put them in the limelight, make you feel your-own-sexy? Beyond what you think looks best, what feels best when touched, which areas are most sensitive, what parts do you like to touch with? What parts feel most uniquely you?

Our bodies certainly have more value and function than merely being sexual. But when they *are* sexual—by ourselves or with others—and when we bring all of our senses to the table and serve 'em what's sexy by our own standards, we can create a sexuality that is authentically our own, one that not only wards off bad body image but also celebrates our bodies to the fullest.

[VIVA LA REVOLUCIÓN!]

Whether or not you feel 100 percent good about your body right now—or ever; this is probably something almost no one will feel very often because we all have our body insecurities, hang-ups, and emotional or cultural baggage on top of all the ups and downs bodies put us through all by themselves—revolutionary body image is about as-is *acceptance,* not perfection. For some people, it's also about love. For others, "love your body" feels like a lot of pressure or just isn't a framework that works for them. If you can't get there, or that feels like it just doesn't fit you, you still can treat your body *with* love, and plain old acceptance is a huge part of that.

So many people are doing everything they can to alter their bodies and their appearance in hopes that those changes will bring about acceptance. Not only will most never be able to make those changes—our appearance, our shape, and our size are determined almost entirely by our genetics—but often those who can *still* do not fully accept and enjoy their bodies, no matter how "perfect" they've made them. Some people who "succeed" at weight-loss programs or have cosmetic surgeries discover, sadly, that they still feel crummy about themselves because they also (or may only) need to work on accepting themselves, full stop, not on "fixing" their tummies or thighs. Your body is not a home improvement project, nor does it exist apart from your mind: mind and body are an inseparable whole.

Nobody's trying to be cute by saying that accepting your body and treating it with kindness, at the very least, can start a revolution. It really can, especially if a whole lot of us can get there. Anybody with half a lick of sense understands that it can be really hard to accept your body just as it is, especially when everywhere we turn a million voices are telling us to do the opposite.

But all those negative messages we take in on a daily, even hourly, basis are so pervasive only because of all the dollars—*our* dollars—that pay for them and all the energy we give to them. What would happen if we all ditched the piles of beauty mags, blew off the diet industry, told the makers of all the "miracle" creams and pills to shove it, scoffed at cosmetic surgery, and kept our dollars out of the hands of everyone who capitalizes on the appeal and power of the superficial image? What if we put our money, our voices, and our real feelings about ourselves out there? What if we refused to let the mass media (and those stinky little voices in our own heads) dictate what we should look like? The whole system that helps keep us down might fall the heck apart.

How you live your life makes a big difference. Rather, *that* you live *your* life makes a big difference. In a nutshell, life's too darn short to waste most of it worrying about how we look. It's easier to get our knickers in a perpetual knot about this stuff when we don't feel accomplished, able, or happy with our choices. So, *live* it. Do things that are actually important to you and that have real value. Follow your heart, your mind, and your bliss. When and if you have sex partners or when you have sex by yourself, with yourself, honor your body and revel in *all* your senses. Spend more time enjoying and experiencing all of your body than you do critiquing it or seeking approval for it. Smile a lot. Be an original. Have an *amazing* life. After all, most of us probably want our headstones to say more than *Beloved Sister, Great Ass, Perfect Hair.*

Accepting your body—both in sexual situations and outside of them—and accepting your whole self, unconditionally, in all your stages and phases, shapes and sizes, when you love them and when you want to kick them in the face, is powerful. It's *revolutionary.* And even if we all never quite get 100 percent there, just being, becoming, and owning *you,* being cool with you as you are and as you look, is powerful and life changing, for you and for all the rest of us.

4

Sex Starts with You: Arousal, Orgasm, Masturbation, and Fantasy

Sex and sexuality don't rely on someone else being involved or around, and they also don't require another person to somehow jump-start them like a car battery or give them to someone like a birthday present. Our sexuality always is just that—*ours,* even if and when we choose to share it, and even though it often is influenced by others. How our body does or doesn't respond to any kind of sex or sexual feelings or thoughts almost always is mostly about us and our body, not what someone else does or "makes" happen. That's why even when we don't have—or want—a sexual partner, we can still have active, satisfying sexual lives and sex.

AROUSAL AND ORGASM: HUMAN SEXUAL RESPONSE COMING AND GOING

Human sexual response is not as simple as many people tend to present it or think about it: it's about way more than just erection and orgasm. If that was all it was about, it'd sure get mighty boring, mighty fast.

Too many people think of sex as a gender-specific set of directions that are a progression toward orgasm. (We know from study that people who think about it differently tend to have a much better time, by the way.) Human sexual response involves a whole bunch of different things, and it's a process in which all the parts can be—and hopefully are!—potentially pleasurable and satisfying. Orgasm usually won't even occur without all the preceding parts of the human sexual response cycle, and it won't feel all that amazing without those other parts in play.

A lot of people believe there are particular things that everyone automatically enjoys, things that should satisfy every person every time. Many people also believe that physical sexual responses dictate, all by themselves, whether someone wants sex or wants to be sexual in certain ways. They don't. Bodies sometimes physically respond—or don't—in ways that aren't accurate reflections of what we want and don't want. The only sound way to find out what someone wants to do—and doesn't want to do—sexually is by talking with them about it and listening to what they have to say. (For more about consent, see page 192.)

These kinds of misdirected ideas tend to make it less likely that people can have sexual lives and any kind of sex they really enjoy and can feel like it is truly about them as individuals. Orgasm is only one aspect of sex and human sexual response, and we don't all function or respond the same way sexually to the same stimuli—not by a serious long shot.

Yet, most of us *do* share certain physical, hormonal, and psychological mechanics and basics of arousal and orgasm, and understanding *those* can give you an awesome foundation for effectively and enjoyably exploring and discovering all the good stuff.

The Basics of Sexual Response

The most commonly used framework for explaining sexual response was first defined by groundbreaking sex researchers William Masters and Virginia Johnson in the 1960s. That framework involves five different stages: *sexual desire, arousal, the plateau phase, orgasm,* and *resolution.* None of these stages is superior to others, and *all* can be, and often are, pleasurable. These stages fall on a continuum, and just as we have to learn to stand up before we can walk, to achieve a particular sexual response stage, at least to some degree we need to achieve the stage preceding it (though we certainly can halt the whole process at any point; not going through all the stages isn't harmful in any way). Someone who doesn't feel sexual desire in the first place is very unlikely to become aroused, and someone who isn't aroused is unlikely to have an orgasm. Here are the five stages in detail:

1. Sexual desire is a feeling, emotional and physical, of wishing or wanting to be sexual in some way. Sometimes desire arises in response to something or someone; other times it seems to come out of nowhere and feels like it is not specific to anything or anyone. When a person says, "I want sex," or "I feel horny," they are expressing sexual desire. Desire for sexual activity is a bit like being hungry to eat: if you aren't feeling very hungry, eating doesn't feel very good. Desire can feel and act like a kind of sexual appetite. Desire can also feel less like a hunger and more like a curiosity or a pull toward someone or something. Desire is: **Want Please *Yes*.** If you or a partner doesn't have a strong feeling of sexual desire—if you don't deeply desire to be sexual—sex of any kind isn't likely to feel good for one or both of you.

Feelings of desire can come up for us in any number of ways, but desire is generally not just physical or chemical; it's also verbal, visual, and intellectual and based in our emotions, personality, life experiences, and individual preferences, wants, and needs. It doesn't exist without or outside of a much bigger context. What things, situations, or people create feelings of sexual desire in people are deeply individual and situational. If you've somehow gotten the idea everyone feels desire based on very similar things, toss it: there aren't any universals when it comes to what turns people on.

For some people, or sometimes for some people, sexual desire just shows up spontaneously—*surprise!*—before anything sensual, sexual, sexy, or erotic is happening. Other times, or for other people, sexual desire is more responsive: it arises, or increases, when something sensual, sexual, sexy, or erotic is already happening. There's this idea about bodies or gender that, for men, sexual desire is almost always, if not always, spontaneous, and for women, it's almost always, if not always, responsive. But the truth is that, although there is some level of gender divide here (and who knows how much of it is learned, how much of it is about social or cultural influence), neither of those ways of experiencing desire exclusively belongs to or defines the sexualities of men or women. How desire works for people varies a lot among people of all sexes and genders, and it also can vary a great deal from day to day or from one time of life to another. Both these ways of experiencing sexual desire are normal and real.

2. Arousal is a physical and psychological state of sexual excitement: it's about feeling more and more keyed up, like how sports fans get during a game when their team keeps creaming the other team. It sends chemical messages to the brain that usually create physical changes and sensations throughout the body. When we're aroused, our blood pressure rises, our heart gets all fluttery, our breathing quickens, our skin may become flushed, and our body becomes more sensitive and receptive to touch. A touch on the neck or face feels more intense when we're aroused than when we're not. The genitals are rich with sensory nerve endings, and arousal sends more blood moving that way, so: arousal usually makes genital stimulation feel a *lot* more intense. We can be aroused by physical, intellectual, emotional, or hormonal stimuli. For instance, we might become aroused by being kissed or touched, but we can also become aroused just by our own thoughts and imagination.

Again, we don't all experience or interpret the same things as "sexual." What is sexy and arousing differs from person to person on the basis of our individual personalities, our sexual history and fantasies, our unique bodies, and what we were raised to interpret as sexually or sensually exciting. It's also very situational: just because something got us aroused, or more aroused, in one sexual experience doesn't mean it will in another, even when that next experience is with the same person or just a couple days later.

But when we are aroused, we all usually have some similar physical responses. One of the primary physical responses to arousal is *vasocongestion,* the increased flow of blood to the genital area (and breasts and nipples), which causes those areas to become swollen with blood. This is how the nipples, clitoris, or penis becomes erect and how the testicles or clitoral hood can elevate as well.

For people who have these parts, during arousal the clitoris and inner and outer labia often become puffy, stiffer, and somewhat enlarged, and vaginal secretions, or a feeling of "wetness," can occur. That's not only normal and nothing to worry about but also a bonus during sexual activities that involve the genitals because lubrication (sometimes called "vaginal sweating") makes any sort of sex a lot more comfortable and enjoyable. As arousal continues in people with these parts, the uppermost third of the vaginal canal also expands a bit, which can result in an "open" feeling inside the vagina. A slight enlargement of the breasts can also happen when some people are sexually excited.

3. If we continue to be all hot and bothered and start or continue sexual stimulation that turns us on and that we enjoy, we may progress to what's called the **plateau phase,** when sexual arousal—both in our bodies and in our minds—continues and increases. Many people experience some of this phase as a feeling of being "on the edge." Our bodies may feel hypersensitive; our skin flushes and we feel our heartbeat more strongly. Vasocongestion continues and increases. The uterus elevates, the cervix pulls backward; the vaginal opening and canal loosen, and the glands in and around the vagina produce more lubrication. The muscles at the base of the penis begin contractions, the urethral sphincter contracts (which is why no one with a penis needs to worry about urinating during sex), and pre-ejaculate is usually secreted during this phase.

4. Orgasm (aka the Big O) is a culmination of sexual arousal that typically begins during and follows the plateau phase. For those with these body parts, orgasm involves involuntary contractions of the pelvis, prostate gland, vas deferens, and seminal vesicles, which usually cause the ejaculation of semen (ejaculation and orgasm are related events but don't always both happen). For those with these parts, orgasm often results in a series of involuntary muscle contractions around the vagina and pelvis that may or may not produce an ejaculate or extra vaginal secretions. For everyone, there is an increase in muscle tension and relaxation throughout the whole body, especially around the pelvis. Orgasms generally last only a few seconds, though it can often feel like longer, and they involve anything from a few to around twenty contractions (the longest recorded single orgasm to date apparently lasted forty-three seconds with twenty-five contractions, for the geeks in the house). Orgasm is all about involuntary response, so no one can "give" someone else an orgasm or "make" someone else orgasm, just like we can't give someone or make someone else get the hiccups: it's more a thing that just does—or doesn't—happen within a person's body rather than something anyone can make happen or externally provide.

It's tricky to describe what an orgasm feels like. Try and describe, in detail, what a sneeze feels like—not so easy, right?

Same for orgasm. Not only does it differ from person to person, just like anything we can experience in life or the body, it often feels different for any *one* person from day to day, sexual experience to sexual experience. Orgasm can feel like a tickle or a hiccup, and it can feel like a very heavy head rush or wave of dizziness through the whole body, a bit like riding a roller coaster. Some orgasms feel practically earth-shattering, and some just feel nice, mellow, and mild. Having an orgasm

Multiple Orgasm

Someone is fibbing about their sex life if they tell you they had forty-seven orgasms in an hour, because that's just not the way sexual response and the body work. It's possible for a really intense orgasm, or an extended state of arousal, to feel that way, but not for that to actually happen. Somewhere along the line, great status was placed on experiencing multiple orgasm. But even people who experience multiples may not always want to. Sometimes, one orgasm is satisfying all by itself, and more than one isn't appealing. Sometimes, after a single orgasm, the genitals or other body parts may feel so hypersensitive, or we may feel so relaxed or wiped out, that more sexual stimulation isn't wanted or even comfortable. For those who do want more and who can be multiple orgasmic, we're generally talking about a couple to several orgasms in a given—and usually extensive—bout of sexual activity—not forty-seven.

Multiple orgasm is generally divided into two types: sequential multiples and serial multiples.

Sequential multiples: Sequential multiples are a series of climaxes that come close together (two to ten minutes apart) but that are separate, with an interruption or pause in arousal between them.

Serial multiples: Serial multiples are orgasms that occur one right after the other, with seconds in between and no lapse or rerun of the arousal cycle.

The difference in how those two different types feel is a bit like this: driving on a road with speed bumps every block or so is like sequential multiple orgasm—there are rests in between the big bumps. If, on the other hand, you're driving on a dirt road or around a block full of potholes, that's a whole lot more like serial multiple orgasm—lots of smaller up-and-down bumps in very quick succession. It's really one orgasm with a lot of little peaks.

Multiple orgasm is generally achieved the same way a single orgasm is: without rushing or a single-minded goal of making it happen, with attentiveness to the whole of the genitals and body—not just the vaginal canal—and with information and knowledge that someone has gained through masturbation and other sexual experience (most people who can reach orgasm with partners can also do so via masturbation, and most people who experience orgasm generally have had it happen first with masturbation rather than with a partner).

Many people—and this is nearly always true for people who've got a penis—find they require a *refractory* period between sexual response cycles to continue genital sex: a period of time that varies from a few minutes to a couple of hours, before they can begin the sexual response cycle in full again (or want to). This doesn't have to be a drag, by the way. This can, and often is, a great time for partners to just be close, hang out, and enjoy the afterglow.

is a bit like being a balloon: your body fills up with pressure and then releases that pressure when it gets to its fullest point, much as a balloon does when it pops. Only you can know if you've had one or not, because no one else can be in your body to tell. However, a partner may sometimes be able to feel your internal contractions when a part of their body is inside or wrapped around yours.

5. The last stage, called the **resolution stage,** is a relaxation of the muscles as well as a psychological relaxation and a sense of all-things-right-with-the-world that usually follows orgasm and results in part from hormones produced by orgasm (mostly endorphins and dopamine). All the blood that has been pooling in the genitals and other sensitive body parts recirculates through the body, and in time the genitals return to their normal "resting" state. It's normal to feel a bit lightheaded, lethargic, or sleepy afterward (which is why plenty of people often feel a desire to roll over and fall asleep after sex, not because they're being jerks). The resolution stage can also happen without orgasm; if we simply stop being sexually aroused, our bodies gradually return

DID YOU KNOW? . . .

There are also other models and ways of viewing and describing the process of sexual response besides the Masters and Johnson model. For instance, sex therapist Gina Ogden's framework expresses the sexual response cycle as three spheres of energy: (1) pleasure, (2) orgasm, and (3) ecstasy, which people can experience separately or together. This framework describes sexual response aspects not just as physiological but also as emotional, intellectual, and spiritual. Sex researchers Beverly Whipple and Karen Brash-McGreer developed a circular model of sexual response in which the stages are described as seduction (desire), sensations (arousal and the onset of sexual activities), surrender (orgasm), and reflection (resolution). If the Masters and Johnson model doesn't work for you, shop around or be creative and make your own based on your sexuality and your experience of sexual response!

Persistent genital arousal disorder

A few people experience sexual arousal at a frequency or level that isn't pleasurable at all. There's a rare condition called PGAD in which some people—usually they are well past puberty—experience constant and persistent genital arousal (for hours, days, or even weeks on end) or spontaneous orgasm, without any real feelings of sexual desire, to the degree that it disrupts normal daily life. Orgasm rarely relieves these symptoms. The causes of this syndrome are still unclear, but medical professionals currently believe the condition results from an irregularity of the nervous system. Current treatments include antidepressants, hormone therapy, or numbing agents. Mental health care is also a big help for people struggling with the stress and strain of PGAD. It's normal during puberty to often be more easily aroused or focused on sex than you might be later in life. But if those feelings seem unusually extreme to you or sound like the above, talk to your doctor.

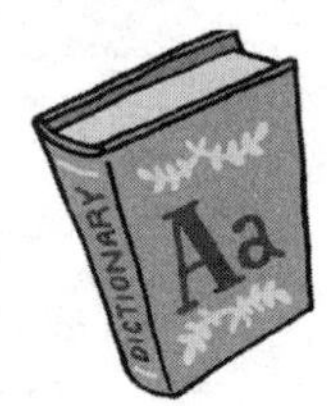

to their normal, nonaroused state. It is perfectly okay for this to happen, and it cannot hurt you in any way—no one is harmed by not having an orgasm.

Ejaculation

Ejaculation and orgasm are not the same thing.

Although they are most often related, and ejaculation during sex often occurs just after or at the same time as orgasm, they are different actions the body does, not two parts of the same thing. Ejaculation is not to be confused with orgasm or seen as "proof" of orgasm. People can orgasm without ejaculating and can ejaculate without orgasm.

To find out the details about when someone with a penis ejaculates—called ejaculation—check back in with the anatomy section about the penis (see page 45).

When someone with a vulva ejaculates, it's called ejaculation, too; some people call it female ejaculation. Many people come of age knowing that people with penises ejaculate, and they expect that to happen with sexual stimulation, but far fewer people learn until later (if they do at all) that anyone can ejaculate, including people who've got a vulva and vagina instead of a penis and testes.

So, in that case ejaculation can and often does come as a surprise to a lot of people, whether it's happening with their own body or the body of a partner.

This kind of ejaculate from the vagina and its related structures tends to be thin and clear or slightly milky. Clinical analysis finds it contains sugars and proteins found in all kinds of ejaculate, leading researchers to believe that the Skene's glands are most likely responsible for the fluid. Like ejaculate from the penis, it comes through the urethra but is definitely not urine. No one who is ejaculating needs to worry they're peeing the bed without knowing it.

Ejaculation does tend to come easier (no pun intended, I swear) to those with penises than it does to those with vulvas, and it's hard to say why. It might be about sexual attitudes, about whether or not people are getting the kind of stimulation and sex lives they need to be able to ejaculate; it might be physiological; or it might be all of the above. But orgasm happens more often without ejaculation

DID YOU KNOW? . . .

Orgasm is totally possible without any genital stimulation at all. Because a lot of what's happening physiologically during the sexual response cycle is a whole-body experience—occurring in the brain and nervous system more than anywhere else—this fact isn't all that surprising. People with little or no genital sensation, as a result of injuries or disabilities, can still experience orgasm. People can experience orgasm by having other places on their bodies touched and stimulated, without genital contact. Some people can even experience orgasm purely through their own imagination; if you've ever experienced orgasm while dreaming, you're one of those people. The idea that orgasm is only about genitals or genital sex isn't based in science but in cultural sexual ideas and ideals, ideas and ideals that can limit how much we really explore our whole bodies with masturbation or sex with partners and that also can limit people's experience of orgasm and the way they learn to experience orgasm.

for people with vulvas and more often with ejaculation for people with penises.

Being able to ejaculate, whatever kind of body someone has, doesn't mean someone is a better lover or has achieved some higher level of sexual awareness. Not ejaculating doesn't mean a partner wasn't sexy or the sex wasn't any good, kind of like not burping after dinner doesn't mean you didn't enjoy your meal. It isn't anything to be embarrassed about either.

How Do You Tell If You've Had an Orgasm? What If You Just Can't Have One, Ever?

Nobody can tell you whether you've had an orgasm. Sure, scientific tests can be done to measure contractions, and these have been used for studies on orgasm, but it's not as if you can just waltz into the doctor's office and ask them to hook you up to be tested for being orgasmic. A lot of people will tell you that if you have had an orgasm, you "just know," and for some people, that's true, but sometimes it is hard to tell, and there just isn't any sense of absolute certainty. It's annoying to hear, I know, but really, we know when we know. We won't when we don't or aren't sure.

If you're not sure you've had an orgasm, or if you haven't had one at all yet, give it time: you will get to know in fairly short order, just like you get to know other body responses and ways of feeling, like you know when you're getting a cold or when you're tired. Over time, you'll even start to recognize those orgasms that happen sometimes that are really subtle. As well, throughout your life, you'll probably discover that even when you are well aware what orgasm feels like, there are times when you're not quite sure if you've had one or not, because sometimes the sexual response cycle is both so fluid and so enjoyable as a whole that the differences in sensation can be subtle and murky.

Most people are, or have the capability to be, orgasmic. (But it's estimated that as many as 15 percent of people have real trouble getting there, and more of those people are young women. For the record, masturbation is what's usually most recommended when someone is struggling in this way, and secondarily—or at the same time—counseling that can address sexual issues that often play a part in this, such as religious shame or poor self-image. But because more often than not people who grew up socialized as girls and women get stronger messages *not* to masturbate, masturbation is probably the big missing link in the gender divide when it comes to orgasm.) Don't let media depiction or others' descriptions of orgasm influence your own discoveries; what we see in movies or what friends tell us tends to be elevated or exaggerated. Some young people who think they haven't experienced orgasm probably have at some point—it's just that their expectations of what it should feel like or look like aren't in line with reality. So, yes, that little ripple, incredibly vague and small head rush, or slight shudder you get certainly *can* be orgasm, and some orgasms are just like that.

And not everyone masturbates to orgasm. It may be that you just haven't figured out how orgasm works for you yet. Orgasm may not be your motivation at all at a given time; you may just want to explore your genitals or your sexual feelings or provide yourself some private comfort time. Whatever the situation, that's perfectly fine. If you just can't reach orgasm right now, don't freak out. Nobody's counting or clocking us, thank goodness. We also shouldn't need to know—nor should a partner or friend—beyond a doubt if we've had an orgasm. We don't need to have an orgasm every time we engage in solo or partnered sex. What's important is that we're feeling good with what we're doing and that we can provide or ask for as much sexual activity as we want, stopping whenever we like, regardless of whether we've had an orgasm.

That's really the crucial point when we say sex isn't about orgasm: when you're really enjoying sex, you aren't focused on reaching or counting orgasms, and you don't use orgasms as stop and go points. It's about the whole cycle, the whole experience, and orgasm is only one, enjoyable part.

Buzzkills

Even people who know what pleases them and who are enjoying sex can have problems becoming fully aroused or achieving orgasm. More times than not, it isn't merely about what anyone is doing wrong physically but about how they feel inside and how those feelings come into play during sex. If we feel that sex is dirty or morally, interpersonally, or religiously wrong or unhealthy, or if we're nervous, anxious, scared, concerned about performance, or emotionally uncomfortable in general, it is going to be nearly impossible to enjoy ourselves and experience pleasure. If we feel unable to tell partners what we like or dislike or how we'd like them to do something, we may be inhibited from feeling the pleasure we seek physically, and we may feel stifled emotionally as well. Relationships can suffer from the lack of sexual communication.

Spectatoring

There's a term for psyching yourself out of orgasm, and that's *spectatoring,* which means engaging in masturbation or sex with partners and being hyperfocused on making orgasm happen. A lot of people have this problem, which isn't that surprising. After all, we're led to believe that anyone who doesn't reach orgasm, all the time or often, isn't having good sex, isn't in touch with their bodies, or doesn't have a good lover—but none of those things may be so. Culturally speaking, we want easy ways to quantify and validate things, so the assumption and assertion that good sex = orgasm isn't all that surprising. Plus, there are times when we just *really* crave an orgasm.

But when it comes to arousal and orgasm, "mind over matter" is a key phrase to bear in mind. If you're overthinking it, obsessing on it, or weighing the whole works down by placing ultimate importance on it, it's far less likely to happen than if you just chill out and enjoy yourself. The easiest way not to spectator is simply to do your best to become aware, and remain aware, that arousal happens in most people without really trying and that orgasm—at least some of the time—is just as inevitable and natural, especially when we can have a relaxed attitude about it.

Other inhibitors to arousal and orgasm include general stress; tiredness or poor health; going without safer sex or reliable birth control methods (and thus worrying about those risks); rushing; worry about discovery (either immediately, such as by someone walking in on you, or long term, such as by parents discovering that you're sexually active); feeling pressured by a partner, yourself, peers, or a situation to be aroused or achieve orgasm; past or current sexual trauma or abuse; some medications (such as antidepressants); and the biggest one of all: psyching yourself out by trying way too hard to be aroused or achieve orgasm.

If you're having very serious and persistent problems with sexual arousal or orgasm, you can talk to a physical or mental healthcare provider. Existing sexually transmitted infections, hormonal imbalances, circulation or nervous system problems or disorders, diabetes, general poor physical or mental health or illness, or the use of alcohol, certain drugs, and medications can be inhibitors that often can be corrected or subdued.

Most of the time, though, barriers to physical sexual enjoyment and sexual response are *not* physical but are emotional, intellectual, and interpersonal (about our relationships, sexual or otherwise). So, if you have a good bill of sexual and general health and your doc hasn't found any problems, and if you feel that you're making sound sexual choices for yourself overall, at the right pace for you, then chances are you might need to look a little bit deeper. If you suspect common culprits such as poor self-image or body image, hidden relationship problems, depression or anxiety, sexual shame, or past or current sexual trauma or abuse, seek out support to address them via a counselor, therapist, or support group.

Even without buzzkills like these, we just can't always reach orgasm or become aroused every time we want to. That's the way it goes, just like we can't always get happy when we want to or burp when our stomach is full of gas. Our bodies are complex systems in which our genitals are a part. Cut yourself a break when that happens, whether it happens to you or to a partner. Do something else you enjoy, sexually or otherwise. If it's a feeling of physical release you're after, go engage in some strenuous physical activity or sport—the feeling of release from extensive exercise or hard physical work is hormonally, physically, and even emotionally very similar to the feeling of release orgasm can create. Honor what your body is trying to tell you it needs and wants. Just as it's not a good idea to eat when you aren't hungry, it's not a good idea to have sex when you're not fully interested or when your body isn't up to it.

MASTURBATION: A SEXUAL SOLO

Self-love. Solo sex. 'Bating. Ménage à moi. Jacking off, jilling off, whacking off, beating off. Paddling the pink canoe, pocket pinball, teasing the kitty, testing the plumbing, fingerbating, jerkin' the gherkin, spanking the monkey, soaking the whisker biscuit, surfing the channel, the sticky finger rhumba.

No matter what you call it—or how goofy what you call it is—masturbation is one of the few things that almost everyone does or has done at some point: about as many people masturbate as play video games, and there are *more* people who masturbate than people who have computers at home or who own cars. In surveys and studies, as many as 95 percent of all people report that they masturbate or have done so.

Most of us, if not all, masturbated before we can even remember: infants and very young children commonly fondle their own genitals and do other things to seek pleasure. That early stimulation and that early kind of sexuality is very different from adolescent or adult sexuality. Although motives and execution may differ, it's masturbation all the same.

There is nothing wrong with masturbation, and it's even clearly good for you in some ways. Most doctors and medical organizations, counselors, sex therapists, and sex educators agree: for our sense of well-being, relaxation, and health; for our sexuality with or without partners; for developing a means for sexual communication; for getting familiar with our own sexual response cycle and preferences; and

FALSE AND TRUE

Masturbation cannot:

- Cause blindness, headaches, or vision problems
- Cause hair to grow on your palms or give you zits
- Make your genitals permanently shrink or grow (beyond the temporary changes brought on by sexual arousal), or change their shape, sensitivity, color, texture, or appearance
- Stunt your general growth or the development of your sexual organs, or make you more or less fertile
- Become chemically addictive
- Cause injury or harm (when done safely—obviously, sticking a penis in a vacuum hose or using an electric vibrator in a bathtub isn't real swift)
- Release "stored up" sperm or sexual fluids (No one needs to masturbate or have sex with partners to get rid of "excess" semen or sperm. Unused cells of the body are absorbed by the body all by itself, and our fluids release themselves as needed without our help.)

Masturbation can:

- Relieve menstrual cramps and muscle tension and be a source of full body-mind relaxation
- Increase circulation
- Increase the ability or ease with which a person can be orgasmic (and is almost always the way people first learn to experience orgasm)
- Enhance sex with partners and help build important knowledge for clear sexual communication
- Help alleviate depression or anxiety by releasing endorphins
- Help improve sexual self-esteem and body image
- Potentially help prevent certain reproductive cancers, such as prostate cancer

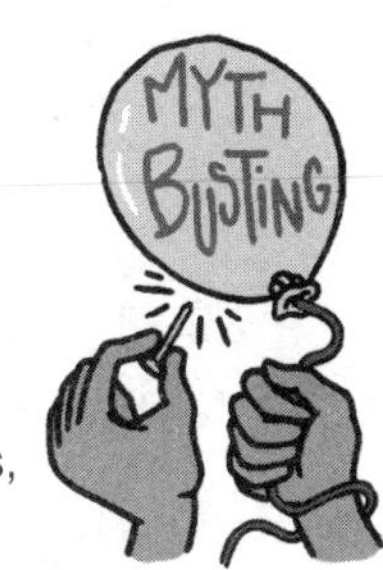

for finding out where all our parts are, how they work, and some of what we like and how we like it, masturbation is the bomb.

How Do You Masturbate?

How any one person masturbates at a given time is based on their mood, what they want, and on their individual psychological, emotional, and physiological makeup. All these variables affect what arouses people, brings about orgasm, and sexually satisfies them. So, although for one person, rubbing their penis or clitoris briskly with their hands or fingers with little lead-up may get them off, another may like to read a book while using a sex toy, and another may enjoy a long soak in the tub followed by a slow and gentle self-massage. What a given person likes can also differ from day to day.

Masturbation isn't just about genital stimulation. Plenty of people also incorporate touching or stimulating other parts of their bodies: breasts, nipples, or chests, thighs, hands or feet, parts of their faces—you name it, somebody's touched it while masturbating. Some people experiment with certain sexual practices alone rather than with (or before sharing with) partners, by using new sex toys or certain types of role-play or sexual fantasy.

For many people, it's common to combine activities like the above rather than just doing one thing or stimulating one particular area. You may also find that it takes a while to discover what really works for you or that something that was satisfying once isn't so satisfying anymore. You may want to mix it up a bit.

What's a good way to get started with masturbation? Start with a space where you feel comfortable and where you don't have to worry about being walked in on or interrupted. Although some people do approach masturbation in a perfunctory way (and that's okay), the truth is that it's like any sort of sex: it's usually far more compelling and enjoyable when you're aroused and going all-in.

Most people have fantasies about what they'd like to do with someone else, and that's as fine a place to start as any. If you're not that most people, and don't tend to feel or experience sexual desire for others, or you're not in the mood for that kind of fantasy, by all means, start with whatever elicits your own sexual curiosity or desire. Although, no, you can't really kiss yourself, you can massage your lips with your fingers, for instance, or run your hands over the sensitive areas of your neck, nipples, legs, or arms. Remember, your whole body is full of nerve endings and sensory receptors, so the genitals aren't the only sexual spaces you've got, not by a long shot. Take your time: when you're masturbating, you are your own lover, so treat yourself and your body just the way you'd like a lover to treat you.

When and if you do want to move the action to your genitals, keep in mind that this is all about you—what feels good to you, what you want—not about what you've seen or heard works for someone else. So, although a lot of people might enjoy stroking the penis with their hands, others might find that rubbing their groin up against something feels good at a given time. Some people want to incorporate vaginal entry into their masturbation; others like to keep things limited to their external clitoris or other parts of the vulva. Because you don't have to negotiate with anyone about anything you do when you masturbate, what you do is 100 percent your call and entirely and only about what *you* want and enjoy.

Keeping It Safe

Although masturbation is the safest sex there is, it pays to bear a few safety issues in mind.

Genital tissue is delicate. So, anything that might cut, scrape, or burn you or anything that might cause electrocution or create very harsh suction is something to avoid. A good rule of thumb is that if it looks like it might hurt you, it probably will, and if anything starts to hurt you, stop. Pain is usually the body's way of telling us to change something up or stop doing something altogether.

Bacteria are a concern with masturbation. Washing your hands before you masturbate is always a good idea because our hands pick up loads of germs during a normal day, and these can cause genital infections. In regard to toys or objects used during masturbation, if they can't be boiled to sanitize them, it's always best to cover them up with a condom or other latex barrier before use to avoid bacterial infections.

Some Common Ways People Masturbate Genitally

People may stimulate the penis, scrotum, perineum, or anus:

- With hands and fingers (usually with a lubricant or lotion), such as by stroking, rubbing, or slapping the shaft and base of the penis
- By using something to surround the penis, such as a sex toy made for that purpose, or household objects like fruit skins, socks, or warm towels, or via penetration with suction such as with a penis pump
- With vibration or pulsation to the penis, scrotum, anus, or general genital area via vibrators or small vibrating objects, by sitting or leaning on larger vibrating items, or with water
- With vibration, massage, or entry of the anus with hands or objects

People may stimulate the entire vulva, or some portions, including the clitoris, inner or outer labia, the vaginal opening or canal; the perineum; and/or the anus:

- With fingers, rubbing, pinching, massaging, or tapping the external genitals (such as the clitoris or labia) and/or penetrating the internal genitals, such as the vagina or rectum
- With general stimulus to the whole genital area, such as by squeezing thighs together rhythmically, by "humping" a pillow, or by sitting or leaning on a vibrating object such as a washing machine
- With objects or items for vibration, such as by applying a water source (like a shower or water jet), vibrator, or massager to the clitoris or vulva as a whole
- With objects for vaginal or anal entry (and usually with lubricant), such as dildos or other safe and similar objects

But Only Losers Masturbate!

If that's true, then pretty much everyone is a loser.

There are still some wacky attitudes out there about masturbation: that people who masturbate do so because they are sexually desperate, don't like the sex they have with their partners, can't get dates, or are just plain losers. In general, a sexually satisfied person—and most people who are happily masturbating are—is not a loser. People with partners masturbate; people without partners masturbate. In fact, many people who masturbate regularly tend to enjoy sex more fully with others, and they're less likely to shack up with the first person available, no matter how unsuitable or uninteresting, because they know how to achieve sexual satisfaction by themselves.

Masturbation and partnered sex aren't interchangeable. They're sometimes interrelated but necessarily different, and one can't usually substitute for the other (partnered sex *especially* can't take the place of masturbation, because you have to consider and pay attention to the other person as much as you do yourself). That's why a lot of people who have current sex partners, with whom they're satisfied, still enjoy masturbation; it tends to fill different wants and needs. (And it is absolutely fine to masturbate when you have a partner—if your partner has a problem with that, have a talk about it. Some partners even masturbate together.)

Often, masturbation can easily fulfill the physical needs and desires we have for sexual gratification. Obviously, partnered sex carries a whole bunch of risks, consequences, and complexities that solo sex doesn't. But most of all, emotionally and intellectually, masturbation and partnered sex are pretty different. When masturbation just isn't cutting the proverbial mustard, that's likely either because we just haven't found what works physically yet or, more likely, because we're craving companionship and shared intimacy. When sexual partnership doesn't feel right, it's likely because the privacy, safety, and self-centeredness (in the good way) of masturbation is more up our alley at a given time.

How Much Is Too Much?

It's normal when masturbating is or feels new to you to want to spend a lot of time doing it, just like when you find a band you really love and want to listen to their latest song over and over in an endless, hypnotic loop. For some, it might start to feel a little compulsive or out of control—maybe you find yourself masturbating in places that aren't really that private or find that your masturbation habits are starting to interrupt or intrude upon other parts of your life.

Generally, it's a pretty simple formula to figure out how much is too much: Is masturbation keeping you from doing other things you enjoy, like being with friends or partners or participating in sports, hobbies, goals, or interests? Is it interfering with your responsibilities (schoolwork, family duties, chores, or a job)? Is it infringing upon your health (keeping you up nights, keeping you from eating properly), causing any sort of injury (such as sore, swollen, raw, blistered, or chafed skin), or creating emotional conflict or distress for you? If it's doing any of these things, then it's time to cut back or ask for help (a mental healthcare provider can help, or you can just talk to someone you trust and respect with something sensitive and loaded like this). If it's not, and it feels good to you, don't sweat it.

[FANTASY FODDER: SEXUAL FANTASY]

Nearly all of us have sexual fantasies, even when we don't recognize them for what they are. We might have them when we're bored to tears during algebra, when we're masturbating, or even when we're having sex with a partner. We may keep them locked in our own heads or share them. We may bring out a favorite sexual fantasy to play in our heads during any kind of sex or may even find some of our sexual fantasies troublesome and try to lock them away. Most people, however, enjoy their sexual fantasies and find them arousing, exciting, and inspiring.

Sexual fantasy might be about engaging in certain activities, such as anal sex or group sex; about having sex in certain situations or places, such as at a concert or in a bar bathroom; or about partnering sexually with certain people, such as with a crush, a friend, an ex or current partner, or a celebrity. Some sexual fantasies may be very visual or tangible, playing out like movies or very realistic dreams, and others may be more like intangible feelings or senses.

Fantasy is extrapolated *from* reality. **But it isn't reality,** isn't often likely to become reality, and isn't usually even based in a whole lotta reality. Sexual fantasy is no different. Fantasy comes from our ideas about, ideals of, or experiences in reality, but fantasy is fantasy and reality is reality. They're separate. And fantasy about sex is often very, very different from sexual realities—and that's what's so exciting about fantasy in the first place.

We all have different needs and desires, and those can change by the moment. Someone who one day is aroused by the fantasy of a romantic and gentle lover may the next day fantasize about being roughly restrained—and both of these fantasies are okey-dokey, even if they might make you uncomfortable or even bored to visualize as reality. They're your fantasies, not your actions: to think is *not* to do.

It's typical to assume that sexual fantasy is our mind telling us what we want in sexual reality, but that's not always so and not always realistic. Our fantasies may sometimes give us clues about such things as specific sexual desires, sexual orientation, sexual ideals, people we're attracted to, or issues or scenarios we're grappling with, curious about, or wanting to explore. Our fantasies may also ensure our safety—we can explore, via our imagination, sexual scenarios that would in reality be unsafe or harmful. Fantasy may also help us to realize and creatively work out sexual conflicts, guilt, shame, or unmet or unspoken desires. And because the fantasy about sex or someone can be so divorced from the reality of that sex or that person, fantasy also lets us experience things in our head that we probably couldn't, or at least couldn't in the same ways, if and when we try to put fantasy in action. Someone's sexual fantasies don't necessarily correlate to what they want to do in reality; sometimes they might, and other times they won't at all.

Which Fantasies Are Okay, and Which Aren't?

Ultimately? *All* fantasy is okay because it only takes place in our head, just as it's okay to *think* you'd like to slap someone when you're mad at them but you know you would never actually *do* that. It's the actual slapping of them that wouldn't be okay, not the thinking about it. Thoughts are not actions and do not somehow make us act on them just because we have them. Some people find that their sexual fantasy takes them places they feel weird about visiting—people have sexual fantasies about things like group sex, casual sex, or sex with a partner of a different gender than they want to be with in real life, even though the idea of doing these things for real may be totally unappealing to them. They may fantasize about being with someone incredibly inappropriate or dangerous, about being raped, about sex with a family member, or about sexually manipulating someone. No matter what your fantasy, it's not going to be a problem as long as you understand the difference between fantasy and reality and don't get all hung up about it.

It may happen that you have fantasies that truly trouble you or that just don't mesh with your ethics or politics; to an abuse or assault survivor, for example, rape fantasies can be deeply disturbing and upsetting. Someone very freaked out about homosexuality may feel tormented by constant same-sex fantasy. A normal and intuitive response to disturbing or uncomfortable fantasies is to try to shut them out of the mind altogether, but that approach usually doesn't work and can even make them more persistent. So, the better tack to take is to talk to a counselor or therapist, even if it feels very embarrassing. In many ways, persistent disturbing fantasies are a lot like persistent disturbing nightmares or dreams: you may just need help finding out what their source is and working through those issues. One form of obsessive-compulsive disorder (OCD) also involves having and getting stuck in and very bothered by "bad" thoughts, which can include disturbing sexual fantasies.

Aside from those types of situations, your fantasies are probably fine just as they are, especially if they feel fine. There's no need to sweat them, put a whole lot of effort into trying to analyze them, or make them realities; you can let sleeping dogs (or bustling threesomes, or amorous teachers, or shiny celebrities) lie (or frolic, or orgasm wildly, or plead to give you more).

For information on pornography and other media that involves or elicits sexual fantasy, see Chapter 6.

[AND YOUR FIRST SEX PARTNER IS . . . ?]

We hear a whole lot about who should be our first sex partner. We're often told it should be someone we love and who loves us back, someone committed to us long term, perhaps even someone we plan to spend the rest of our lives with.

It totally should be. **And that person is *you*.** You, all by yourself, have all of those qualities and abilities, more than any other person. You're the awesome sexual partner you've been dreaming of.

Claiming and recognizing yourself as your first and foremost sex partner is freaking powerful. Your sexuality is yours, it is totally about you, and it mostly comes from *you,* not from anything or anyone outside you. Feeling like it isn't yours, isn't mostly about you, and can only come from or be about someone else can do everything from really limiting your sexual life and your enjoyment of it to making you more vulnerable to predatory people or plain old jerks. No one else is ever going to be able to get to know your body well unless you do. Knowing yourself sexually equips you with the tools you need to build a healthy sexuality and balanced relationships for the rest of your life: the ability to determine when it's the right time for you to have solo sex and when it's right to take a partner. Getting to know your own body and sexual identity through self-evaluation, through masturbation, enables you to find out a great deal of what you like and dislike sexually and physically, to see and feel what your genitals and the rest of your body are like in a healthy state, to discover how your individual sexual response works, to explore your orientation and gender identity, to check out your fantasies, and to gauge your sexual expectations realistically. It's something that supports your sexuality and sexual life like they are really yours.

That isn't to say that it's too late to start regularly masturbating even if sexual partnership has already begun for you, because it isn't. It doesn't mean that you're immature or that you'll have lousy partnered sex if masturbation doesn't interest you. Rather, the point is simply that masturbation is a great way for a lot of people to explore their sexual selves in a very safe, open setting.

It's not called self-love for nothing, you know.

5

So Much More Than Either/Or: Gender Identity and Sexual Orientation

Two big facets of sexuality and personal identity for many people are gender—how we self-identify as well as how we conceptualize and experience gender as a whole in our lives and our world—and sexual orientation—who revs up our sexual or romantic interest or desire, particularly when it comes to their gender identity and presentation.

Gender and orientation are hardly rocket science. But, ironically, because of our world's massive oversimplification of them, making sense of them—and the roles and statuses often based on them—and finding your place within, around, or outside of them can sure get complicated. People's ideas about them vary widely, yet the most pervasive of those ideas are often superbinary and superlimited and limit*ing*. However we interpret and experience these things, and however relevant (or not) they are to us as individuals, they are a big deal in our world, and they do tend to get a lot of real estate in our sexualities, sexual lives, and sense of ourselves and others as people.

GENDERPALOOZA! A SEX AND GENDER PRIMER

You already know what sex is: the classification and assignment of someone based on how their genital anatomy looks or what kind of reproductive systems or chromosomes they have. When you were born, it was the assignment of sex (just based on a glance at your genitals, not your internal organs or chromosomes) that brought a doctor or midwife to holler out, "It's a girl!" or "It's a boy!"

It's typically assumed that sex and gender are the same. They're so not.

Gender is another way to classify people or to classify ourselves. It's a giant batch of varied ideas and concepts people—as individuals but also as communities and cultures—have come up with or have about masculinity and femininity; about who's a man, who's a woman; and about what it is or means for someone to be, or be treated as, one or the other. Gender can be something experienced as external, such as how someone is treated as a woman in the world; it can also be experienced as internal, such as when someone talks about how they feel like a man or don't know which if any gender they feel like. When we talk about gender roles, we're usually talking about how we or others think or insist people of a given gender are supposed to look, think, feel, act, or interrelate based on their assigned sex or their own gender identity, when gender is not the same as the sex someone was assigned.

Gender isn't anatomical: it's intellectual, psychological, and social (and also optional in most ways). If our doctors or midwives were to assign and call out our *gender* at birth rather than our sex, they would be shouting "High heels!" or "Sneakers!"

Say *women* or *feminine* and many people are likely to define those words pretty similarly in terms of appearance and behavior just as they would if you said *men* or *masculine.* But seeing such big groups of people so broadly and narrowly has more to do with people's *ideas* about gender than it does about the realities and diversity of gender in people's actual lived experiences, including our experience of ourselves. Even just those two categories differ with staggering variance. Think about how our cultures don't have a problem with subclassifications or variations within most other big groups, such as food: we've got food groups, then more specific classifications within a food group, and even more specific classifications or subdivisions within *that* group. Gender is the same way, but it is something many people choose to think about in ways more limited than gender actually is.

In many ways, the spectrum of gender is much like the spectrum of sexual orientation. Very few people are at the outer poles of the line that runs the length of the continuum traditionally or currently defined as from "men" to "women." Realistically, we're talking about a spectrum, like the color spectrum, not a line, with people all over the place, even if we just stick to men and women. If we expand gender to include **everyone,** not just people who feel like or identify as men or as women, or just people who feel a harmony between their gender and their assigned sex, all of what gender can be and feel like fills every point on that spectrum and colors outside *its* lines.

It'd be tough to find someone who hasn't been exposed to gender roles and who hasn't experienced status and privilege (or a lack thereof) about or with their sex or gender. Maybe growing up you got a big message that "real" boys weren't supposed to love the ballet or that "good" girls weren't supposed to ever sit with their legs open (*the scandal!*). Maybe you've experienced how much emphasis is put on how women look or what men have in the bank. You may have gotten the message that only weak men cry or only unhinged women are loud, that women are "natural" caretakers and touchy-feelers and men are "natural" fighters and thinkers. In your family or community, certain duties may be assigned to members of your household only on the basis of gender. You may notice that the media and advertisers present women as being concerned primarily with romance, family, and appearance; men with sex, money, and sports. Those kinds of stereotypes are all about gender roles.

If you've studied history, you know how women have had to fight for the same rights men have been afforded (mostly by other men), such as voting rights, fair pay, and the right to simple legal autonomy. If you are globally aware, you know how many women worldwide are still viewed as property or are required to be submissive or subservient. These facts are about gender and status, or privilege.

DID YOU KNOW? . . .

Not all cultures and communities see or treat gender as binary. In many Native American tribes, a gender called two-spirit (a person who considers themselves neither male nor female, determined by identity, not by their genitals) was known and respected. In India, a "third sex" called *hijra* is recognized. *Xanith* is an Arabic term that recognizes persons whose gender identity is not in accord with their assigned sex.

When it comes to sexual behavior, gender expectations, relationships, roles, status, and identity often loom large. Many people decide who they will and will not date or sexually partner with based on gender, assigned sex, or both. Often, "feminine" men are assumed to be gay, "macho" men to be heterosexual; "masculine" women are often assumed to be lesbian, and "femme" women heterosexual, even though those assumptions are often incorrect. Gender is the core of the classical concept of sexual orientation: what gender we identify as and what gender people are for whom we feel sexual desire.

Gender—both how we identify with it and how others identity us through the lens of gender—also plays a part in the way we have any sort of sex, how we present our sexuality to others, how we feel comfortable or uncomfortable in our sexual behavior and attitudes, and how we might expect the dynamics of our sexual relationships to work. This is obvious in heteronormative relationships between two straight, gendernormative people. There are so many assumed norms and roles between men and women: about who should do the asking out, take sexual leadership, claim sexual responsibility, set sexual limits and boundaries, and be "outwardly" sexual. Gender norms can even dictate the "right" way to have sex, such as ideas that it's not "manly" for men to enjoy receptive anal sex or not "feminine" for women to ask for sexual activities to bring them to orgasm after their male partner has had his. Queer people, relationships, and communities are not immune to typical gender roles either: lesbians and gay men have often—some voluntarily, but some involuntarily—been divided based on appearance and behavior into binary masculine (butch or top) and feminine (femme or bottom) categories whose attributes are often based on heteronormative gender roles. Sometimes people even ask, "Who's the man?" about a relationship that doesn't have any men in it. Sigh.

Whatever-normative

When there's a *-normative* at the end of a term, the term is describing a way of being or thinking in ways considered "normal" or which are particularly common. For example, *heteronormative* describes behaviors or attitudes that suggest that heterosexuality, or certain common dynamics of heterosexuality, are what's normal and how everything else should be.

Although many young people now see themselves as being more flexible when it comes to gender than their parents or grandparents were, some studies and a lot of behaviors have shown that, despite what we might think, many "traditional" or stereotypical gender roles and norms are still assumed. Plenty of young people do still think that asking someone out, making the first move sexually, and providing condoms are things guys do, and that saying no to sex, setting and enforcing sexual limits, and bringing up or providing birth control are women's required roles. Some people think it's right—the only right thing, even—for young women to abstain from sexual activity but don't feel at all the same way about young men.

Many of us have at one time or another experienced what is called *gender dysphoria:* discomfort with our sex or gender identity and the gender norms and roles out and about in the world. You may have found that certain clothing picked out for you by parents conflicted with your gender identity—not all girls like ruffles; some boys prefer sparkly shoes to sneakers. As a young boy, you may have wanted a doll and been told that wasn't okay, or perhaps as a young guy, you find that ideas such as sexual initiation (or uncontrollable libido or sexual dominance) don't fit with how you see or experience yourself. Growing up having been assigned female sex at birth, you may have found that your world changed radically during puberty, when you had more visible "markers" of your biology and were perhaps told that activities you once enjoyed were no longer appropriate for you. You may have once been comfortable with more stereotypical gender roles and expectations, but now feel a new discomfort. For instance, someone who felt that traditional gender roles fit them just fine and dandy may feel differently the first time they face job discrimination or harassment based on their sex or gender. Sexual relationship problems may crop up when people are faced with the assumption that only women need to take responsibility for birth control or safer sex or that men should be the only ones to initiate sexual encounters. You may even feel funny about being gendernormative, because you have a hard time figuring out if you're really being you or just identifying with what you've been told you're supposed to be.

It's not exactly accurate to say you can pick your gender roles and status. You may be able to to some degree in your own home or in a given relationship or community, but out and about in the world we don't always get a whole lot of choice. How others perceive us based on how we appear, what our gender is thought to be, dictates much of our status and our roles. Few of us can completely escape or ignore those expectations, especially if and when a group we're not a member of or have less power in has more influence over them than we do. For instance, women can't just decide they're going to be paid as much as men for the same work and make it happen; men can't just decide that strict ideas about masculinity won't be applied to them and get instant freedom from those constructs. So, it's common for our gender identity—and how we present ourselves—to be largely or entirely determined by the overt and covert messages we're all bombarded with from a very early age that tell us how we should be valued (or value ourselves), act, and appear.

Some people assume that presentation is a given: they figure you're born male or female, so you will or must look a certain way or act a certain way, and any appearance or behavior outside expected norms is a deviation rather than a variation. Many assume that you either accept or deny looking or acting "male" or "female" rather than recognize that gender roles and presentation are active—not passive—choices we all should get to make and that those distinctions are largely arbitrary. There is nothing at all essential or universal about them. Those assumptions and assertions cause very real problems for many individuals and groups—everything from being called Mr. instead of Ms. to the overt violence of hate crimes (such as rape or the murders of queer and trans people). The collective cultural notion, for instance, that men should be physically "stronger" than women has caused numerous social and interpersonal problems for men and women alike (as well as simply is untrue). The notion that biological attributes must and automatically do "match" gender identity creates a world of confusion, conflict, and imbalance for many of us, and for some, it creates serious emotional and interpersonal distress.

But you *can* choose a great deal of how *you* present your gender (how you behave, dress, groom, and carry yourself) and how you identify (what you call yourself and what that means to you).

You can also cast a wider net and work to change the status of your gender as a whole or challenge large-scale gender roles with activism, especially when you are of a sex or gender with greater agency. For instance, a man could speak out about how traditional ideas about masculinity have really messed with his life and his head or work with an organization to prevent rape.

Challenging cultural gender roles, status, and assumptions isn't always easy or successful, even when we just want to change them in our house, our relationship, or our own head. But often it's easier in the long term to live with the discomforts we experience when we reinvent or defy assigned gender roles than to try to live out roles that don't feel true to us or that we can't or don't want to support.

You get to—and should—explore, challenge, and ultimately understand whatever gender identity suits *you* best, whether it's a good fit and match with existing gender roles or it isn't, even if the rest of the world isn't ready for you yet. It's just like that glass slipper in Cinderella. If the shoe doesn't fit, don't wear it or try to shove your foot into it when it's obviously just *not* the shoe for you. You can still go to the ball and wear whatever you want, and only what fits the person you are and want to be seen as.

As with most aspects of identity, as you continue into and through your adult life, you'll likely find that your personal gender identity and your feelings about gender change and grow, becoming more clear (and more murky!). With time and life experience, you will probably realize that gender isn't anything close to binary, but like most things is a wide, diverse spectrum, a varied, veritable genderpalooza.

[BEYOND THE BINARY]

Plenty of people find that gender roles, status, and expected behaviors don't suit them and create problems, challenges, and even a world of frustration. But for some, those disconnects and conflicts are even more unsettling or upsetting. Here are some terms that describe some more challenging gender identities:

▶ **Transgender (TG):** Those who experience their gender identity or expression in profound conflict with their sex assignment. *Transgender,* or just *trans,* is an umbrella term that can include people who may or may not pursue medical interventions such as hormone therapy or surgeries, who transition between gender identities, or who transgress or transcend them altogether.

▶ **Gender nonconforming:** This is a big tent term used to describe a person who does not experience, follow, or identify with the most common ideas, systems, roles, and frameworks of gender and whose identity and sense of self disagree with how they or others are "supposed" to look, behave, or essentially be, based only on the sex they were assigned at birth.

▶ **MTF (male to female), trans woman, transgender woman, or just woman, all by itself, like many women use it:** These are the most common current terms used by and for people assigned male sex who identify as women.

▶ **FTM (female to male), trans man, transgender man, or just man, all by itself, like many men use it:** These are some common terms used by and for people assigned female sex who identify as men.

There's no right or wrong term to use. To know what term someone uses, as with almost anything else about a person, we've just got to ask them. What terms you want to use for yourself is up to you.

▶ **Genderqueer (GQ):** Those who identify as genderqueer generally reject binary systems of sex and gender outright, often express or seek a place for themselves within the gender spectrum, and/or participate in endeavors, behaviors, or activism that queer up traditional gender approaches. Genderqueer folks may also consider themselves covered by the trans

Language and terms that address gender, specifically gender identities and experiences beyond or outside of the narrow binary, are in a constant state of flux. They're shifting and changing all the time, and given how big and diverse the spectrum of gender is and how unique people's lived experiences of themselves and gender are at any time, a good many people can feel like none of the current terms are a right fit for them. It's always okay to get creative and make language or terms for yourself that do feel right. Inventing or refining language is how, after all, we have the terms we already do.

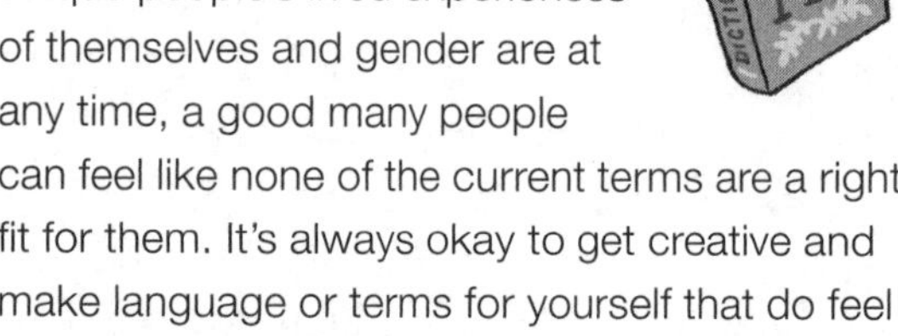

umbrella because they *trans*gress or *trans*cend gender altogether.

▶ **Cisgender:** A term often used to refer to a person whose gender *does* feel like a fit with their assigned sex. For example, someone assigned female sex at birth who identifies herself as a woman.

Trans-lation

Transgender or other gender-nonconforming people are not all alike; we can't assign certain appearance, behavior, lifestyle, or sexual attributes to people who are trans or otherwise gender nonconforming any more reliably than we can for young people, people of color, poor people, or any other group.

Just like it is for cisgender people, the sexual orientation of everyone who's gender nonconforming varies. Transgender people can and do work most of the same kinds of jobs as people who aren't trans (and when they don't have some of those jobs, it's usually because of discrimination), have the same wide array of hopes and dreams, have the same diversity of political, religious, and social beliefs. The way gender-nonconforming people present themselves when it comes to gender varies as much as it does for anyone else; same goes for the way anyone thinks, feels, expresses themselves in words, and otherwise behaves.

There's nothing "weird" or wrong with being transgender or otherwise gender nonconforming, just like it's not weird to be brown instead of white or to feel that you're an atheist when you grew up with Catholicism as an assigned belief system for you.

There's also nothing new about it. It's not like gender-nonconforming people were dropped from a spaceship twenty years ago and were never part of the world before. There's just more visibility now than there was in the past.

Transition

Some transgender people choose to physically change their bodies from having the kind of body that feels and looks like the wrong sex or gender to having a body that looks and feels like the right one. But not everyone who is transgender engages in hormone therapy or surgical procedures. People who identify as transgender may, in fact, not look any different from what is usually expected of someone with their biological makeup.

For those who do seek to physically change their bodies and who have access to what's needed for that change (including the hefty price tag), the procedures vary. For some, this involves lifestyle, external appearance, and legal name changes; for others, those things and more: psychotherapy and counseling, hormone therapies, and even gender confirmation surgery for those who wish to adopt the physical characteristics typically expected of their gender. Those who opt for surgery usually do so to feel more comfortable with their own bodies and to get the social benefits of doing gender in a way that is clearly understood by everyone in a society in which binary gender is a social norm.

Gender Confirmation Surgery

Also called sexual reassignment surgery (SRS), gender confirmation surgery (GCS) isn't something a person can just walk in and have done; it is often very difficult to even qualify for. Presently, those who wish to qualify for any medical interventions related to gender often must be diagnosed with a psychiatric disorder. In other words, transgender identities are still, quite unfortunately and inaccurately, considered to be "disorders" by medical standards, even though being gender nonconforming is not an illness or disorder but just a way some people experience and understand themselves. Qualification for these kinds of surgeries can require an extensive procedure that begins with long-term counseling and personal interviews about gender development and history, family background, general lifestyle, interpersonal relationships, and aspects of sexuality. If those issues don't appear to be problematic, hormone and other therapies can begin. Hormone therapy is typically continued and monitored for a couple of years, as is the person's experience of transitioning.

If surgery is wanted and okayed—and is also within reach, financially and otherwise—genital and/or nongenital procedures may be performed. These may include surgery that changes the genitals and/or internal reproductive system, breast implants or reduction, facial surgery, voice surgery, and/or other cosmetic surgeries. Just as the words and terms for transgender and other gender-nonconforming identities are in a pretty constant state of flux, all of these medical protocols or standards change a lot, too. If you want to keep current and see healthcare protocols created and endorsed from a more modern and less biased perspective, check out the World Professional Association for Transgender Health (WPATH) standards of care, which you can find easily online.

[TRANSPHOBIA, DISCRIMINATION, AND BIAS]

Despite all the recent strides we've made in many parts of the world, gender discrimination is still rampant for cisgender people, especially women, and it's more prevalent still for gender-nonconforming people, especially when they're *also* women. Those of us who are disadvantaged in one or multiple ways by the gender binary are oppressed: disadvantaged socially, politically, and economically. Those who benefit from the gender binary are thus privileged—through cisgender privilege or male privilege, for example. Privilege can be understood as all of the things you *don't have to worry about,* which can make it hard for some folks to identify when they possess or leverage it. The invisibility of privilege leads those who wield varying amounts of it to believe that the playing field is level and that their lives are "normal" or standard. This in turn can contribute to both victim blaming and the choice to ignore the violence and discrimination that others suffer. And, sadly, people benefit—though our world certainly doesn't—by taking the power of others because it gives them power themselves.

So, it's no surprise that transgender individuals—and especially transgender women, who get a double-whammy in this department—often experience profound sex and gender discrimination. As with any bias, misunderstanding and lack of exposure often breed prejudice and contempt. A lot of people who talk about transgender, transsexual, intersex, or genderqueer persons negatively have never actually spent time with any of them (or have, but don't know they have) and instead form their opinions from the media, gossip, or subjective assumptions. Often, they feel threatened by anyone who questions or contradicts a system and understanding of gender they feel benefits them.

There are plenty of people who feel satisfied with sex and gender systems, roles, and norms just as they are. There are plenty who've never thought about it much at all. For those people, the idea of gender dysphoria may not make much sense. They may be unable to understand it and may label gender dysphoria as a mental illness (as some schools of thought and medicine have done). Some may politically or philosophically object to concepts of transgender or genderqueer, just like some people politically or philosophically object to reproductive choice, sex outside of marriage, or homosexuality. Some may be transphobic—scared of or hateful toward those who are transgender or intersex—and perpetuate or even believe the myths that all transgender people are sexual deviants, are homosexual, are simply trendy people who want to change their bodies the way others change hairstyles. Many of us have heard, seen, or experienced similar intolerance for other groups—toward women or feminists, people of color, people who are homeless, queer people, senior citizens, or youth.

Others argue validly that current gender roles, statuses, and norms, even the whole concept of gender, are oppressive and problematic but nevertheless dismiss transgender people or disapprove of or are even abusive toward them. The problem with that position—besides bigotry, which is never anything but a problem—is that gender is applied to everyone. If behaviors, roles, and statuses designated purely on the basis of assigned sex or gender are oppressive and problematic, then they are problematic for *everyone* because they are applied to everyone, not just one group.

Families often have a hard time seeing gender dysphoria and treating gender-nonconforming people compassionately. They may refuse to hear or understand the feelings of someone gender dysphoric and/or gender nonconforming within the family. Schools and workplaces can also be unaccepting, and what are simple acts for some of us—such as buying a pair of shoes, riding the bus, or using a public washroom—can force other people to face biases great and small more frequently than many of us can imagine.

All too often, there is no community that will truly support or include transgender people. Even queer or progressive communities often reject them, diminish their issues, or see some or all transgender issues as in conflict with their own. That isolation compounds the emotional distress of gender-nonconforming people in a very big way.

If you are gender nonconforming or questioning, or even just struggling with or about gender period, seek out support. There are some excellent online communities for gender-nonconforming folks (see the Resources section). There may be support groups in your area, and you may find that some queer communities or alternative gender communities are welcoming and supporting, even if some people within them don't fully understand your issues. You may find that some of your friends and family can provide support and back you up when you advocate for yourself.

Gendermending

We're all lucky in that some aspects of gender have become less binary, less limiting, and less strictly enforced than they have been throughout much of our known history. Gendernormativity is becoming more of a choice than a mandate for many. Thanks, activists! Even though, as a culture, our progress is a bit slow, people coming of age now are often given more latitude when it comes to gender identity—and what's expected on the basis of assigned sex—than the generations before. Just a hundred years ago, for instance, women who did something as simple as wearing pants or cutting their hair short or who made bigger strides by directly challenging higher male gender status could nearly always find themselves victims of intense violence, social isolation, or even execution. Advancements in research also continually show that many gendered attributes once assumed to be biological are actually the product of socialization.

Our society could certainly still stand a whole lot of improvements: the shifts we've experienced recently and throughout history are a start, not a finish. Women are still greatly oppressed as a class; men who challenge their gender roles or presentation are often still met with disdain, fear, aggression, and violence. Many men are still being reared to instigate or enable violence or aggression to uphold a gendered status quo. Many gender-nonconforming people are isolated, cast out of homes and communities, abused, sexually or physically assaulted, and even murdered, over nothing but their gender identity and appearance. And we can know just how binary most of our cultures still are by the fact that we talk so much about men and women specifically in terms of rights and roles assigned to or afforded them. In a world that was more accepting, equitable, and less polarized between two groups based on sex or gender, we could do a lot more talking that's just about *people*.

If rigid ideas about sex and gender weren't so pervasive and so widely and strongly enforced, a lot of us would be safer, happier, healthier, and more whole. But for now, many people still accept,

HOW TO BE TRANSFRIENDLY AND SUBVERT CRUMMY GENDER AND ORIENTATION STEREOTYPES IN FIVE EASY STEPS!

1. Don't assume to know someone's gender identity or sexual orientation based only on your perception of them or the gender you think they are. We find out someone's gender by asking if and when we do need to know (which we actually won't very often). Call people what they want to be called, identify them as they want to be identified, and find out that information by either asking or listening for their cues. Many women don't like being called *ladies* or being addressed as "Miss," "Honey," or "Ma'am." Plenty of people who self-identify with terms like *dyke* or *fag* aren't comfortable with just anyone calling them that or with being identified that way in every setting. Some people don't dig gender or orientation identifiers at all and just like to be called their names: "me" is a totally acceptable gender and sexual identity. When in doubt about someone's gender, sexual orientation, or identity—and you do actually need to know—just ask politely.

2. Turn off the switch in your brain that makes you say things like "All men are jerks" or "Women just want money"; "Only gay guys talk like that" or "She looks/acts/sounds like a boy." There are *no* real sex, orientation, or gender absolutes, and the less we fall for and support them, the less power they have to keep all of us down.

3. No staring and whispering, please. When someone looks or acts in a way that you feel is in conflict with their sex, orientation, or gender, check *yourself* out, not them. How you feel is about you, not them. Think about *why* you think that way, where your ideas about gender or orientation come from, and whether your attitude and definitions are really reasonable or fair to apply to everyone. Question why it's even your business or feels like your issue; take a few minutes to wonder how much the criteria you're thinking about even matter. It's okay to be curious and to ask respectful questions. What's not cool is making someone else feel unsafe, insulted, or demeaned because you're uncomfortable with your own lack of knowledge or understanding, inflexible in your ideas about gender or orientation, or insecure about your own identity.

4. Subvert—or, heck, outright overthrow—the status quo. If there's something in your school or workplace that is unfairly closed to a given sex, orientation, gender, or gender identity; that is based on gender appearance or heteronormativity; that unreasonably excludes others on the basis of orientation, sex, or gender, question it. If, in your relationships, you have a partner who is holding you to an identity, role, or status that isn't okay with you, speak up. Challenge sex, gender, and orientation discrimination directly when need be, and gather your forces to do so. Write letters. Engage others in discussion and awareness. Be visible. Don't accept gender or orientation norms, roles, or status at face value (even if they are just fine for you). Question them.

5. Work on tolerance and compassion. You don't have to agree with someone, or personally understand where they're at, to be kind, humane, accepting, and fair. Imagine yourself walking a mile in another person's shoes—including the blisters you'd wind up with wearing their heels.

support, and encourage a very limiting view of sex and gender, so gender identity tends to be pretty important, as does the body we're born with and the sex we're assigned. Our challenges based on those things may be great or small, but only a rare few of us will face no challenges.

As with anything else, though, gender is only one part of you, a whole person with a million facets. How you identify and whatever kind of body you were born with is only as important and relevant to you as you want it to be. Even if you can't identify and present the way you'd like to yet, when you're out and about, what goes on in your head is all yours. The relationships you're in and your roles within them are up to you, and the way you define yourself—as well as the latitude you hopefully give others in choosing and presenting their gender identities—is your choice.

THE RAINBOW CONNECTION: THE SPECTRUM OF SEXUAL ORIENTATION

Everyone has a sexual orientation or a sexual identity, not just people who are homosexual, bisexual, or queer; not just people who are sexually active; and not just people who give names or great importance to either or both of those things. Everyone.

As with a lot of terms developed to describe an "other," "them," or any group of people outside a current or accepted norm, it's common to hear orientation terms used within or about queer culture, and it's more rare to hear them when talking about everyone else. That's a bummer because questioning, sorting out, and learning to embrace our sexual orientation and identity can be a big help when it comes to our sexuality as a whole: by ourselves and with partners, in reality as well as in our ideals and fantasies. Because there is no orientation default setting, just a lot of variation, exploring and identifying our sexual orientations are pretty darn important.

First things first: let's just define some terms.

Sexual orientation: This term describes the gender or genders or people to whom someone is sexually, emotionally, and/or romantically drawn or who have a pattern of eliciting sexual or romantic feelings in someone; which gender or genders (including none) someone can be in love with or want to be actively sexual with in some way. There may be varying degrees of attraction or ways someone experiences attraction—for instance, a person may be very physically attracted to men but more emotionally attracted to women, while some people find that they don't experience some kinds of attraction or ways of feeling attraction at all.

You may be wondering: **Why is sexual orientation all about gender, like gender is *the* big deal when it comes to sex with others?** Because for a lot of people, and certainly in most cultures, gender *is* a big deal, and as you know, gender is one of the most common ways people classify themselves and others as they grow up. But how big a deal it is—your gender, other people's genders, and what part gender plays in your sexuality and sexual life—is individual. So, if gender is a major player in your sexual identity, okay.

If not, that's just as okay. It's only one part of a person, after all.

The most common terms used to describe sexual orientation—heterosexual, homosexual, bisexual—are limited in meaning. Same goes for the idea of sexual orientation as binary, linear, or something completely permanent and never shifting. Most people's lived feelings and experiences, especially over a whole lifetime, reflect the fact that sexual orientation is way bigger than binary categories and more fluid and shifting than one lifelong way of being and feeling.

JUST BECAUSE THERE'S A *T* IN LGBT DOESN'T MEAN ALL—OR EVEN MOST—TRANSGENDER PEOPLE ARE QUEER.

Although transgender (the *T* in LGBT) is often considered and treated as part of queer issues, it's a mistake to make any assumptions about transgender people's sexual orientations, just like it's a mistake to do that with anyone. The range of sexual orientation that exists for transgender and other gender-nonconforming people is the same (read: ginormous) as for those who find that their gender fits their assigned sex, and orientation is usually mostly about gender, not which organs a person's body has. A trans woman who is attracted primarily to men usually identifies as straight; a trans man attracted to men usually identifies as gay.

MYTH BUSTING

There are a lot of words and terms for something as diverse as sexual orientation and identity. Here's a handful to start with:

Heterosexual (or straight): Someone who solely or primarily (mostly) experiences sexual or romantic feelings with and/or desire for people of a different gender than theirs, such as men who feel attracted to women.

Queer: Generally, queer is an umbrella term that describes a person who is not heterosexual. Someone may use the term *queer* as the way they identify, period, or they may use terms like those below and also identify as queer.

Homosexual (gay or lesbian): Someone who solely or primarily (mostly) experiences sexual or romantic feelings with and/or desire for people of the same or similar gender as theirs, such as men who feel attracted to men.

Bisexual: Someone who finds they experience sexual or romantic feelings with and/or desire for people of more than one gender—men and women or people of all gender identities—or who doesn't experience gender as a major factor in their attractions, period.

Pansexual or omnisexual: Someone who experiences sexual or romantic feelings with and/or desire for people of all gender identities or who doesn't experience gender as a major factor in those feelings and desires, period. People sometimes use *bisexual* and *pansexual* interchangeably.

Asexual (or nonsexual): Someone who has not experienced or does not experience sexual feelings about or with others or who does but does not feel any desire to be actively sexual with others. In other words, someone who is not sexually attracted to anyone of any gender. Like all things gender and sexuality, asexuality also has a spectrum, which includes orientation subsections such as *demisexuality;* those who use that term are often describing their experience of sexual attraction to other people as something that only happens or mostly happens only after forming some kind of close emotional bond.

Androsexual, gynesexual, ambisexual, or skoliosexual: These terms are a different framework for orientation than the framework of heterosexuality, homosexuality, and bisexuality, one that can be more inclusive and expansive than hetero/homo/bi and that doesn't require the gender of the person who is feeling the attraction to be defined in a given way or at all. If you're not sure about your own gender identity, or you find it seems irrelevant with all this, but you have a sense of where you're at when it comes to attraction to *others* based on their gender, these terms might work better for you. *Androsexuality* refers to someone who is attracted to masculinity; *gynesexuality,* to femininity; an *ambisexual* is someone who can be attracted to both or either or who experiences gender as a nonissue; and a *skoliosexual* is someone who is attracted to noncisgender or nonbinary people in general. Asexuality is also included in this framework. This framework doesn't make rigid assumptions about the other person's gender either: here, a person can be attracted to masculinity in women or femininity in men, for example.

Pomosexual: Someone who rejects or does not identify as or with any categorization of sexual orientation as a form of identity. *Pomosexual* is basically a term for someone who feels that giving a name to their sexual orientation feels limiting or otherwise like a bad fit for them.

Questioning (or* –curious *or* –flexible, *as in bicurious or heteroflexible): Someone who isn't sure right now or who has never been sure of their sexual orientation and who is in the process of figuring that out. Terms like *bicurious* are often used by someone who feels a sexual interest or curiosity about a given gender of people but is still in a process of questioning. Terms like these are sometimes used to describe an interest in people of a given gender that's there, but not felt as so central to be part of someone's overall orientation.

Sexual identity: This is an umbrella term used by someone to sum up the big gist of

GLBT...Q...A...I...WTF?

GLBT (or LGBT) is a commonly seen acronym that addresses sexual orientation, sexual identity, and gender identity, and sometimes it has even more letters tacked on to it.

G = Gay
L = Lesbian
B = Bisexual
T = Transgender
Q = Questioning or queer
A = Asexual
I = Intersex
P = Pansexual (attracted to all people of all sexes and genders)
O = Omnisexual (like pansexual) or other

their sexuality in terms of how they identify and present themselves. It may include sexual orientation, politics, affiliations or interests, relationship models, status and experience, gender identity, sexual preferences—the whole enchilada. *Queer, dyke,* and *straight* are terms for sexual identity, as might be *kinky, polyamorous, slut, asexual, vanilla, tutti-frutti,* and so on. Because sexual identity is so personal, some people get creative and come up with combination phrases, such as "genderqueer granola dyke" or "heteroflexible kinky poly switch." Sexual identity is also mighty big, so no one term or handful of terms is likely to cover all the bases for any given person—terms we use to express our sexual identities are usually just a blurb, not the whole story.

Sexual identity is fluid. Although research has found some portions of our sexuality to be, and experienced as, at least partially fixed by the time we're in puberty or even well before—including sexual orientation, parts of our gender identity, and some of our sexual or relationship patterns—many aspects of our sexual identity develop, shift, and evolve throughout our lives. For instance, during one period of our lives, we may explore a certain type of sexual activity, such as role-play. At the time we're doing that, it may become a prevalent part of who we feel we are. Later, we may lose interest in that or decide that it really isn't the thing for us and isn't a part of our sexual ID anymore. Some other recent research has found that people who identify as women may be more fluid in their sexuality than those who identify as men, including with sexual orientation.

While we're single, our relationship status of being single or multipartnered may not be a big part of our sexual identity, but if and when we become monogamously partnered or married, it may then become major. That said, a lot of this isn't something a person can just snap their fingers and change, if they can change it at all. We know that, for instance, sexual orientation or gender identity can and often does change or shift in some ways throughout our lives, but we also know that those shifts and changes are often outside our control. Someone queer can't "make" themselves straight—nor can someone else do that to them—and someone can't force themselves to feel like they are a different gender than they experience themselves as being.

As well, sex and sexual relationships are only part of our lives. If every part of us is completely wrapped up in sex and sexual identity, we're likely to miss out on other equally enriching and fulfilling parts of our lives. So, although your sexual identity is often an integral part of who you are, and a very big deal while you're seeking out the whole of your self-identity so intensely, there's never any hurry to claim or label it or to carve it in stone and make your current sexual identity your *whole* identity.

Sexual preference or sexual "lifestyle": These are terms people sometimes use when they talk about orientation, and almost always they are talking about orientations other than heterosexuality. Usually, these terms are used from a place of ignorance or bias, and they're very problematic. Sexual preferences are things like feeling sexual desire more for people who are tall rather than short or who are brunette rather than blonde. Sexual preferences can also refer to preferred sexual activities or dynamics with them, such as certain sexual positions or kinds of sexual language. Sexual orientation is not a sexual preference. Sexual "lifestyle" or something like "gay lifestyle" are language most often used to suggest that people of any one orientation (and usually only queer people) have a universal way of living or having a sex life. This is, of course, totally ridiculous: there's **no** group made up of millions of people who all live, have sex, or love the same way.

Feeling, Not Just Doing

Sexual orientation is as much about feelings as it is about actions and behaviors.

It's not something anyone needs to—or can—prove with their behaviors, and people's behaviors don't always match their feelings for a whole bunch of reasons. Someone can date and have sex with a ton of people outside their stated or felt orientation; that doesn't prove or disprove how they feel or who they feel the most sexual desire for, and it does not dictate their sexual identity. You don't need to have sex or romantic relationships with anyone to have your orientation validated: how you feel and how you identify yourself are all that's needed for that. Of course, most people will want to, and if they can, choose to pursue sex, romance, or both with people to whom they feel sexual and romantic attraction. By all means, there certainly isn't anything wrong with anyone of any orientation pursuing those desires! But it's not a *requirement* anyone needs to meet to be allowed to have or claim a sexual orientation.

You might also find that at some point you feel like you can't really be sure of your orientation unless you go out and do some field research by having sex with others. Again, if you have these kinds of feelings, chances are you might want to explore them in action with someone else—not to try to prove anything, but because you have that desire to do so. But sexual behaviors don't and have never proved sexual orientation: orientation is about *feelings*; behavior is about *actions*. And people sexually behave in ways counter to their feelings all the time, for example, by being sexual with a gender of people you're not attracted to, faking orgasm, or having a kind of sex you know isn't a kind that you want. So, no sexual behavior you can engage in can prove—or disprove—your orientation.

But it is okay for people to experiment sexually, exploring orientation or figuring out whether they like oral sex or trying on a new name to call their genitals. Really, all sex we have is an experiment in one way or another. Experimenting is fine; treating people with a lack of humanity as we'd treat something dead we're dissecting in biology class is not. Like any kind of sexual exploring or experimenting, we just need to be mindful about it and sensitive to and about the other people involved. Do make sure that any sex or romance you have with someone else isn't *so* much about you, your own curiosity, or figuring out yourself for yourself that there's no room for that whole other person to really be a whole other person, too.

How Do I Know If I'm . . . ?

Sorting out what your orientation may be, what—if anything—you want to call it, and what you want to do with it is a constant and lifelong process. It can feel frustrating not to "know who you are" when it comes to this area of identity and might feel like you have to have it all figured out *right now* because everyone else seems to (they don't, by the way). You don't ever have to have it all figured out, and to a large degree, you won't ever really be able to have it all figured out once and for all because our lives, sexualities, and who we are as people are all so fluid and ever shifting. But if you want help coming up with some kind of answers, even if they're just for you, a self-assessment tool can come in handy.

In the late 1940s, sex researcher Alfred Kinsey devised a tool called the Kinsey Scale to help codify sexual orientations and see how we really look as a whole people in this department. The scale was revolutionary at the time, but it only considered sexual behavior, not feelings or wants. In the 1980s, another researcher, psychiatrist Fritz Klein, developed a new tool for sorting out orientation, the Klein Grid. It takes actions, feelings, *and* wants into account and a person's past, present, and future. It's not perfect either (is anything?), but it's awfully good. Check out the chart on page 103 to see a version that makes room for more than just binary sex and heterosexual or homosexual identities or experiences.

Ultimately, what you call yourself, how you identify, and when and even *if* you identify are all your choice, and it isn't a choice you get only one chance to make. Just like with what you call the way you eat, what your spiritual beliefs are, or what name you like to be called, there should always be room for revision.

Who we are throughout our lives often shifts in a million different ways. So, we often adapt and adjust how we describe ourselves as we go. That's just as okay for a person to do about sexual identity as it is for someone to do about relationship status, where they live, religious beliefs, or how they choose to eat. And it may change over time: experiments of today are not necessarily identities of tomorrow. Claiming an identity, using certain words to describe our identity, including to others, or having any kind of sex with someone else is not some kind of lifelong contract or commitment. All it needs to be—and all it possibly can be, unless you've got yourself some psychic skills with which to predict the future—is about what we know so far about our present selves, up to and in this very moment.

The important things are that you do what you can to make yourself comfortable and at peace with yourself; that you are honest with yourself and your friends, family, and/or partners in a way that feels right and safe for you; that you realize you have as much time as you want or need to become and discover who you are; that you know you always have the option of changing it all up to fit you best.

To Be or Not to Be: Is Sexual Orientation a Choice?

Generally, sexuality research on sexual orientation suggests that orientation is hardwired to some degree (and more

THE KLEIN GRID

How Do You Experience . . .	In the Past	In the Present	And Want to in the Future
Sexual Attraction (sexual desire and/or physical arousal)			
Sexual Behavior (sexual activity with other people like kissing, oral sex, or sexting)			
Sexual Fantasies (sexual thoughts or daydreams)			
Emotional Preference (love or emotional intimacy)			
Social Preference (what place gender has in your friendships and the communities you have chosen to be part of)			
Self-Identification			

To use this tool, think about your feelings and experiences in each of the areas related to the gender of others in the past, present, and wanted future. It's okay if everything doesn't seem to match up right: who we are, how our lives have been so far, and what we want are often full of contradictions in this area, just like in any other part of life or identity.

You can either just think about or write in your own answers in a way that works for you uniquely, or use numbered codes to keep it simple, such as:

0 = With no one, so far, of any gender

1 = With people of a gender different from mine only

2 = With people of a gender different from mine mostly

3 = With people of a gender different from mine somewhat more

4 = With people of a gender different from mine *and* with people of a gender the same as or similar to mine pretty equally

5 = With people of a gender the same as or similar to mine somewhat more

6 = With people of a gender the same as or similar to mine mostly

7 = With people of a gender the same as or similar to mine only

The last row, self-identification, is about how you have, do, and want to identify yourself in terms of your sexual orientation using whichever words you have, do, or want to for that, whether they're existing terms—such as *queer, straight, questioning, asexual, gynesexual, or even "anything but straight"*—or words or terms you've created or creatively combined for yourself.

flexible or fluid in certain situations). Some aspects of our sexual orientation are probably fixed pretty early in our lives on the basis of a combination of genetics; early familial, platonic, romantic, and sexual relationships; and the environments in which we're reared. Orientation is also both fluid and based on active choices. We all make conscious choices about whom we take as sexual partners, what we call ourselves, and what communities we participate in.

The American Psychological Association makes clear that "sexual orientation emerges for most people in early adolescence without any prior sexual experience." (In other words, like we mentioned before, most people do **not** have to experiment with partners of various genders to discover their orientation.) The APA continues, "And some people report trying very hard over many years to change their sexual orientation from homosexual to heterosexual with no success. For these reasons, psychologists do not consider sexual orientation for most people to be a conscious choice that can be voluntarily changed." The APA also states officially that "conversion" therapies are unethical.

There's a lot of argument about this issue. Some folks use the notion of choice in how we *enact* our orientation as a way to support certain personal or political agendas, stating, for instance, that if a queer person has the ability to choose to partner with whomever they like, they can choose to be heterosexual. That's false logic when we understand orientation as both attraction and action, obviously, but the argument is made all the same. Approaches like that make looking into the why of orientation a loaded issue, and they can bias the way even academic or medical researchers look at sexual orientation (see page 100 for discussion on the term "sexual preference").

Asking about choice in orientation is tricky because we just don't have one absolute answer yet, and we probably won't ever have one. We do have enough research and real-life knowledge and experience to know that orientation, and how people express it, is a combination of both choice and some hardwiring. But it doesn't really matter very much what the exact combination is, and it also doesn't make any difference whether our orientation stays exactly the same through all of our lives or changes for us every five minutes: how we feel is valid, however long—or briefly—we feel that way.

What matters is that, whatever our orientation, including when we don't know what it is, the way we act on it feels right and okay with us and with our partners. Whatever phase of our life we're in, however we experience and identify our orientation, and whether that does or doesn't shift or change over time, we should be respected as should what we know so far and say we feel right now about our orientation or any other part of our present sexual identity.

When so many parts of your identity are in flux, it's understandable to be in a hurry to affix a label to your orientation, especially if ambiguity or false assumptions are causing you grief. But determining sexual orientation can't be rushed, nor

IF SOMEONE TELLS YOU "IT'S JUST A PHASE. YOU'LL GROW OUT OF IT."

Young adults are often involved in big stages of personal and sexual development, physiologically, emotionally, and in their relationships. The nature of personal development of any kind is that it is a process that takes time rather than being complete in one step. It's always been common, for instance, for people to have crushes on best friends, or sexual fantasies about same-sex friends, or even to engage in same-sex activity during childhood and adolescence, no matter a person's orientation in the long run. It's typical for many people who are gay or lesbian to have partners of a different gender during their developmental years and sometimes beyond, especially given the pressures most queers experience to be straight. It's also normal for some young adults to be less choosy about their sexual partners than most older people are.

In other words, many young adults sexually explore and experiment with partners (same gender or of another gender) they might not choose later on the basis of factors like availability, peer and community pressures, safety or privacy, sexual or personal compatibility, and basic care and respect.

When you're a teen or emerging adult, honest, consensual sexual experimentation—whether it's in your head or out and about with others—is normal and helpful. There isn't a thing wrong with whichever sexual orientation you feel belongs to you. People who are queer aren't necessarily more cool (a lot of us are total dorks!), sexually available, or enlightened; people who are straight aren't necessarily prudish or narrow-minded. Having attractions or relationships outside what ends up being your orientation base doesn't mean you're flighty, nor does it mean those relationships aren't or weren't important.

is the process of determining it something you need to "just get over with." It takes time, and it's common for many adults in their twenties, thirties, and even forties to be uncertain about theirs or to experience gradual or even radical shifts in orientation. So, yeah, it's possible that what feels like your orientation at times may be a phase, but orientation is often phasal for everyone, young and old, gay and straight, and everyone in between. But even when it is a phase, there's no "just": it's still meaningful, still relevant, and still 100 percent who you are.

WHAT DOES IT MEAN TO BE QUEER, BISEXUAL, OR PANSEXUAL?

As basic frameworks, homosexuality and heterosexuality are pretty straightforward: gay people are primarily or solely attracted to people of their same gender; straight people to those of a different gender. Bisexuality, pansexuality, and other queer or more complex frameworks that include more than either/or aren't so clear-cut.

A bisexual person is someone who can or does experience attraction in our

binary gender system to either gender; a pansexual person is someone who is or *can* be attracted to any gender, any sex, and any combination of gender and sex. Sometimes the terms *bisexual* and *pansexual* are used interchangeably. Like gay and straight people, bisexual and pansexual people can be monogamous—feeling sexual or romantic desire for or with people of more than one gender isn't usually about a need or desire for a partner of each or every gender at the same time, nor is it about feeling like something huge is missing if and when we date someone of any one given gender. Also, many bisexual and pansexual people do not experience a 50/50 split of attraction between people of different sexes or genders. A bisexual person may be, for example, mostly attracted to women and only occasionally attracted to men.

Bisexual, pansexual, and other queer people often have to deal with a lot of bogus misconceptions about their orientation. Some people may assume they are just greedy or indiscriminate or even that they're so sexually "out of control" they'll sleep with just anyone. Gay or straight people can be reluctant to date those who live in the murkier middle for fear—often quite invalid—that a bisexual/pansexual person will be dissatisfied having a partner of only one gender, even if the bisexual/pansexual person is more interested in monogamy than they are.

If you do identify as bisexual, pansexual, or another way of being queer that involves people of more than just one gender, it's good to be prepared to do a little mythbusting now and then and to try—though it can certainly be hard sometimes—not to take it too personally. As with any sexual orientation or identity that isn't considered a norm, there isn't a lot of accurate public awareness out there, so every person who has the patience to do some sincere and honest educating, even just among friends and family, can help to make those misconceptions and stereotypes fall away.

DID YOU KNOW? . . .

Not only are bisexuality, pansexuality, and homosexuality natural in humans, they occur commonly in other mammals and animals as well, including chimpanzees, bonobos, guinea pigs, ducks, ostriches, cats, dogs, insects, gorillas, horses, sheep, monkeys, and a plethora of other creatures. It also is nothing new. Though through much of history many homosexuals and bisexuals have not been "out," most anthropologists and biologists agree that different sexual orientations have occurred in humans for just as long as heterosexuality has.

Psychological and sexual research clearly shows that orientation in and of itself is not a cause of emotional or social problems. More often, when such problems are associated with homosexuality, bisexuality, or pansexuality they are rooted in the nonacceptance of the orientation or taunting, scolding, or punishment resulting from perception of these nonconventional orientations.

"Bad" Words

Certain terms for sexual orientation and identity vary in use and acceptance from place to place, from person to person. So, whereas for one person self-identifying as a "fag" feels right, it may not to another. Even those who do self-ID with "fag" may not like others using the term to identify them; in other words, they may be hurt or insulted by being called a fag, especially when it's intended to be an insult or a slur.

Over time, it's common for some negative terms to be revisited or reclaimed, even those that were once considered insults. Terms like slut, queer, dyke, straight, or poof are good examples; many people now use them as positive or even cheeky self-identifiers. However you choose to identify yourself, whatever feels best to you, is fine. It's also fine to object to how another person identifies or describes you, even if you do use a word yourself that they're using to describe you.

Your sexuality is with you through your whole life, so you get to take all the time you need to explore it on your own and figure out what, if any, names you want to give it at any time or in any given circumstance or situation. You can research various orientations online; attend youth groups for gay, lesbian, bisexual, and questioning teens; or see if your school has a Gay-Straight Alliance (GSA). You can talk to teens and adults of various orientations to get an idea of how much diversity there is and what living with a given sexual orientation might be like.

Ultimately, you're the person you have to live with every day. Trying to make yourself into something you aren't or fighting who you feel you really are may seem like the easier thing to do in the short run, but in the long run it's incredibly stressful and can have serious ill effects on self-esteem and all your relationships.

No matter who you are, or in which stage of understanding your identity you are, the real goal is to accept yourself as you are and to allow your identity and actions—sexual and otherwise—to come from that place. If you're sincere, open,

Homophobia

Homophobia, like any phobia, is an irrational fear or hatred, in this case, of people who are gay, lesbian, or bisexual/pansexual (*biphobia* is also a term in use) or of the mere idea of such sexual orientations. Because discrimination against or ignorance about queer people isn't always based in fear—or phobia—some people call prejudice against these orientations *homonegativity* or talk about *heterocentricity* instead. Unfortunately, just like sexism, racism, and all the other *–isms* that indicate some sort of discriminatory belief, homophobia is still frequently perpetuated by public figures, by the media, by a lack of visibility, by generational prejudices. Homophobia is often at the root of hate crimes against queer as well as transgender people or those assumed to be. Many hate crimes go unreported and unpunished, or they do not get media attention, and this lack of exposure of the issues helps to perpetuate homophobia.

Homophobia is not exclusive to heterosexual people; some GLBT people have internalized levels of it themselves—about themselves or other portions of the queer community—which can lead to serious self-esteem problems and severe emotional distress or self-hatred. Those feelings often contribute to self-destructive behaviors such as cutting, substance abuse, risky sexual behavior, and suicide.

honest, and caring, if you live with integrity, you're someone to be proud of, no matter your orientation.

[COMING OUT]

Although plenty of things about orientation and gender apply to everyone, the process of coming out—voluntarily making your sexual orientation or gender identity public—is mostly relevant for those of us whose sexual orientations or gender identities are something other than the presumed "default" settings (even though that's a foolish and flawed presumption in the first place). In other words, coming out is something that primarily concerns people who aren't straight, who aren't gendernormative, or both.

Coming out is totally optional. No one *has* to come out. It's not a requirement to get your queer or trans seal of approval or to validate your sexual or gender identity. How private or public any of this is, to the degree that that is within your control, should be completely up to you. Everyone's wants and needs are different, as are our circumstances. It's much less safe for some people or some people in some places and some communities to come out than it is for others. And some identities are certainly met with more acceptance, support, or plain-old-belief than others. You also get to decide where and when to come out if you do: it's perfectly fine to be out with your family, but not with most friends, or out online, but not at work.

No one is more of a "real" gay, lesbian, bisexual, or asexual person or a "real" man, woman, or otherwise because they're out or coming out—everyone is already real all by themselves. Coming out shouldn't feel like something you have to do to prove yourself. It's something you just choose to do—if and when you do—to be able to feel like yourself with and be treated like yourself by others and to feel like you're able to be honest about who you are when that's something you want, as it often is. No one owes anyone else information about their identities either; if a potential or current sexual or romantic partner wants to know, but you're not there yet, you get to tell them it's not something you're ready to share, and they should leave it at that. If they're not comfortable staying with you in those ways because they feel they need to know these things, so be it—it might be time to just part ways and move on.

There's also no time limit for coming out or a specific schedule: you get to take as long a time (or as little) as you need to feel comfortable. How "out" you are is also up to you: whatever level of private or public works best for you and/or your partners is just fine. You can also choose to come out in some contexts, but not in others, depending on safety concerns or personal comfort. Nobody has to cover themselves in pride pins, feather boas, or leather chaps—or, in that case, *not* cover themselves—to be out (but if you want to, knock yourself out). You may not even need to come out in any formal way; sometimes it's casual and incidental.

But at a certain point, life in the closet can do a real number on you and your partners. When you're with someone, being reluctant to even hold their hand in public can put a painful strain on a relationship, and feeling like a dirty secret doesn't help anyone's self-esteem.

When it starts to become clear that their sexual orientation or gender identity is more than a curiosity or a passing crush, many people become nervous or scared, worried that they might not be "normal." (You might not be, by the way, if "normal" means you are like a majority of people. But not being normal is not automatically a bad thing. It's good—and certainly a lot more interesting—to be weird in some ways. I say this to you as a lifelong weirdo myself, so I acknowledge I may be biased in this respect.)

Others strongly suspect or know for sure that they have certain gender attractions or gender conflicts, but they are afraid to say so, either because they feel they will be branded in some way or simply because they fear being rejected by their friends, family, or community. For example, in the United States, during the 2004 elections, exit polls indicated that 4 percent of all voters publicly self-identified as gay or lesbian, yet an overwhelming number of people in the world, despite solid evidence to the contrary, still think of homosexuality as an illness or perversion. Transgender people are even less generally accepted, even among "alternative" or progressive communities, than those who identify as gay or bisexual. In the United States alone, over seven thousand hate crimes are reported every year, with a great number of perpetrators and victims younger than the age of twenty. In many schools, teachers and school administrators fail or even refuse to intervene when orientation-based abuse or harassment occurs, and in some situations, teachers and administrators themselves have been responsible for the attacks on students or other staff. Being nervous or afraid to come out when you're about to come out as anything

Straight and About to Skip This Part?

Please don't. *I am literally begging you.* Not only may you find that, over time, your own orientation or sexual identity shifts but also queer people, like transgender people, like all young people of any stripe, need allies. In many places in the world, it is still really awful and hard to be queer. The suicide rates, for instance, of queer and transgender youth are two to three times higher than rates for heterosexual, gender-conforming youth. *Suicide Attempts Among Transgender and Gender Non-Conforming Adults*, a 2015 report from the Williams Institute and the American Foundation for Suicide Prevention found that between 42 percent and 46 percent of transgender individuals reported suicide attempts. A 2011 report from the United States Department of Health and Human Services *(Sexual Identity, Sex of Sexual Contacts, and Health-Risk Behaviors Among Students in Grades 9–12: Youth Risk Behavior Surveillance)* found that queer youth are four times more likely and questioning youth are three times more likely to attempt suicide as their straight peers are.

Rates of homelessness, abuse, and depression are also much higher. So, even if this isn't about you, have a read and prepare yourself to be a great source of support to a friend or family member who may need it from you more than you will ever know.

other than heterosexual or gender normative is completely valid.

If and when you do want to come out, you'll probably find that doing so selectively and in gradual steps makes it feel less terrifying and makes it go more smoothly and safely for you. And most people who come out overwhelmingly report that they are glad they did and that it's helped them to feel more at peace with themselves and more free to live their lives as they want to.

A Basic How-To

Being a young person is stressful enough. Although it's typical to keep some aspects of your sexual life or identity private from some or all people (like not telling parents you're sexually active, or not telling a friend what sexual activities you've engaged in), feeling like you have to *hide* your sexual and personal identity or experiences can really limit your quality of life and the quality of your relationships. Here are some points to keep in mind:

▶ **Take whatever time you need.** Consider the positives and the negatives. Ready yourself for the sorts of questions you're likely to be asked, even the stupid ones (and there will be stupid ones). Expect friends and family to ask if you're sure you're queer, or sure you're the gender you're telling them is yours, or how you know; how important it is to you; whether someone else is pushing you to be out or be queer; how out you need to be in your town, school, or extended family; how you want to handle it; what you expect from them; whether you're dating—and if so, whom you're dating, and what you're doing with them sexually (don't be surprised by the infamous "How can two women have sex, anyway?" question). It's normal for people who are straight or cisgender to have basic, earnest questions about orientation or gender, so prepare yourself to be able to address the questions calmly, or refer friends and family to groups or resources for more information. Have a good idea of what you want and need from the person or people to whom you're coming out.

▶ **Start small.** Start with someone you have a pretty good idea will be supportive and accepting. (If you don't have even one person like that in your life, try starting with a support group, in person or online.) Testing the waters first is a good idea. For example, you might bring up a current event that involves queer or trans issues, such as marriage equality (or how marriage asks queer people to assimilate in some ways), how typical incarceration protocols put transgender people at a tremendous risk of violence, or hate crime law. Talking about queer or trans issues in a general way—rather than personal issues—can give you a good idea of how to gauge someone's feelings and if they're a safe person to come out to.

If you get a good feeling about them, you can move a bit further. A good opening for coming out is something like, "I have been going through something important and challenging for a long time. I want to share it with you, and it feels very necessary. I'm not sure if you'll understand, but I trust you, and I'm asking for your support and acceptance, even if you can't give it to me right away: I'm queer/bisexual/asexual/lesbian/gay/transgender/genderqueer."

▶ **Expect surprises.** It can be a terrible blow when someone you were sure was going to be behind you all the way turns out to have some reservations or some prejudiced ideas. Soften it by communicating, over time, both by talking and by listening. If what they say to you is hurtful, let them know that. If they say things that simply aren't true, especially for you, gently correct them. For more on dealing with this, see Chapter 6.

Most people with any kind of bias developed it when they were pretty young. They have so far managed to go through life without having those attitudes challenged. Most prejudice is based on ignorance and lack of personal experience. If you have to deal with it, you may feel validly pissed or sad to have to take responsibility for a situation that you did nothing to create and that does you harm. But try to think about that differently, for your own sake. An opportunity to teach, to work to undo prejudice and intolerance, is always a good opportunity, because even one person can foster change that has a ripple effect in the long run. It's hard, and certainly very upsetting and frustrating at times, but I do think we are always helping ourselves and others in big ways when we can and do make ourselves more visible and insist on being seen, which includes being seen and understood without ignorance, fear, or prejudice. Plus, people with bias are often much more likely to start to shift their thinking when it becomes clear their bias is hurting people they care about.

Once you've got an ally in your corner, figure out where you want to go next. If it's your parents you want to tell, first call on family members you know will be the most supportive. Choose neutral settings for coming out: places that are conducive to calm communication and that aren't stressful. Family gatherings, holidays, public restaurants, or workplaces are usually not good choices. If you want to come out at school, see if you can start with a GSA (Gay-Straight Alliance), or form one with friends. The more support you have at every stage of the game, the better.

Chances are, there will be stops and starts. A friend or family member who is supportive at one point may backpedal or stall a bit with certain issues or at certain times. Many good people have blind spots, hidden biases they aren't even aware of. They may find it hard to recognize these or may become angry and resentful when your issues bring them to light.

Of course, sometimes the surprise we find is a nice one: plenty of times people have come out cautiously to a parent or friend only to be told that the person already knew all along and was completely down with it, that they were just waiting for us to figure it out for ourselves!

▶ **Be fair to your parents, even when they're hyperventilating.** For many, coming out to parents is the scariest part, and the fear of rejection is intense. But, for the most part, parents are cool people who usually love the heck out of you. That doesn't mean it's always easy as pie to come out to them. Your parents may go through a wide range of emotions: some may cry, others may yell, others may get very noncommunicative for a bit, even very angry. Your parents may suggest therapy for you. Some parents feel that having a homosexual, bisexual, or transgender child means they were lousy

Coming Out as Asexual?

It can seem like asexual is the new bisexual: finding people who believe you're even for real, let alone who are supportive, can be a struggle. Asexuality is uncommon and also not well understood, so lots of people haven't even been exposed to the idea or concept of asexuality or may not have ever met anyone who identifies as asexual, who doesn't experience and express feelings of sexual desire for others and the desire to be sexual with people. (From a bisexual who's been there, my deepest sympathies.) So, you may just want to especially ready yourself for that and approach discussions with people with information or suggested reading they can do to educate themselves rather than grilling you.

parents or that you're betraying them by being different. Some may hold typical misconceptions or strong beliefs, such as that homosexuality is sinful or unnatural. Some who aren't homophobic or transphobic, who are perfectly accepting or who are queer themselves, may still have strong emotional reactions. Queer parents, for instance, may feel upset about a child coming out because they have faced a lot of discrimination, rejection, or violence in their lives and feel scared their child will face this, too.

Your folks have been through a lot during your adolescence. They've watched you change in so many ways (and so quickly, from their perspective) that they sometimes have to sit down just to fend off motion sickness. So, even the most accepting, open-minded parents may not want to throw you a party the minute you come out to them, and they may choke on their carrots instead of saying "congratulations" when you announce your sexual or gender identity at the dinner table.

As it is, most parents have a tough time adjusting to and keeping up with their teens' sexual development, maturation, identity, and relationships. (You can probably understand this: for a lot of us, thinking about our parents having sex is at least slightly squicky.) If you've known about your orientation or identity all along, or had that niggling feeling, then being queer or gender nonconforming may not be a change for you at all—but your folks may not have seen this one coming.

So, when you lay it on your parents, do your best to be kind. Be patient. Be mature. Be compassionate. When you are, you're more likely to get the same treatment from them. Be the change you want to see (in your parents). Offer to answer any questions they might have, and be ready to listen, even if what they say isn't so great to listen to. Make yourself available to talk about it. Let them know that you're okay with it if they're not elated right now. Give them the time they need to absorb it all before you hang a rainbow flag on the front lawn or expect them to do battle with you with your homophobic uncle. In time, most parents really do come around.

▶ **Think before you pull out a megaphone.** When you first come out, you may feel like you want to tell the whole world. It's exhilarating to feel that you can be honest and forthright about your sexual or gender identity, with yourself and with others. Just be sure that you're doing it *in places and with people who are safe for you.* And it's okay to be more private with all this, if that's what you want or for your safety. There's nothing "better" about people who are, literally, proud very out loud.

Basic sexual and interpersonal safety smarts apply to being queer just as much as they apply to being straight, and in many places, more so. Being more marginalized always means being more vulnerable.

Not every place or situation is the right place or situation in which to be sexual or to discuss sex or sexual identity, especially when your sexuality is controversial or titillating in the eyes of some or completely objectionable in the eyes of others and considered to make it open season to abuse or harass you. When you

CLOSED DOORS

It will take some family members a much longer time to accept having a queer or gender-nonconforming kid. Some, sadly, won't ever be okay with it. That's a harsh reality that really, really hurts. Sometimes bias and prejudice are unsurpassable, even in people we love.

Some parents kick young people out of the house when they come out, cut off college-age kids financially, disown them, or ship them off to therapists or communities that claim to be able to "convert" GLBT people. By the way, those approaches—often called "conversion therapies," even though they're anything but therapeutic—have never been proven to transform people who aren't straight into people who are. In fact, they've been found to engage in serious abuse and to cause very real and enduring harm. Most credible psychological organizations have issued strong statements against conversion therapies, and we're even (thank goodness) starting to see some legal intervention and restriction. The state of California, for example, now has a law that bans outright this kind of abuse.

If that happens to you or you suspect it might, call on your support system of friends or extended family to help. Make your safety your top priority. Remember that parents are people, and like any other people, sometimes they're really messed up.

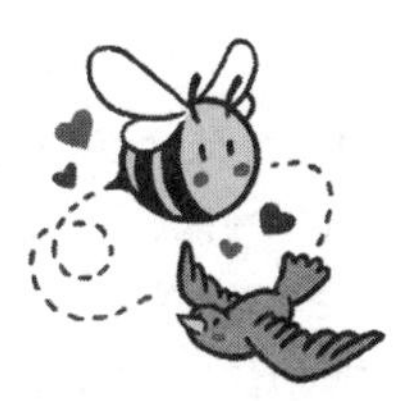

Do what you can to not internalize their bias or assume it's right. Bias is never right, not ever. It's the biased person who is always the problem, not the person whom the bias is against. If non-acceptance of your sexuality turns into any sort of abuse—physical, verbal, emotional, or sexual—treat it as abuse: get help and do what you need to to get and keep yourself in a safe space. If you suspect you may face abuse in coming out while still living at home, it may be safest to wait to come out until you're in a safer setting. (For more on abuse, see Chapter 11.)

With parents who don't take it to the absolute extreme but who really aren't happy about or accepting of you coming out, you may find that to keep the peace you have to agree at some point not to discuss the issue. If you find that that simply doesn't feel right, you may have to come up with some other solution.

MENTORING IN THE QUEER COMMUNITY

It's unfortunate, but a lot of queer youth find that the only "in" to the queer community and to queer mentors or support is through dating or sex. Thing is, while sexual or romantic partners may love and care for you, they're not always the best mentors when it comes to queer life and community because they may be very temporary, their love is likely conditional, and if you do seek out support via sex, you may find that it leaves a bad taste in your mouth.

If you're seeking out the queer community via a website or app, for instance, make clear you're looking for *friends,* not lovers. Don't make any lover your whole support system. Remember that you're a whole person and that your sexual orientation and identity are about more than the sex you're having; they're about you as a whole person.

If you're having a hard time finding community outside dating or sexual relationships, see if you can't broaden your horizons. Many cities have queer and gender-nonconforming youth groups, on campus and off. Hook up with a queer activist community. The queer, questioning, or straight-but-supportive friends you don't date can also be great, nonsexual support and people you can go with to places where you can all broaden your community. If you're having a really hard time of it, many counselors and therapists who are queer-friendly or transfriendly advertise in print and online publications for the queer community.

do choose to be out or sexual in public, be sure you're making safe choices. Be alert. Know the risks you are taking, and do what you can to minimize them. If where you are doesn't feel like a safe place to be out in, you're probably right. If someone you're thinking about telling or inviting into some part of your sexuality or sexual identity just doesn't feel supersafe, trust your instincts. (For more on hate crimes and sexual assault, and protecting yourself, see Chapter 11.)

▶ **There's a difference between holding the door open for someone and pushing them through it.** Once you're out, past the toughest parts, and feeling all the relief of being out, you may want others you know to experience the same thing—even if they aren't quite sure they're queer or gender nonconforming in the first place. Well intentioned as that may be, it's never a good idea to pull someone kicking and screaming out the closet door. You also may want some company in being out, which is understandable, but never something to try to drag someone into when they don't want or don't feel ready for that.

You can talk to your maybe-definitely-in-the-closet friends about how great you feel right now and about how much being out benefits you. You can share the things you did that helped make the process easier. You can let them know that, if they want to come out, you'll be the first in line to be part of their community. Just be sure that you're also respecting their pace and allowing them the same sort of time you had to come out when you were ready. When they're ready, they'll likely let you know, and then you can be the supportive, wonderful friend that you are and tell them about all the mistakes you made coming out yourself. Maybe by then these will be funny.

▶ **Celebrate yourself.** Amid all the complexities of getting used to your sexual or gender identity and all the mistakes you'll make—because we all do— please don't forget to take time out to really appreciate the good stuff. It takes serious guts to be honest, real, and at all public about our sexual or gender identity when it's not easily accepted or a norm. It takes a lot to make yourself more vulnerable for the sake of living honestly and to have the patience and energy to work through all these issues with others while you're still learning to understand them yourself—but it's a truly great thing. Although it's got its rough spots, it usually feels really good.

Do nice things for yourself. Have a coming-out party with some close friends. Pamper yourself. Get a new haircut; buy some new books. Explore it all: write about what you're going through, talk to close friends you know are supportive, listen to music that makes you feel good about this journey and this part of who you are.

Coming out isn't usually something we have to do only once in our lives; it's a lifelong, constant process. Because you'll be entering into new situations, new partnerships, new communities throughout your whole life, you'll probably have to make choices about coming out more than once and go through it more than once.

As time goes by, as your support network grows, all that gets a lot easier, and your sexual or gender identity through the years will become a more integral and effortless part of your entire personal identity. Even amid coming-out chaos, be sure to take care of and enjoy yourself and who you are. Sexuality is supposed to be about joy and about pleasure and about feeling good. Honor it—all parts of it—and you honor yourself.

DID YOU KNOW? . . .

In 1977, when Harvey Milk became a city supervisor of San Francisco, he was the first out homosexual to be elected to public office in a large city in the United States. Milk knew that as an openly gay man in public office, his safety was precarious. Sadly, he was right: he was assassinated only a year later by a fellow official. However, Milk had prepared for his possible murder and recorded several tapes of his words to share with the world should he not get the chance to pass them on himself. In those tapes, he said that if everyone who was gay, lesbian, or bisexual told their friends, family, coworkers, and fellow students the truth about who they were, none of the stereotypes about queer people could stand in the light of reality. One of Milk's last recorded passages was, "If a bullet should enter my brain, let that bullet destroy every closet door in the country."

One of the first transgender rights activists, the amazing Sylvia Rivera, said something very similar when she said, "I was a radical, a revolutionist. I am still a revolutionist. . . . I am glad I was in the Stonewall riot. . . . I thought, "My god, the revolution is here. The revolution is finally here!"

The revolution is finally here. And it's about freaking time.

6

You, Me, and Everyone Else: Big Outside Influences on Your Sexuality

I don't mean to creep you out, but when it comes to our sexuality and sexual lives, even when we are all by ourselves, we're never *really* alone: much of what we think and feel about sex and sexuality, what strongly influences our sexual choices and sexual lives, and even how we experience our sexuality and sex lives, comes from other people. The most impactful of those outside influencers are usually our families, our peers, and, more recently in history, media, especially mass media.

Sometimes that outside input is positive and supportive and empowers us. We're likely to get something good from having a friend or family member tell us they love and accept us when we come out to them; from a movie that shows sexual interactions between young people that are both healthy and fun for them and that doesn't end in epic tragedy of one kind or another; from a television show that gives positive visibility, without stereotyping, to the sexual or love lives of LGBTQ people; from a sex ed class that leaves us feeling empowered and informed. Sometimes the messages and input we receive make us feel able to be ourselves and more comfortable with ourselves.

Sometimes outside input is negative, disempowering, or nonsupportive. A movie that presents someone with a disability or who is transgender expressing their sexuality as some kind of joke, a friend or family member who shames us for masturbating or wanting a sexual relationship, or a sex ed class that makes us feel ashamed even for having a pulse let alone a sexuality is more likely to result in negative impacts rather than positive ones. Sometimes the messages and input we receive make us feel *un*able to be ourselves and *un*comfortable with ourselves. Often, people develop different personas within relationships or groups to try to fit in them because they don't feel like a fit for the whole person we are.

How big and enduring an impact these outside influences have has a lot to do with how important the source is to us, how prevalent the message is (or we perceive it to be), and what degree of power and influence that source has for us. On the whole, messages from family members, especially parents, tend to have strong influences on people's sexualities and sexual lives and how they feel about them. The same goes for our friends and peers. And with the growing number of all kinds of media and their pervasiveness and influence in most of our lives, the media have made their way onto that list of major influencers, too.

Getting a real awareness of these influences, knowing how to make sense of them, learning how to keep them in perspective are essential. A sexuality or sexual life that has more to do with what others think, feel, or say than with what *you* think, feel, and say and what's really right for you as your own person, with your own life, isn't good for anyone. Some outside messages or modeling can really help us out and help us to create and feel supported in a healthy, happy sexuality and sexual life; others can do the opposite, setting us up for or keeping us in sexual lives that are stinkers or sexualities that we know are our own but that we feel like we have to hide out in.

[YOUR FAMILY]

As Aline P. Zoldbrod points out in *Sex Smart: How Your Childhood Shaped Your Sexual Life and What to Do About It,* you've been learning about sexuality from your family from the minute you were born, whether you were aware of it or not. How your parents or other family members touched you and treated you, from how affectionate they were or weren't to how they handled gender, power, and your sexual or interpersonal development, and what they showed you about sexuality and relationships through their own interactions with others and their own sense of self have a huge impact on your sexuality and all your relationships, including your relationship with yourself—there's just no getting around it.

We know from many studies that parents or other primary care providers have, hands down, the biggest impact on us as we develop our sexuality and make sexual choices. How we were raised to think about and handle our bodies and sex and sexuality plays a huge part in the formation of our sense of self and body image and where these two conceptions overlap. When family influence is positive, it's amazing: having the support of your family as you develop and enter this part of your life makes even the really challenging pieces, even trauma or unwanted outcomes, much easier to deal with. Learning it's okay to talk openly about any of this and experiencing and seeing healthy relationships and interactions help people immeasurably develop healthy sexual lives.

Getting the message from family that it's okay to have not just a sexuality or sexual identity but *your specific* sexuality and sexual identity, whatever they are, and feeling that acceptance and respect are huge.

Suffice it to say, if things aren't so great—or worse, if they are downright awful or abusive in any way—the impacts can be equally strong on the flip side, making what's usually a challenging part of life and growth way harder or traumatic, setting people up for unhealthy ways of thinking, acting, and seeing themselves that can make sexuality and how you choose to express or explore it less likely to be or feel beneficial. These are things that, when people become aware of them, and if they choose to try to resolve them, can take a lot of hard work and time to turn around.

You probably have a sense of the overall impact of your family on your sexuality, an idea about whether they've made sexuality feel like something that is or isn't okay. You might also know about the impact of your family on specific aspects of all this, like if you've found going through puberty to be pretty comfortable because they've been supergreat about it, or if you've experienced growing feelings of sexual desire much harder to deal with because someone in your family talks about sexual desire like it was some kind of monster that could eat people alive. You've undoubtedly experienced which parts of sex and sexuality your family will or won't talk about and how they talk about them when they do; you've seen how members of your family show you, in words or actions—and sometimes by the absence of either—how they feel about their own bodies or sexualities and any of their own sexual relationships.

One thing I hear a lot from users at Scarleteen is how concerned—sometimes even to the point of developing a great deal of ongoing anxiety—many young people are about what their families do or might think about their sexualities or sexual lives. Fear of nonacceptance or of disappointing family members by making a "wrong" choice or by having a sexuality or sexual life that family members, especially parents, have given clear messages they don't or wouldn't approve of looms large. Even in families in which it seems likely parents or guardians would handle sexuality-related news well and with care, many young people still keep their sexualities or sexual lives (including solo sex) hidden, often less out of a desire for privacy and more because they are just that scared of disappointing their families or of facing judgment. Those kinds of big fears happen in part because we know the impact our families can have, and we know it can be giant.

Our families are also one of the primary places we learn values and are shown cultural or religious beliefs (see page 374 in To Be or Not to Be . . .), and they also are the primary and most powerful place any or all values and beliefs are reinforced, enforced, and challenged. All of those beliefs, ethics, and values already play a big part in our sexuality, sexual choices, and who we are as a whole, and when family is part of that—as it most often is—both the impact of our family *and* the impact of those things are amplified.

Working out the impacts our families have on our sexualities and sex lives is a lifelong process. It is something we understand only in steps and stages, usually more and more deeply over time. When those impacts have been negative, it tends to take a good deal of time and personal growth work to make sense of them, put them into context, and resolve them. It's just not something anyone can tackle in any big way early in life, especially if you're still living at home and soaking it in every day.

But what you can do now, whether you're still living at home or not, is try to gain and keep an awareness of the impacts your family has had or is having on your sexuality. Evaluate for yourself which of those impacts has been positive and which negative. You can start to put any negatives into perspective and do things for yourself to try to resolve them, such as choosing to create sexual or romantic relationships that have real equity in them and other

WHAT MAKES A FAMILY?

Who your family is—who *you* call and consider family—is very much up to you. It's sadly common for people to experience big rifts, including rejection and abuse, with family when it comes to sex and sexuality; in this department, plenty of people have been or are still traumatized by their treatment by family. This is one of the big areas in which people either surrender to what family wants or allows, suppressing their own wants or sense of self, or separate from their families. (Religion and power struggles among family members are other big influential issues; both are often part of conflicts over sex or sexuality.) And if separating from some or all of your born-into family now or later is ever something you want or feel you need to do, it is okay to do that, and that doesn't have to mean you don't have any kin. If in any area of your life, including your sexuality, you feel like your family hasn't acted like family should, and you want family, you get to and can make your own family.

Family can really be anyone we call, consider, and treat like family on the basis of our own definitions of family. "Family" can be people we share genetics with, such as a group made up of a biological father, mother, and their children, but it doesn't have to be; there are other ways of defining family. Who is "family" can be as simple as who makes us feel like we're at home in and with ourselves—people with whom we feel both accepted and acceptable and who we want to feel the same way with us.

For example, if your current family is not supportive of you as someone who is queer or gender nonconforming or as someone having a sexual life or pregnancy outside marriage, you can conceptualize and create a family who *is* supportive. This can mean separating from your existing family entirely or just a little bit or adding more members to your family so that it includes people who support you. Family can be created of friends and sexual or romantic partners, neighbors, mentors, or anyone else you can think of (including pets!); family doesn't have to be just people we're related to and doesn't have to be something someone can make anew only if they reproduce. Family also doesn't have to be a force that keeps having a negative impact on our sexuality or sexual lives. We can always build a family or extend a family so that it benefits us and positively affects our lives instead of causing us pain and suffering. ■■

healthy dynamics or focusing on more positive messages or relationships that make you feel good about yourself, your sexuality, or your sexual life, whether that's finding information that supports masturbation as something healthy, not dirty, or friends who will celebrate your giddiness about a new girlfriend instead of making you feel scared or ashamed. You can seek out support for areas in your life where you feel those negative impacts; finding other people or sources you know are sound, trust, and value to give you more positive messages and emotional support goes a very long way.

Sometimes, we can create—but certainly don't always—sexual lives that are some kind of reaction to or rebellion against our families or messages they have given us, whether or not we even know we're doing that. If this happens, and if the way it's part of or motivating our sexual lives and choices feels like a great fit for us and positive, it isn't usually a problem—it's often a very good thing for everyone. *Rebellion* isn't a bad word. Positive resistance of authority, control, or convention is a very real and beneficial thing, whether it's something we do in our sexual lives or something we do in activism that's larger than us to change the world for the better.

But if any sexual rebellion doesn't *feel* positive, isn't leading us to things that are healthy or beneficial, but instead is making our lives worse in some way, what's probably going on is that our sexual choices or sense of sexual self are *more* about our family or our issues with our family than they're really about ***us***. We're probably creating or enabling more strife and conflict than we're already dealing with. So, try to keep an eye out for ways your sexuality or sexual choices might be a reaction to your family, and about them, rather than being based in hearing and responding to *yourself* and creating and expressing a sexual life or identity that comes more from you and is mostly about **you**.

If your home is a safe place, where talking about sex and sexuality and any ways you're feeling crummy because of how those topics have been or are being treated at home is something you know you can do without any kind of abuse, you can try to address conflicts with your family (see page 169, conflict resolution) and see if you can't work together to remedy trouble spots now, before they dig in deep in your sexuality or create permanent or longtime rifts between you and your family when there could, instead, be peace and connection. Those conversations still might feel scary or nerve-wracking even in a safe home, but when there's a real possibility of resolution, it's usually totally worth some awkwardness or temporary discomfort for everyone involved to work through them. Often, parents or other family members don't even know when they're sending negative messages—especially because these messages often come from family members' hardwiring, sexuality baggage they're unaware they have, including from their own upbringing—and they *want* to know when they are and they *want* to fix it.

[YOUR FRIENDS AND PEERS]

What friends or peers think—or even *might* think—or how they react or might react, really can feel like *everything* sometimes. Sometimes it *is* everything, and that everything is wonderful and what we need in our interactions and relationships with each other. Our friends and larger peer groups can really have our backs sometimes, or they can make us feel more okay about a part of ourselves we don't feel okay about yet. They can, and often do, help us let out feelings of loss or frustration, help us get out of dangerous or crappy situations, give us needed perspective, or support us in being resilient by helping us laugh our butts off about something we're taking much too seriously.

Those feelings of what friends or peers think as being everything aren't always positive, though. You know what peer pressure is, and you know about the very damaging impacts of peer harassment (aka bullying; for more, see page 220). Most talk about sex between you and other people probably happens or has happened between you and your friends. That's how almost all kinds of sex information—the good, the bad, and the ugly—get spread around and the most quickly, whether it's accurate and sound and helps people or it's presumptions that will undoubtedly hurt someone.

Many people in their teens and early twenties feel a lot of pressure about or with sex and sexuality, like the pressure to conform to the actual or assumed sexual norms of a friend or peer group or to be in the exact same sexual or romantic place and circumstances—like starting to have a certain kind of sex with a partner (or refraining from a certain kind of sex with a partner), or being bisexual—at

Pluralistic ignorance

When a majority of people assume that something is true for most people when in fact it's not, and then they start to think or behave in a way that matches that not-norm—sometimes to the degree that it becomes a norm—that's **pluralistic ignorance**. It's basically like life imitating art except that it's usually not something as grand as art it's imitating; in the case of sexuality, pluralistic ignorance takes the form of what's said or shown in the media and what peers say is going on when in fact it really isn't going on . . . until it is, but only because everyone falsely assumed it already was. Some common examples of pluralistic ignorance around sex, sexuality, and young people are the idea of "hookup culture" being prevalent in high school or college (it's not, actually: my generation was having far more sex outside ongoing relationships than yours is or has been), the idea that "everyone" or "those kids today" are having sex in high school or college (realistically, young people are having sex with partners later, not earlier; people who say things like "those kids today" probably had sex *before* you did or will), and the notion that because a lot of current pornography contains violence or sexism people want that or are doing that in their real-life sexual lives. A lot of the trouble we have in the world with people being bystanders when sexual or dating violence occur is also related to pluralistic ignorance: people often assume nothing is wrong just because no one else seems concerned.

the same time as their friends. A desire to fit in with the people we consider our tribe is a very big deal for human beings everywhere (and many other animals, no less). It can play a big part in sexual choices, how we make them, and how we develop and learn to feel free to express our own sexuality that belongs to just one person—us—not to a friend or a group of people. It can also make it trickier to claim and feel good about our sexuality if any aspect of it feels far outside the norm. In that situation, it feels like a choice must be made among exclusive categories: the sexual self, sexual life or relationships you want, or your friends and peer acceptance.

Pressure or peer pressure might not even come from someone else for us to experience it. A whole lot of what people experience as peer pressure is often more about perceived pressure or wanting to avoid that pressure or conflict. In other words, it is pressure that comes from our own fears regarding people and that we put on ourselves rather than pressure someone else is putting on us. It's okay not to fit with what a friend or peer group thinks or says: in our relationships and communities, it should be okay that everyone isn't exactly the same and sometimes is even really different. Unless we're all just clones of each other, that's going to happen at least now and then, if not an awful lot. We can all not fit in, or be alike, as much as we want and still all be accepted and accepting. But often people are so scared that it won't be okay that they act in ways that kind of assume pressure or nonacceptance would happen.

Sometimes, your friends—and if you make a family with a partner, then some of your family—are or become your sexual partners. That can be fantastic (and I hope for anyone that their lovers are also their friends), but it can also increase the impact of any pressure.

HOW TO ASK FAMILY OR FRIENDS TO TURN DOWN THE VOLUME

Setting healthy limits and boundaries can make room for everyone to think what they think and feel how they feel but without expressing those thoughts or feelings in a way that is hurtful, harmful, or otherwise not cool or to someone who might be hurt by them.

▶ **Set a limit or a boundary:** It should always be okay to ask for a certain conversation or way of communicating to just go dark or for someone to leave out certain statements they're making that you really disagree with or that make you or someone else feel like dirt. You can make this request in person, with words, or if you don't feel confident or emotionally safe enough to do that, you could also do it through an e-mail or handwritten letter, a phone call, or even a text message. A note about texting, though: use a different medium for any big, serious conversations—text just isn't a good format for loaded conversations. It's way too easy for people to take shortcuts and misunderstand or not hear each other and for the quick-by-design nature of text messages to make people's responses to your big deals feel like blow-offs. (For more on resolving conflict, see page 169.)

▶ **Close the door if your limits and boundaries aren't respected:** Let's say you've asked a parent or a close friend to choose someone else to discuss their feelings about certain reproductive choices or sexualities, because those conversations with you just aren't something that you want or that you feel is healthy for you. You set a clear limit and boundary. But they keep doing it. When they do, restate your limit or boundary, and then just do what you can to get gone—walk away from the table, go to another room, close a phone conversation, whatever you need to do to make clear that if they're not going to respect your limit, you're going to do what you can to separate yourself from them and hold the line.

▶ **Gather allies:** Perhaps there's someone in your family or friend group who can help gently remind others of the limit you've set and validate that limit with you. Like saying, "Hey, remember when she told you that misgendering her is hurtful and asked us to use the pronouns she uses for herself?" or "I'm very uncomfortable with this conversation because Sol asked all of us not to go there again last time, so please stop."

▶ **If you've done all you can to encourage your friends or family to be supportive, emotionally healthy, and kind and it's not working, do what you can to separate yourself from, or dump entirely, people who aren't or clearly don't want to be:** Again, with family, especially if you still have to live at home, separating or dumping is not always doable. But we can emotionally protect ourselves more or leave, full stop. Usually, we can at least create some extra space or distance, like by sharing less with anyone who's not being a positive influence, sexually or otherwise, or more strongly holding our own lines rather than just surrendering to their yuck. Friends, on the other hand, are almost always completely elective: who your friends are is totally up to you. As people go through adolescence, it's common for some old friendships to end, for new ones to begin, and for friend groups to shift and change

TECH TIP

Unfortunately, a lot of people feel more free to act like jerks online or through mobile technologies than they do in face-to-face interactions. Particularly, when people can be anonymous in any way or feel more secure because they're part of a bigger group, they tend to feel like they can say or do inappropriate things, which unfortunately often translates into making someone else feel bad. If an online social network of any kind is toxic for you, either dump it entirely or do what you can to make it better. You can remove certain friends or followers, better protect your privacy by keeping more things to yourself, or ask for outside help from someone you trust and know has your back (and/or who can just let you rant about what jerks people can be online until you can let go of the big impact it's having on you!). If any mistreatment has moved or is moving into full-blown harassment, see Chapter 11 for information about abuse and what to do about it. And by all means, don't take part in this yourself, like by insulting someone's body or participating in making any part of someone's private life public. When we act like jerks ourselves, we send a clear message that says that's okay. So, we're not only more likely to wind up surrounded by other jerks, we're more likely to have people be jerks to us, especially if the kind of people who act like jerks are people we've made our friends.

a lot. Sometimes that's precisely because some friends don't learn how to be supportive—or just stop doing it—with very sensitive, personal issues related to difference; in a word, they lack the emotional maturity to maintain healthy intimate relationships, which includes accepting difference and resolving conflict in healthy ways. It may absolutely be best for you to leave old friends behind because not only do they just not fit with who you are anymore but also they can't even deal with healthy limits and boundaries. It's hard, and it sucks, but it usually beats the alternative, big time.

[MEDIA]

Before I get to perils and problems with media and our relationship to media, especially mass and sexual entertainment media, I want to be sure to make clear that the media, just as with most things, are not essentially bad—or essentially good.

What's "Media"?

Media just means instruments or methods of conveying something; in our context, instruments or mediums used to communicate to other people in some way, often in words, sounds, or images. "Mass" media means media that, usually by intent, reach a large number of people. "Mainstream" media are mass media that reflect popular or prevailing thought, influence, or activity. "Alternative" media are media that put forth views that stand *counter* to, or that challenge, popular thought and what's typically found in mass or mainstream media. Differentiating a kind of media from another has gotten a lot harder, because more and more of them have become more and more enmeshed. News is often on sites that are actually tabloids, and tabloid media are all mixed into news sites: the same place you might seek out instructions on how to max your gains at the gym can also be a place to find sexual entertainment in the sidebars. Popular culture is also often part of media, especially mainstream media and sexual media. If you're in or have been in junior high and high school, you probably know how this works. Just like popularity in those settings, *popular culture* is a term that generally describes highly influential media or ways of thinking that are often the lowest common denominator for any big culture at a given time.

Media vary as much as the people who make it do. There's no one way all media are. Media include *all* of art, music, film, and literature. Reporting or activism through or with the help of media has created some of the most needed, powerful, and positive change in the modern world. Media include radio and television broadcasts that warn people of serious dangers and save thousands and thousands of lives. Media have broadened our world considerably so that everyone can know and understand more about the world, the people in it, and its diversity way more than we could just knowing our own communities.

Sometimes the media present healthy and less visible sexualities, identities, or sexual lives we might never otherwise see, for example, showing people enjoying more kinds of sex than just intercourse, someone asking for a kiss instead of just giving one without permission, and showing an

Be Stingy with Authority

Giving something authority—whether it's a friend, a family member, someone in the media, some media, or even someone like me—means either letting them take the driver's wheel for us in some way or allowing them to have a very big influence on our ideas or actions. We should think of it as a pretty big deal and not something we want to give just anyone or give someone just because they told us we should or because they communicate in a way that makes it seem like they know what they're talking about or what they're saying or showing must be important. Take your time with picking who you give that kind of trust to and how you involve them in your sense of yourself and what you do. Make anyone you give authority to earn it first.

identity so infrequently seen that someone who felt so isolated because they were sure they were the only person like them on earth gets to feel giant relief and solidarity. There's no way that marriage equality would have finally started happening so broadly and when it did without more and more queer visibility and acceptance occurring in mainstream media. Media have provided ways for people to find needed support that's helped them to survive. Media include this book and the Scarleteen website.

There are and have been so many good, even truly great, things media have given us—both tools to make our own media and media others have made—it boggles the mind. Suggesting "media" are bad and we'd do better staying away from them would include staying away from all of those good things, too, and we can probably agree that no one would benefit from that.

But.

Mainstream media has a *lot* to say about sex and sexuality a whole lot of the time, to the point that if we are paying attention to just media, it can make sex and sexuality feel like a way bigger part of life than either is for most people in reality. A biennial study released in 2005 by the Kaiser Family Foundation found that the number of sexual scenes on television had substantially increased in less than 10 years. This study found that during the 2004–2005 season, 70 percent of all television shows aired included some degree of sexual content and averaged 5.0 sexual scenes per hour (a lot more than the average mere mortal could manage to fit into an hour!).

The media mirror culture. We're all living in a world that, overall, isn't very healthy or forward-thinking sexually, so what's in our media reflects that and is very often negative, factually incorrect, abusive and otherwise inhumane, or just crummy and one-dimensional. A lot of what most media have to say about sex and sexuality is as oversimplified, commodified (made into a thing to be bought and sold or exchanged for something), uninformed, unrealistic, and just plain messed up as what a lot of *people* have to say about it.

So, the ways a lot of people are thinking about these things—things that are part of sex and sexuality or how people experience it, such as gender roles, bodies, privilege, and power—are usually reflected in the media.

We don't always recognize when media are giving us messages about sex or sexuality or when our ideas about them have come from media: by the time you're in your early teens, you will have already had many years, including in early childhood when you probably didn't have any critical awareness of media, of taking in many highly influential messages from the media. Studies have found that the rigid gender stereotypes some people hold on to, for instance, are often strongly linked to how much media (particularly television media) they consumed as young children.

Where we expect to get messages about sex or sexuality—like in pornography or a sex scene in a Hollywood movie—or where we engage our sexual selves with media, the messages can be easy to see. But when we're just glancing at celebrity gossip while we wait in line, absentmindedly playing a video game, we can also be taking in equally powerful messages about sex, sexuality, and all the things that are parts of one or both. Sometimes those kinds of subconscious messages are even more powerful and sticky because when we don't know they're there or that we're taking them in, we don't even know to question them.

When the subject is sex and young people, what the media choose to say or represent is usually even more out of touch with the real world. More times than not, what is shown or reported about sex and young people is reported as being common or the norm, but in reality it is usually the very rare exception. Over the years, the media, particularly mass media, have sowed or cultivated the seeds of misinformation and panic that have caused an awful lot of (perhaps well meaning but often highly misinformed and overblown) adult freakouts about sex and young people. Some recent media-based sex-and-youth urban legends have included things like rainbow parties or jelly sex bracelets or sexting as sexual activities only young people do (nope) or that all young people are doing (also on the nope), things that may have happened in some way for a small number of young people but that were talked about and reported more sensationally or sexually than how they happened, or are represented as widespread when in fact they aren't at all.

The fallout from this can be pretty massive. For one, accurate or not, when widespread media send a clear message that there is something *all* young people are doing, it's easy to then believe that to be true and to then feel sexual pressure about that thing. Most people are pretty concerned about what is or isn't normal or common, and young people, in particular, feel a lot of pressure to try to conform to norms. It's also harder to get a realistic idea about what really is common and what isn't when you have little real-life experience with sex and people's sexualities. Too, young people as a population—though plenty of older people as well—have a bad track record of being dishonest about their sexual behavior, often saying what they think peers want to hear and what they guess will result in the least amount of blowback.

The impacts media have are equally broad. Just because the content of or messages in media are about sex or sexuality doesn't mean that they're all bad, all good, or all neutral; that we all interpret them the same way; or that we are all equally influenced by them or in the same ways. We also don't all give media—or all media—the same level of authority in our lives and over our ideas, use all the same media, or use them all the same ways; how much time and energy we put into keeping up with media vary. All of that diversity influences media's impact on us.

Not Just What, but How

A study released in 2015 by Common Sense Media (*The Common Sense Census: Media Use by Tweens and Teens*) found that American adolescents use an average of nine hours of media every day, not including media used for school or homework. That's more hours than most people spend each day sleeping, in school or at work, or with friends or family. But I actually found another bit of data more troubling: only a small minority of that time (only around 3 percent) is spent using media to *create* something. In other words, young people's media use was found to be almost entirely about what *others* (and mostly adults, based on this stat) have made and said through media rather than about using media for self-expression, to say something for and from themselves. That makes media much more about consumption than creation, about the feelings, thoughts, voices, and personal agendas of others instead of your own.

It's sound for any of us to have concerns about media, just like it's sound to be concerned about anything that takes up a lot of our time or emotional energy and that strongly informs and influences our thoughts, feelings, or behaviors. And if we want media to be something positive for us, we have to think about and consider the actual or possible impacts or influence of media on our sexualities, sexual self-image, or sexual behavior. This includes, but by no means is limited to, sexual or sexualized media, whether that's porn or reality TV. And we do this with media just as we do it with anything else that can influence or inform sex and our sexuality. We have to be sure we're approaching media alert on the road rather than asleep at the wheel. Consuming most media is less often a problem than consuming it without thinking about it and making intentional choices.

Unless someone goes and stays utterly off the grid, there's just no escaping at least some forms of media as some part of our lives. Although what we're exposed to is sometimes out of our hands—like a video that just wasn't what we were looking for at all, a show someone tells us to watch without us knowing what it is first, or a billboard right in front of where we have to wait for the bus—more often, it is under our control to at least some degree, often a pretty big one. We and others mostly get to choose what media we make a part of our lives and how we interact with and about it. And if and when media seem to be playing a part in ways of thinking or behaving that aren't good for us or other people, we can usually adjust or make changes to help remedy that, like by limiting how much time, attention, or power we give a certain kind of media or by talking with a partner to work out a way we feel we can keep media from messing something up between us or from keeping us from what could be really fantastic.

SEXUAL ENTERTAINMENT MEDIA

For as long as entertainment and media have existed, there's been sexual entertainment and sexualized media: media or performance created to try to get or keep someone sexually excited or curious. Modern technologies have made sexual media and entertainment way more widespread and much easier for everyone to access than ever before, but sexual media aren't new. They were discovered in ancient civilizations and in texts that are thousands of years old. The term *pornography*—which literally means "to write of prostitutes," from the Greek words *porne* and *graphien*—was coined when Pompeii was first excavated and sexual media was found. Porn is literally as old as dirt.

People have always created art, literature, and other materials from their life experiences and imagination. Sex and sexual fantasy are often big parts of our lives and our individual and collective imaginations. What's much more recent—and can make a lot of this much more thorny and problematic—is for sexual entertainment to be mass media and very, very big business, generating profits in the *billions* of dollars every year. (If you want something interesting to chew on, think about how industries with similar—but higher—profits are the diet, cosmetics, and wedding industries, all of which also have quite a lot to do with sex and sexuality.) Putting ginormous amounts of money into the mix changes everything with this, just like it does with anything else.

Because of mass access and the mainstreaming of porn—including cultural shifts toward porn being thought of as normal or common rather than as evidence of perversion and porn becoming one of the most profitable industries there is—what's also more recent is porn's strong influence on culture as a whole, particularly the perceived or expected sexual norms and expectations of the people within that culture.

The dictionary definition of *pornography* is any material that is used or intended to arouse sexual desire in people. Although many people use the word *pornography* to refer only to explicit visual material—such as photos, illustrations, and videos—pornography can also be textual or performed. Pornography may be explicit, but it may also be subtle. Just as all depictions of naked genitals aren't intended to be or usually used for pornography (think of photos of breasts for the purpose of breast cancer study), all pornography doesn't show people having sex or being naked. It may or may not contain explicit sexual language or depict sex acts graphically.

What is or isn't pornography for someone—or what someone does or doesn't "use" as pornography—could be anything from an XXX video to Elizabethan love poetry, from a romantic comedy to a catalog of kitchen gadgets. Anything—*anything*—can potentially arouse feelings of sexual desire for people. If it exists, even only in the imagination, at least someone, if not another few thousand or even billion someones, can be or has been sexually aroused by it.

People of all genders, ages, and social strata seek out or are exposed to sexual media.

Erotica

Sometimes, media or material intended to sexually arouse people is called *erotica* instead of porn. Often, things classified this way are less sexually or visually explicit than, for instance, what you might think of as *hard-core* porn, or they may aim to be more subtle, artistic, or literary. Some people define erotica as suggestive, and porn as directive. Some people say that's a bunch of hooey, and *erotica* is just a word people use because they don't want to call their porn what it is. (I propose both schools of thought are right sometimes and wrong other times.)

Some people have the idea that men look at or use porn and women don't, or that all men do and no women do. None of that is true; though there are some gender divides, most of them are not based in biology but in economics—who has the money to spend on it when it costs, as it often does, and more often that's men; and who has the most cultural permission to look at or use it, which is also more often men. People in romantic or sexual relationships, including relationships where they're having fantastic sex, and single people are exposed to, seek out, make, or "use" it. There are also both single and shacked-up-with-somebody people who aren't or don't.

Some people use it as a masturbation aid to incite or inspire sexual fantasy. Others use it to experience arousal or feed fantasy that they want to bring to partnered sex later. They may or may not share or use the material with their partner. Some seek it out to explore their own feelings about sexuality. When young people first seek out sexual media, they are most often just looking out of simple curiosity, which includes trying to find out what's normal or common (pornography is a very unreliable source of that information, but many people don't know that) and to get some sense of what sex even is.

Some people enjoy sexual entertainment that closely resembles or mimics their sexual reality or their actual wants; more are usually wanting something that's all fantasy. The media that turn someone on may contain depictions of people who look or act like their partners or sex lives that are like their sex lives; more often it won't because sexual entertainment is about fantasy in how it's made and for whoever the audience is. Fantasy—whether we're talking porn, Harry Potter, or a role-playing game—is all about getting at least a little bit away from, if not a land far, far away from, reality.

Pornography: Not Realistic Since Ever

Rarely in sexual entertainment do you see a couple disagreeing on whether to have sex, plainly discussing what kinds of sexual activities to engage in, negotiating safer sex and birth control, or just hanging out and snuggling before, during, or after sex. It's unusual to see porn in which someone isn't seriously groomed or made up, has stubble on their legs or a giant zit on their nose, is wearing their ratty laundry-day undies, isn't in the mood, has a bad head cold, or isn't okay with sexual language a partner uses. We're probably never going to hear someone in porn say,

"Please don't call my vulva a pussy, okay? I *hate* that word."

Sexual entertainment is usually very intentionally both fiction and fantasy. Even a video of a real-life couple having sex in their own home or someone's sexy selfies (lots more on selfies here: page 65), created without a production department or a fancy website, it's still something that was intentionally created and most often intentionally distributed. It is often based on a given set of sexual ideals or fantasies that are either really narrow—and don't represent most people's sexual realities—or very subjective—which might represent what one person thinks is or will be found to be sexy but which doesn't represent what everyone finds sexy.

Even amateur photos or videos of "natural" models or "regular" people usually have plenty of adjustments made: lighting, editing and retouching, or sexual behavior that's more about who is or might be watching rather than who's being watched or seen. We very rarely see active consenting in pornography because it's all done off-screen and wasn't recorded or made part of what we're seeing or reading. The majority of material produced as pornography, like most mass media, portrays pretty unrealistic body types and appearances: the penises and breasts we see in porn are usually much larger than

To think about and evaluate sexual entertainment media clearly, it helps to keep some basics in mind:

***All* sexual media or entertainment created as entertainment:**

- is an intentional performance
- is fantasy of some kind
- isn't intended to be education
- can't tell or show you very much about sex in real life

***Most* sexual media or entertainment:**

- is made by the people involved as if anyone, or even everyone, could be watching; there's nothing private—behavior or otherwise—about it
- has more to do with someone making money than anything else: it is usually mostly, and often only, about profit
- isn't often reflective of most people's sexual realities or contexts (for most people, their doctor provides professional health care, not oral sex; their teacher makes assignments, not sexual advances; and they don't go to sleepovers with their friends dressed like lingerie models)
- is very heterocentric, including in material or entertainment that includes sexual activity between people of the same gender
- enables or even purposefully sexualizes bias and marginalization like sexism, racism, classism, fatphobia, and ableism
- gives messages about sex and sexuality that don't square with physically and emotionally healthy sexual practices, interpersonal dynamics, or relationships

***Some* sexual media or entertainment:**

- contains, presents, or celebrates sexual violence and abuse or presents sexual violence as consensual sex

average, and when we see diversity with race or ethnicity, it also often comes with a heavy dose of racism or tokenism. How people in porn style themselves—including their pubic hair—isn't very reflective of how people (even those people themselves) look or present themselves in their daily lives or their off-screen sex lives. It's rare to see actors in pornography who don't reach orgasm, who have orgasms that are quiet or subtle, or who aren't turned on by (or are totally turned off by) typical "porny" stuff—yet all of these reactions are normal and common in real-life sex. People who don't realize this or who expect their partners to live up to porn's fictions, ideals, and fantasies are in for a rude awakening. Even porn stars couldn't—and often don't want to—live up to those expectations in their real lives.

The Worst of Us, Sexified

A lot of current sexual entertainment—just like a lot of other media or popular culture—unfortunately presents some of the most unhealthy aspects or patterns of our culture as normal or okay, and as something sexy.

Media designed to turn us on—whether meant to be porn or an ad for a car—often present people (or one gender or other group of people) as objects, only sexual, or as sexual commodities rather than as whole persons whose sexuality is

- is not made or distributed ethically or humanely (it might be made without everyone's explicit, informed, and enthusiastic consent or without humane labor practices and policies) (and some is)
- is about someone trying to show you their personal sexuality
- is made creatively, thoughtfully, or independently and tries to do porn in a way that leaves out a lot of the Big Bads—like *-isms* and bias, sexualized violence, heterocentricity or gender stereotyping, lack of active consenting, and poor labor treatment
- can make people feel supported in their sexualities or sexual lives and good about themselves and others; others do the opposite; and some have no seeming impact; this depends on what the entertainment is, specifically, who is watching or otherwise taking part in it, and how they feel about it

Plenty of what's out there also currently contains and even celebrates violence or coercion, presenting those things as normal, hot, or sexy. Some pornographic material contains fantasy scenarios in which resistance from one person is shown to turn into an enthusiastic sex session—without any discussion whatsoever about consent and that apparent total change of heart. Depictions of abuses of power or nonconsensually inflicted pain, hate speech, or slut-shaming have become increasingly common in a lot of sexual media and entertainment.

Sometimes, the making of pornography *itself* is an abuse or exploitation: as with any other kind of work, abuse, assault, and harassment happen to people working in pornography. Media distributed as porn where anyone involved didn't consent to that—such as "revenge porn" or content that was hacked from someone's personal files—are abusive and exploitive, and by design, the invasion of someone's privacy or personal safety is part of what's supposed to get someone off.

just a part of them. One word for this is sexualization, a term meant to describe when someone—or a group of people, such as girls or women, who are far more sexualized in all kinds of media than boys or men are—has had sexual desires, values, or motives put on them, as individuals or as a group, and where their sexual value is presumed to be their whole or central value as people.

At a symposium in London in 2011, Onscenity, Australian researcher Alan McKee put porn, as a whole, though the filter of core components of healthy sexual development to get a sense for which ways porn generally supports, counters, or says nothing about healthy sexuality and sexual interactions. He mentioned that some positive, healthy things porn can and often does support are presenting sex as something joyful and fun, not joyless, and the presentation of sex as something pleasurable. Some areas most sexual media don't support or where they send the wrongest of wrong messages are about things like good communication, how sexual bodies or response actually works in reality, consenting, and safety. More does tend to wind up in the bad pile than the good when we run porn through that filter—if you check out the healthy sexual development list on page 176, you can consider it by all those bits for yourself. Some of that is about any kind of pornography, just by virtue of it being something performed and constructed, and some of that is about some kinds, but not others. Whether porn is good for us or not, as a whole people or as individuals, not only depends on who we are and what sexual media or entertainment we are talking about, very specifically, but also isn't so simple as being all good or all bad.

How Should We Feel About Sexual Entertainment?

You feel how you feel.

People have different opinions about whether it's okay for people to like porn or to dislike it, just as they do about whether it's okay for people to like or dislike organized religion, country music, or bacon. People hold very strong opinions about pornography or other sexual media or entertainment for all kinds of reasons. For some, it's an ethical or political issue; for others a more personal or interpersonal matter (or both); and for others, still, it just boils down to whether they get turned on by it or not. You get to hear and figure out how you feel about those opinions, who they come from, and how much they play a part in helping you form your own opinion. Your opinion is what matters most for you and is going to be based on whether it feels okay—whatever the "it" is and however you are or aren't interacting with it or having it be part of your life—for ***you***.

Just like you get to choose how you feel and what you'll do for other ethical and lifestyle decisions that affect you and others, like eating meat, making certain reproductive choices, reading tabloids or otherwise taking part in gossip, and where you get your clothes from, the same goes here.

Your own wants and do-not-wants with this kind of media and how to have it be a part of your life, if it is, in a way that feels healthy and good for you and for everyone else is something you'll just need to figure out for yourself in the unique context of your life and relationships as you go. There's always going to be some balancing to do, like there is with any kind of media or any other part of your sexual life, and there's always going to be some thinking and evaluating to do when it comes to your sexual media choices. If it ever seems like it's not good for you, then it's time to make some changes, whether by changing the kind of material you're taking in, how much of it or how frequently you use it, or how much of a role it plays in your sexuality or sex life. If your sex life includes other people, now or later, and porn is part of your sexual life or theirs, that's something you can talk about. That talking might just be a yay—like talking about porn you both like or want to explore in your sexual life together—or about hard feelings or conflicts—like insecurities you might feel about pornography, sexual misunderstandings, pressures or expectations that porn is at the root of, or ethical or political differences about sexual media and entertainment as a whole.

If we immerse ourselves in anything that celebrates or shows the worst of us rather than our best selves—whether that's sexist porn or tabloid media—or becomes some kind of ideal, we aren't very likely to experience the positive impacts of that medium. If we're soaking in anything, including media, full of sexual yuck, it's harder to feel supported in creating or living a sexuality and sexual life that makes us and others feel good about ourselves, where we interact in ways that are healthy and positive. The opposite is also true: when we take in a lot of good stuff, things that present the best of us—and that doesn't mean not being sexual!—it's easier to feel supported and empowered in a healthy sexuality and sexual life that make everyone involved feel good, including emotionally. It can help to think about media choices, for sexual media or any other kind, like the choices we make with eating: if we eat nothing but junk food, we're going to get sick or feel like crap a lot of the time. If, on the other hand, we make most of what we eat foods that support our well-being and health, we're more likely to be healthy and more likely to feel good.

It's always a good idea to be mindful about what we make part of our sexual lives and to think and question our choices—including the media we use and

Is Looking at Porn Cheating?

Whether we consider looking at pornography as cheating on our sexual or relationship partner really depends on what, in a relationship with exclusivity agreements, you and someone else have made part of that agreement. What is or isn't "cheating"—or, to put it more clearly, what is or isn't outside the boundaries of any given sexual exclusivity agreement—isn't something universal but is something individual, personal, and situational. For more on making choices with someone else about sexual exclusivity and what to consider in those agreements, see page 149.

purchase—even when our culture tells us something is a no-brainer. Simply being thoughtful and really considering your choices in media—sexual or otherwise—always makes for more ethical consumption and makes it more likely we'll seek out media that we feel best about and that feels best in our lives.

"They Saw It in Porn, So Now They Want and Expect It from Me"

No one's sexual wants or expectations—no matter *where* they come from—are something anyone ever is obligated to meet or try to meet or anything anyone ever has to do unless they also have their own desire to do it and *want* to do it.

Whatever our sexual expectations are, we must always make room for the *actual* people involved and what is *actually* going on, not our fantasies or what we might want them to be like or want from them. We always need to regard the reality of any person we're with much more than our ideas about them, what we do together sexually, or how that plays out. Same goes for the whole of our reality, like what's actually even possible, safe, and sound: fantasy media often shows us things that are not possible in real life or that would be unsafe for someone in some big way. In the real world with any real-life people, what's real and what's actually going on always needs to inform what we do or ask for. If those realities stand counter to any expectations, then it's clearly time for an expectation adjustment.

Someone whose expectations and ideas about partnered sex are so out of whack that they don't even get that they need to square them with sexual realities is showing you they're just not at all ready for sex with another whole, real person, period. You don't need to worry about where their ideas are coming from or how to change them; you just need to move the heck on to a partner who is that basic kind of ready. If you're more like, "But I saw it in porn/a romantic comedy/on YouTube and I expect it from *them*," just take the above and please apply it in reverse. And don't forget that "I saw it in porn, so everyone must want it!" is about as sound as "A potato can kill zombies in my game, so clearly it's an excellent weapon for self-defense in real life."

Do You Want to Be in Porn?

If you're thinking about creating sexual media to share with someone else—such as photos or sexy texts—as with any other sexual choice, you must give it some big thought to figure out whether it's both something you really want to do and something you're okay with. I talk about the important legal considerations of this choice, especially for minors, for whom being part of sexual media is almost always unlawful, sometimes in ways that carry some huge and possibly even lifelong legal and social consequences (see page 218).

But the law isn't the only thing to consider. You also want to think about other kinds of risks, including the emotional risks and the big risks to your privacy and safety, and what you can do to reduce them. Obviously, you also must consider whether creating or sharing sexual media you (or a partner) have made of yourself is even a thing you want to do. (Yep: these are all the exact same things we want to think about and think through with any sexual choice.)

It might not feel like taking a couple pictures and clicking them over to someone's cell is making and distributing porn, but it actually is—legally, in many cases, and practically pretty much always. Making or sharing this type of pornography opens up someone to a lot of the same emotional and social risks as are the people who do porn for a living.

In most places, whether it's your job or just something you're doing for fun, participating in any kind of porn opens you up to some cultural stigma, can give someone who wants to harass you an easy vector to do so, and presents personal safety risks—the more widely the porn gets shared, the bigger those risks become. These risks are less manageable than any risks we encounter when we share our sexuality with others in ways that don't create any kind of record of it outside our memories. You could lose out on a job, leadership opportunity, or something else you really want in your life. Your participation might also influence how you feel about yourself, especially if you took part in porn as a result of any kind of pressure—coming from you or someone else. When we make, and especially when we share, any kind of digital media, we need to always remember that it's permanent in some ways, including ways that can be totally outside our control.

All this risk is one thing that can make doing porn feel exciting. But, of course, what gets us excited in our heads or by doing it isn't always what we want to actually do or what's safe for us to do. So, the thrilling idea alone isn't ever going to answer the "Should I?" of all this. (Again: just like with any sexual choice.)

As with other sexual choices, if you know that being in porn or being involved in any part of it is so not what you or someone else wants, or you just aren't sure, it's best to just nix any of this unless your feelings change radically. This is just one of those things where it's better to be safe than sorry and where it pays to choose carefully. We all have imaginations we can use to visualize people we're into. We can paint our own pictures, so no one should ever feel like they need to literally make those pictures when they don't want to or the possible cost feels way too high.

Exhibitionism and Voyeurism

In sexology, *exhibitionism* is a term that basically describes when someone feels turned on sexually—or responds sexually, like with orgasm—by being seen or watched publicly (like on a city street) or semipublicly (like in self-made media shared with partners) being naked, sexual, or engaged in some kind of sex, whether it's masturbation or sex with partners. Exhibitionism is about wanting someone or more than one someone to watch you doing what you're doing rather than being an in-the-flesh part of what you're doing. The on-the-other-side-of-things term and situation to exhibitionism is *voyeurism*, which is when someone wants to watch another someone doing something naked or sexual.

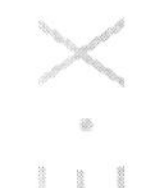

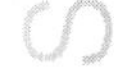

Should anyone ever ask you to make sexual media for them and pressure you in any way, know that caving in to that pressure isn't the way to go. Someone behaving that way is showing you a big red flag for (and sometimes of) some kind of abuse, so the very best thing you can do is to get gone from them, full stop. Sexual pressuring of any kind is never okay and is never the hallmark of anything good.

Ultimately, only you can decide whether and how you use or take part in mediated sexual expression and what, if any, type of sexual media is supportive of your heart and mind, well-being, relationships, and sexuality; and what feels like the right thing when it comes to your life and what you do and don't want as part of your sexual life. As with most other aspects of sexuality, you also get to change your mind or adapt your thinking and habits at any time.

MAKING SENSE OF EXTERNAL MESSAGES AND HEARING YOUR OWN VOICE

When it comes to making sexual choices and figuring out your own sexuality, the person's voice who needs to be heard and regarded the most **has to be** your own. If and when you add sexual partners to the mix, their voices must be incorporated and given big priority, too. But when we're dealing with our sexuality by ourselves, with the sex we have with ourselves, and there aren't partners in the mix, it gets to be and should be all us. If it's not, it's going to be pretty hard to create a sexuality and sexual life for ourselves that we feel good about and that are really right for us because they won't really be about us.

We can't just tune out family's, friends', and media messages and statements when it comes to this stuff or somehow not see what's being shown to us. But what we can do is our best to stay aware of what is and isn't our voice and make choices that are based less on what we think we should be doing or feeling, or what someone tells us we should be doing or feeling, and more on what we actually want to be doing and feeling.

One thing that helps is thinking critically about messages from people you know or media, focusing on what the person, people, or media are saying—including how and for what intended purpose—rather than only on what impact it has on you.

When you think about any of these messages and the places we can get them, try thinking about them like this, which is an adaptation of a tool called the media literacy ladder:

1. The form: Through what medium is the message delivered? Through a statement, printed words, video, song, or picture? Did the person who is most directly delivering the message—whether it's something said, written, or shown in images—actually make the big decisions about it, or is someone else (like a production company or screenwriter) actually in charge of the message or media and who that message or media tell us the most about?

2. Its intended purpose: Who created or gave the message and why? Do they mean to make something happen or to try to influence your thoughts or behaviors. Or did their mouth just run off without them even thinking? Was something created as purely a creative expression or to sell you something, whether that is a thing—like a razor—or an idea—like shaving—or both? What does the person who created the message seem to want anyone who gets the message to do with it?

3. Your own interpretation of the message or media: How does the message make you feel? What do *you* think about it? What do you think the other person or media are saying: what are you hearing or seeing, whether it's actually being said or shown?

4. The reality of the media or message: (Hint: our interpretation isn't the reality of the media; it's *our* reality.) What's the actual point of view—the reality—of the person or people who made the message, not what *you* think it is or says?

Some other helps with making sense of powerful external messages and managing their place, impact, and power in your life can be:

1. Finding supportive people for honest conversations and questions in safe places for you to be you: Seek out people and places that you know have a positive impact on you and that feel like safe places for you to challenge any messages or media that don't.

2. Put it where you can see it: Journaling or practicing some other kind of personal creative expression that's just for us—not to share in any kind of social media or otherwise—to get our thoughts and feelings out, expressing them instead of bottling them and putting them in a more tangible form, makes it easier to get a real awareness of them, process them, put them in context, and deal with them when they're not-so-awesome.

3. Keep desires for and efforts to get approval in balance: We all want to be accepted to some degree—that's just part of being a person. But if our desire or need for approval (which isn't the same thing as acceptance) gets out of whack or takes the lead in our sexuality or sexual choices, we can lose ourselves in these messages and in our attempts to conform to all of them, which is usually impossible anyway because we get different messages from all the people and media in our lives. Instead, see if you can't stay focused on who *you* are, what *you* think and feel, what *you* want and don't want, what *you* are and aren't okay with. Figure that if people or some media disagree, that's okay. If it isn't, the problem isn't with you

TECH TIP

A wide range of both opinion and study of pornography and its impacts is available online. This section provides just a very light overview that includes what I think are the most important things to know and bear in mind. But if you want to dig deeper or just want to see an array of perspectives to try to get a better sense of how you think or feel, open up a search engine. Obviously, it'd be pretty easy to wind up with nothing but actual porn when searching for things about porn, but if you use more academic search terms, such as "pornography studies," "data on pornography and sexual behavior," or "impacts of sexual media," you'll find your way to the kind of information about pornography and sexual media that you're looking for.

Want more help with media literacy? Check out your local public library. Librarians aren't just generally awesome, smart people, they literally have a degree in this, and they usually love to help with this kind of education. Many libraries also have librarians who are specifically young adult (YA) librarians, and they tend to be particularly gung-ho about helping young people in this arena.

being your own person who thinks, feels, or wants differently; it's with those messages or their sources not leaving enough room for you.

4. Try to create at least as much as you consume and speak for yourself as much as you take in the words of others: It's pretty hard to hear your own voice when you aren't using it. That can even be a positive way of engaging in media as a two-way communication rather than just as an audience or market for it. For instance, the next time you see or read something in media that does something hideous, such as blame a rape victim, hold up a harmful sexual myth—like erection equals consent—or present an ethnic group as a sexual commodity, media-back: create something of your own to process, counter, or challenge it. The next time you see, hear, or read something you think is amazingly positive and of great value, bounce it yourself either by penning a great cheer or creating something different entirely that you were inspired to make because of what that powerfully positive creation gave you.

5. Pay attention to how media or messages from others make you feel: If they make you feel terrible, see what you can do to get away from them or to at least minimize their place in your life and your head. If they make you feel great and truly great about yourself, stick with that and see whether you can't keep finding more of that. Strike a good balance: do what you can to stick with what's positive and of benefit to you, and steer clear of what isn't.

7

On Board the Relationship

It's common to assume that *relationship* only means an exclusive romantic and sexual relationship between two people and that that sort of relationship is automatically the best, most intimate, and most important anyone can have.

But *any* ongoing interaction we have with another person is a relationship, and *any* kind of relationship can be intimate, important, and wonderful. A nonsexual friendship is a relationship. We have relationships with parents, siblings, teachers, bus drivers, healthcare providers, counselors, boyfriends, girlfriends, and even casual sex partners. There need not even be another human being involved for a relationship to exist: we have relationships with animals, with our culture, and with the planet we live on. How important, intimate, or "best" any of the relationships we have are, what kind they are, and what place they have in our lives isn't assigned to us, nor are those things universal. Relationships are individual and about what we actively create and build, not things that just do or don't happen to us without our participation.

If and when we enter into a sexual or romantic relationship, or one that's both, with another person, we usually can't make many—if any—assumptions about what the word *relationship* means and what the specifics or aspects of that relationship are without discussing them with the other person. The specifics of a relationship are things we need to think about, examine, discuss, agree upon, and actively do together. Just like there's not just one or two kinds of or ways of doing gender, there are way more than just one or two kinds of relationships and ways of doing relationships.

[*RELATIONSHIP* SHOULD BE A VERB]

Healthy relationships that benefit us and others require our time, energy, attention (including attention to ourselves and our own feelings and behaviors), and shared, active participation, especially in communication, time management, and integration into all the other parts of our lives. I'm not a big fan of framing these requirements as "work," but if you are, figure that no relationship should take so much work to maintain that most of the time it isn't pretty easy to just be and enjoy yourself and the other person or people without trying too hard. Intimacy should feel good; it should be pretty comfortable and beneficial for everyone involved. After you spend time with someone you're in an intimate relationship with—even just thinking about them—you should usually feel seen and cared for, happy, and energized, not physically or emotionally exhausted, stressed out, dissatisfied, or riddled with doubt, guilt, or fear.

The reason to be in a sexual relationship—or one that isn't yet but that may be in the future—is to explore and express your sexuality with someone else. They're about—or, at least, should be about—being with and getting closer to someone who makes you feel good, who is hopefully a friend as much as they are a lover, and who supports you and appreciates who you are **as is,** and vice versa.

Because this is a book with a focus on sex and sexuality, this chapter primarily addresses relationships that are or that can be sexual and those in which sex is one part of the relationship. But please know that, although some people think only relationships that involve sex or romance can be big, important, and intimate or the kind of relationships where the people involved consider each other partners, I don't think that at all. I think what makes a relationship have value, importance, and intimacy is how we actively do that relationship together, and how important it is to us, not what kind of relationship it is. I also talk a lot here about romantic relationships. That's not because I think only romantic relationships can be (or must be) sexual but because, most commonly, people in romantic relationships are sexual together, and people in sexual relationships are often romantic with each other.

An intimate relationship being fun and joyful—as any healthy relationship should be—doesn't mean it's childish or not serious, nor does a relationship being a constant struggle or drama mean it must be true love (in fact, that's a good sign that it very much isn't). For people of any age, intimacy should be about celebrating, sharing, and enjoying life with someone else—for however long it lasts, in whatever model works best for the partners.

The Scariest Thing on Earth (or So You'd Think)

Rejection: something that can feel so scary that the fear of it—even just the mere possibility of it—is probably the biggest thing that keeps people from pursuing and exploring relationships or interactions they want, asking for what they want in relationships, sexual and otherwise, and being who they are, in like, love, sex, and the rest of life.

I get it: being accepted, especially early in life, is huge. Wanting to be liked or loved often takes a backseat to just wanting acceptance; even when we don't care much about being liked, or even loved, we usually still want to be accepted for who we are. Also, getting what we really want obviously is a very big deal. So, the prospect of not being accepted, the possibility of not getting what we want, when the stakes are high can feel scary as hell.

But here's that catch-22: if we don't take the positive risks we must; if we're not open in the ways we need to be to be seen so that someone can even know who we really are to accept us; if we don't speak up and say what we want so that someone can tell us if they want to give it to us or do it with us, then we're a lot less likely to get what we want, acceptance included. And in the event that it seems like nothing could be worth risking rejection, then you have to ask yourself if you had any designs on actually living this life rather than just phoning the whole thing in. If you want to live fully—or, let's be real, much at all—you're going to have to risk rejection sometimes.

What can you do to go for what you want, even if the fear of rejection has you quaking in your boots?

1. Do your best to make sure the level of risk or the context of that risk is safe and sound and that you're mostly taking positive risks: Sometimes when we feel terrified of rejection, it's for good reason: at those times we might be choosing to take risks that are more likely to endanger than benefit us or we're taking risks when we're just not stable or okay enough to handle

Romantic

What does *romantic* mean? It's an excellent question—alas, I wish I could give you a clear answer. For some people some of the time, a romantic relationship and a sexual relationship are one and the same, or romantic and sexual feelings feel inseparable. Historically, though, we didn't even have a *concept* of romance until around the seventeenth century in Europe: the basis of "romance" as most people know and think of it is the troubadours system of courtly love, or chivalry (which involves a whole lot of sexism). For troubadours—and in an awful lot of romance novels—romance was about unrequited love, lust, mutually assured destruction, or a mashup of all of the above.

But some people experience sexual feelings and romantic feelings as very different or as separate (many asexual people, for example, still experience romantic feelings or desire romantic relationships), and some frame sexual or romantic relationships or concepts quite differently. Some have concepts about what romance is for them that didn't come from a bunch of lovesick dudes walking around with lutes; other people's ideas of romance center around those ideas and traditions. This is—sorry!—one of those murky concepts for which you need to figure out what, if anything, romance means to you and how it's different, if it is, from what's sexual.

the unwanted outcomes if they happen. If a situation would set you up to be truly unsafe in any way—like by telling someone abusive what you want when you know it will trigger abuse, or by putting yourself out there in other ways when it's much more likely to harm you than to do you good—that fear is probably trying to tell you not to go there. On the other hand, if the possible pros outweigh the possible cons, if unwanted outcomes stink but they're safe and you feel able to handle them, and if what you're choosing to risk rejection over makes you feel like you're really living, I suggest you go for it.

2. Seriously, often it really is them, not you: When we want something and someone else doesn't, or we want to be with someone in a way they don't want to be with us, the former is about you, the latter about them. You want a thing: that's about you. They don't want a thing: that's about them. Just as when someone *not* wanting a thing doesn't mean there's something the matter with them, there's nothing the matter—or substandard, broken, not good enough, wrong, perverted, prudish, pathetic, or whatever judgy word your psyche pulls up when you're dealing with or fearing rejection—with you because you want a thing someone else doesn't. And even if they did want what you want, that doesn't tell us as much about how awesome you are as it tells us that two people just happened to want the same thing, at the same time, in the same place, with each other. Someone nixing a hookup, a romantic relationship, the kind of sex you want, the kind of relationship model you want is nixing those things; they are not nixing *you* as a whole person, even though it can feel that way.

3. Steer clear of the usual rejection or fear-of-rejection bad self-talk: When we get in a fear spiral with rejection, or after we have just experienced rejection, the way we talk to ourselves often is not only earnestly cruel but also usually makes us feel more scared and less brave, and it has no basis in reality. Talking to ourselves in a way that communicates that we feel we're worthless, stupid, or hideous only ensures we feel that way and get stuck feeling that way. (If you ever made funny faces and your mom told you your face would get stuck that way, figure negative self-talk is the real version of that myth—if we keep it up, we're going to get stuck feeling that way, even when we are getting what we want.) Be kind and talk with love and care to yourself when you have rough feelings, and see what you can do to keep it mostly positive around or with rejection.

4. As long as you let it go when it happens, rather than internalizing it, it will get easier the next time: And the next time. And the next ten times or one hundred times, because as long as we're checked in to life and going all-in, rejection is just going to be something like it or not we have to deal with, just like taxes and our relatives saying asinine things on our social media pages.

[DATING: DIFFERENT, NOT A DINOSAUR]

"Dating," as a lot of people think about it, has never been all that common. People very formally asking one another out has happened, for sure, but more informal ways of connecting and getting romantically or sexually involved have always been more common. The definition of *dating* is always changing, and dates more often now—especially at the start of relationships—are happening in groups and more casually and with less hoopla (which is great news for everyone who breaks into a cold sweat at the prospect of having to ask for a formal date). Too, right now, it's common for the start of more serious relationships to happen a bit more organically and fluidly than with someone asking a partner to "go steady."

Dating isn't extinct; it has just changed over time, like most things. A basic definition for now might be: when someone has casual outings or spends time with one or more people in whom they have some romantic and/or sexual interest to discover whether or not they both want to pursue that interest and *how* they want to pursue it.

Dating is, in a word, a lot like shopping, and then living with what you got for a bit to see if and how you like it: you're trying on different pairings and dynamics with different people before (or without) deciding whether one is just the right fit to pursue or continue a sexual and/or romantic relationship with, and then, if you decide you want to keep seeing each other, figuring out how you each want to do that. When you're just dating, you're not usually making a commitment to any one person; the aim is to first test the waters, getting to know people in different settings and social groups and spending time with them to see if you'd *like* to develop a deeper romantic or sexual relationship with them over time, and if so, how you both want to develop and do that relationship. And if you'd like to make any kind of commitment to each other, you get to decide whether that commitment is to some kind of exclusive relationship or to continuing to hang out or hook up regularly. *Or not.*

Dating can be everything from hanging out at a concert with a whole group of friends and your "date" to stepping it up a notch and going it alone with a date to dinner or lunch, on a beach day or hike, to a dance or other more formal social gathering, to a night on your couch with a pile of movies. You may already know the person you're going on a date with, or you may find yourself on a "blind date," where friends or family have set you up with someone you're meeting for the first time. Someone in the process of dating may or may not be engaging in sexual activity with the people they're dating; some people consider an ongoing booty call to be dating. Obviously, established couples can also have dates, even when they're past the stage of dat*ing*.

It sounds totally cheeseball, but for real, all you have to be is yourself when you're dating, with at least some of the person you consider your best self to be in tow. There's so much talk—and so many rich talk show hosts and self-appointed dating-advice gurus!—about game and other dating strategies, but a whole lot of them boil down to acting like someone you're not, which doesn't make a whole lot of sense when you're looking for someone to be with *you,* not someone else. If you're not yourself, the other person can't actually date *you*. If someone doesn't want to date or hook up with you, they don't

NRE: New relationship energy

Wheeeeee! You're in a brand-new relationship, or you have just met someone you're seriously into—you're head over heels. Just thinking about them makes you restless, anxious, dizzy, or giggly. You feel like you've found the one person in the whole wide world who was made for you and you alone. That's what new relationship energy often feels like.

NRE feels fantastic, but it can do quite a number on your critical thinking. Very few of us can be particularly objective when we're weak-kneed or superlusty. So, when making sexual and relationship choices in a brand-new thing, you can rest assured that your judgment is bound to be a little wiggly.

When you're in that space, you need to use a little more caution than usual to make big decisions. Additional factors may also be at play: body or self-image issues, feeling pressured to be sexually active or have a sexual or romantic partner, fear of being alone, performance pressures, rebellion or conformity issues, and even simple curiosity.

Don't ditch the rest of your life when you're in a new relationship. Keep up your platonic friendships and family relationships, and be sure you also get some quality time all by yourself, at least a couple of days or nights a week. Just add a little perspective, some limits and boundaries, and a wee bit of distance to the mix as needed. There's absolutely no reason you can't enjoy a new love and keep your head screwed on right at the same time.

Too, know that NRE always has an expiration date: the way we feel at the start of things isn't going to be how we always feel, and it's most common for the intensity of our feelings to dial down gradually over time. When NRE is over, that doesn't mean something is necessarily wrong with a relationship or that the relationship is over; it just means you're past the point where it's all brand-new and you are moving into another phase, which may feel less exciting in some ways but which can be richer in other ways (and give you your attention span back).

want to date or hook up with you, period, and that's just how it goes sometimes (and sometimes how it goes for a long time). You're probably going to feel that way about some people you date, too.

If you aren't into a date—or whatever you want to call it—or into dating as you go, if it isn't fun, or if it doesn't feel right, you don't ever have to continue or move forward with it. (Which is one reason why always having cab fare is a good idea: it's harder to end a date if you need a ride from your date.) No one is ever obligated to stay through a whole outing or keep seeing someone just because they did once or twice already. Dating should be like a subscription that you can start but then cancel anytime, for any reason. Have and keep an open mind. Be kind. Have a good time and, if you like, let the boring or eye-rolling times be fodder for hilarious (but anonymous so that you're still being kind) blog entries. Don't agree to things you don't want or feel comfortable with.

CHEAP DATE!

YOU DON'T NEED BIG BUCKS FOR AN AWESOME DATE, JUST A LITTLE CREATIVITY...

SHARE A MEAL!

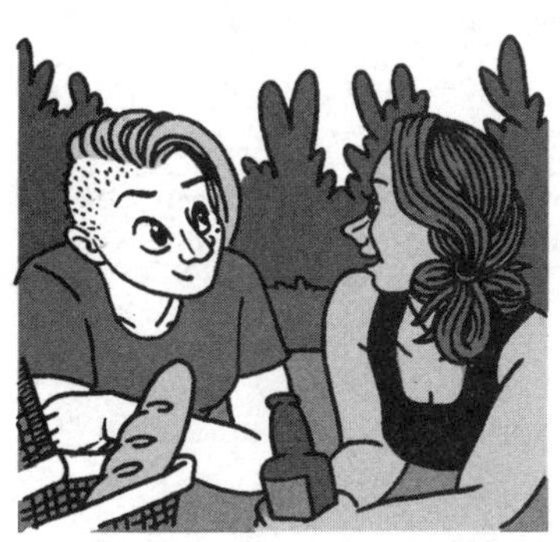

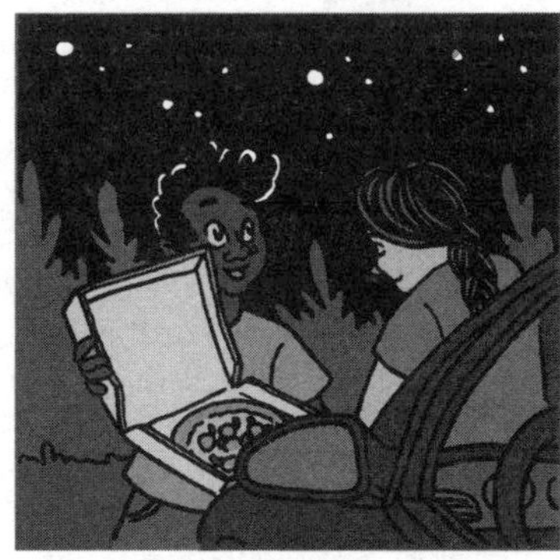

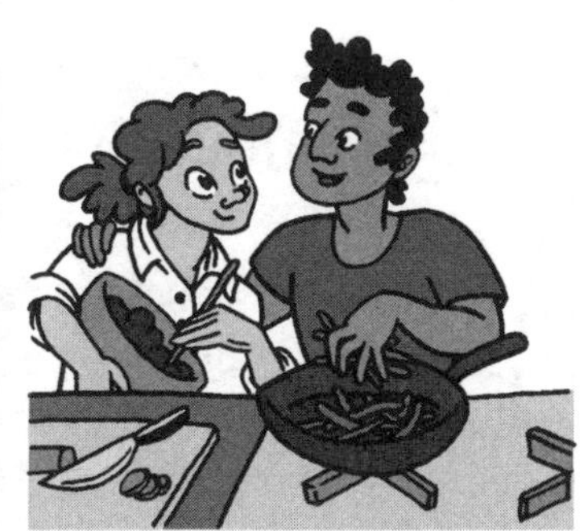

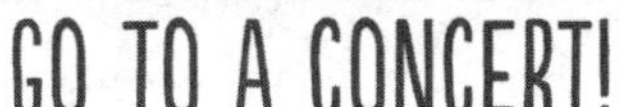

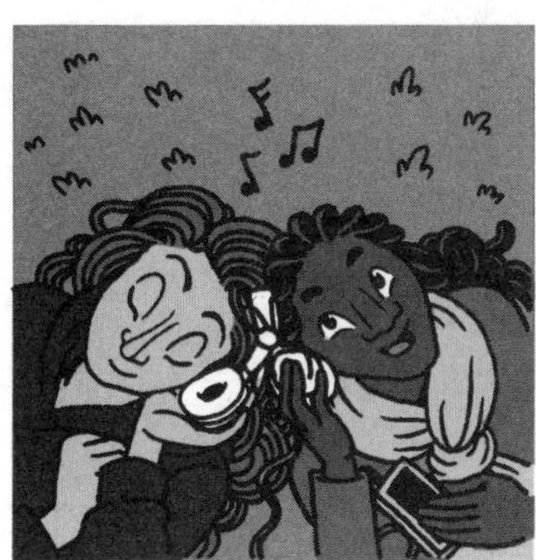

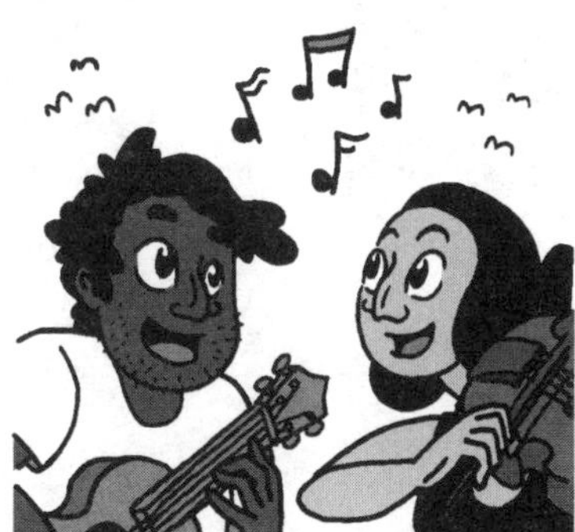

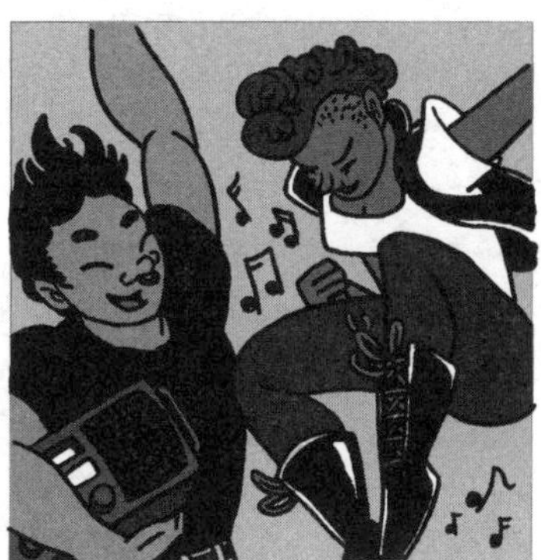

OR ENJOY A NIGHT ON THE TOWN!

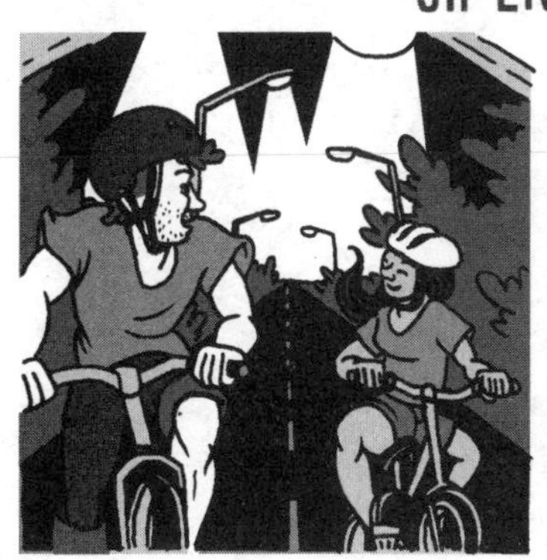

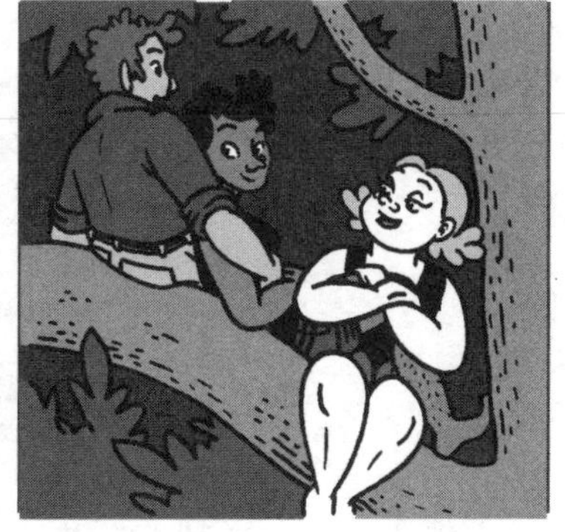

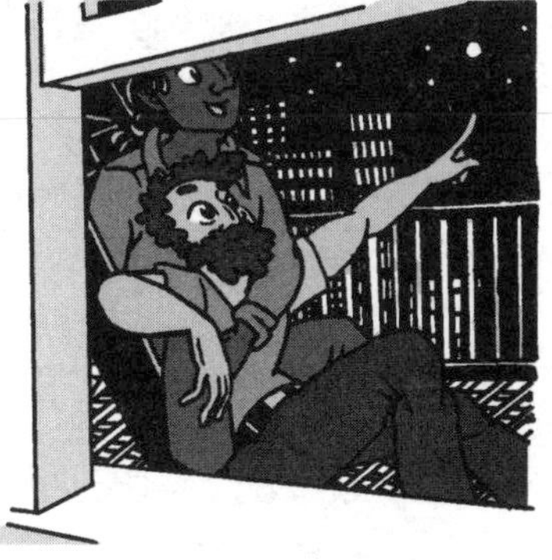

There's no rule in terms of sex or gender identity for who is supposed to ask whom out. Asking someone out on a "date" also doesn't have to be formal or require background music. It can be as simple as, "Hey, I'm going to the bowling alley with some friends later. Want to come with us?" or "Do you want to go to the movies or do something together sometime? How about next Friday?" You also don't have to do this face to face if that freaks you out. Texting can be a great, lower-pressure way to ask someone if they want to hang out with you. That doesn't mean you're not allowed to be nervous. But asking for a date really doesn't have to be a big, honking deal. Clichéd as it sounds, the worst someone can do is say no.

Serial monogamy

What a lot of people do currently instead of more casual, gradual dating is what we call **serial monogamy,** going from one serious partner to the next without spending substantial time single in between partners or spending more casual time with a person before making a commitment to them. That's not the worst thing on earth, but it does have some pitfalls.

It's easy to get sucked into this sort of pattern, especially if we feel lonely, if we feel like we're the only one of our friends who isn't part of a couple, or if our friends and family only approve of or recognize "serious" relationships. But hopping from serious relationship to serious relationship, without a breather or any downtime, can also skew our character judgment and make it harder for us to pay attention to negative patterns we keep ending up in. It can become difficult to keep the rest of our lives balanced with our romantic lives, allowing us less of the time we need to figure out what we really want in relationships.

Know how you're supposed to wait at least twenty minutes after eating before you go swimming? Apply a similar rule to intimate relationships and you'll do just fine.

It's good protocol, when dating, to inform the people you're on dates with that you *are* dating—that you're just feeling things out for now—rather than making any sort of commitment yet. They don't need to know the name and Social Security number of every single person you've recently dated or are dating, but informing them that you are considering others is polite and considerate. Everybody's got a different theory about when is the right time to say, "Hey, by the way, I don't know how you're feeling, but right now, I'm still testing the waters here," so it is really a matter of personal preference and feeling things out as you go.

Let's face it: some dates are *great* dates, some dates are total yawners where you and someone else find out you just don't connect, and some dates are just plain awful. (Even bad dates, believe it or not, can be fun in their own weird way. The girl with the bizarre pet ferret she smuggled into the ballet in her jacket and the person who accidentally tripped a waiter while showing off their dance moves make pretty excellent stories on a rainy day, after all.) Some dates turn into an ongoing relationship, whether that's romantic or sexual or platonic friendship.

Some dates never even make it to a second round.

Dates aren't synonymous with commitment, and how many dates you have with someone is up to you (and the other person). If the first couple of dates are lackluster but something tells you to give it a bit more time, go ahead and give it another shot. If a date is so painfully bad you know you do *not* want to go there again, there's no need to. In those cases, a simple (albeit sometimes awkward) statement at the end of the date—or at whatever point you decide is the end—that you just aren't feeling it suffices. If you've had a few bummerful dates or attempts to feel out a possible sexual or romantic relationship, know that that's more the rule than the exception, not some sign you're doomed to be without those kinds of relationships for the rest of your life. We often have to have at least a few—and sometimes way more than a few—tries before we wind up finding people with whom we feel a mutual connection and the timing is right for wanting similar things at the same time.

Dating is also a good way to find out whether you feel ready or able at a given time to pursue relationships at all. Sometimes, a few dates—or a conversation about stepping things up a notch that just doesn't feel right—can make clear that it's really not what you or the other person is up for.

SAFETY MATTERS

When you're out with people you don't know well or at all, or when you're in a new relationship, do keep your safety in mind. Tell your folks, a sibling, or a friend where you're going and with whom, just to be on the safe side. Seeing someone new first in a group, where you have at least one wing person around you know has your back, is a great safety help (and awesome if a date is just a stinker and you want an easy escape route). The United States has the highest rate of date rape in the world, and date rape is especially pervasive among young people. To find out how to protect yourself, see Chapter 11.

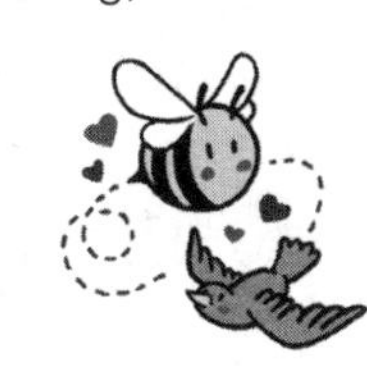

On the other hand, at a certain point, you may discover that after a couple dates with someone your feelings *are* growing, and you *do* want to pursue something deeper with them, and they with you. You may even feel you want to stop dating others to focus on them and go all-in. You both get to talk about and decide as you go what relationship model you want and what pace feels right.

I say: reclaim dating. Call it hanging out if you want, or call it something else entirely. But dating is usually a good thing—even for people who are shy or feel socially awkward, even when you wind up on a date with pocket-ferret-guy. And, ideally, gradual dating can be the best way to start *any* kind of romantic or sexual relationship.

[RELATIONSHIP MODELS: WHAT WORKS FOR *YOU*?]

When you enter into a sexual or romantic relationship, it's time to think about what's going to work best for you and yours. There really is no one model or type of relationship that is best for everyone, no one label, no one set of rules and regulations, wants, and needs that fits all. Think it's a simple matter to define when someone is a boyfriend or a girlfriend? Not so much—even among people who are boyfriends and girlfriends *with each other.* Mediamark Research found that in one large group, 38 percent of the girls said they had a boyfriend in the group, whereas only 29 percent of the guys said they had a girlfriend in the group. That's a pretty major divide. It's not sound to simply assume you have a relationship with someone based on arbitrary criteria; what kind of relationship we have is something we need to actively decide on and make shared agreements about with each other.

There's a lot of noise out there that healthy sex or love can *only* happen within a certain context: within marriage, between heterosexual people, within a certain time frame, at a certain age, only if two people are "in love" and in a romantic relationship. But healthy, beneficial sex and quality sexual relationships happen not in one specific framework but in an environment that is tailored very specifically to best fit the people involved. Realistic expectations, a solid friendship, healthy boundaries, constant communication, and negotiation may be key, but trying to fit every person and every relationship into one ideal model is like everyone in town trying to fit into the same size jeans. A whole lot of people are going to wind up with painful muffin tops or their giant jeans falling off on the bus.

Active communication needs to be a constant in any relationship. You may find that, over time, the needs and wants of one or both of you have shifted—the longer a relationship goes on, the more shifts or changes that tend to happen—and you may need to discuss those things and renegotiate your agreements. Deciding on a relationship model, on the specifics of your relationships, and on how you live in them tends to be ongoing, not something you choose once and agree to for life. Don't feel the need to go on a first date with a monster checklist in your hand; you can start talking about the relationship at a pace that feels comfortable to you both when it becomes clear that you are going to spend more than one or two dates together. When you are in constant communication with a partner, when you're fostering intimacy, a lot of this stuff comes up in casual conversation.

Relationships are active, not passive. Over time, the nature of some relationships does change because people and circumstances change. Someone who has been a romantic or sexual partner for a while may start to feel more like a platonic friend, or vice versa, or one portion of a relationship may become more or less important than another. Much of the time, people don't have great conflicts or feel devastated when a friendship or more casual relationship starts developing romantically or sexually; however, many people feel far differently when the opposite happens. That's not too surprising—our culture puts a lot of status on romantic relationships, often deeming them more important than other kinds of relationships. Plus, romantic and sexual relationships tend to be highly charged at the front and include friendship and other aspects of intimate bonding and relating, so when those intense feelings start to fade or change, we may feel that we're losing something rather than simply evolving and growing. It's entirely possible to move from a romantic relationship into a platonic friendship; often, it just takes time, some mental adjustments, and a person we still care for and want to keep in our lives, even though it may be in a different way than we're used to.

[CLOSED OR OPEN?]

People often have *very* strong feelings about romantic or sexual exclusivity, about monogamy and nonmonogamy. Many people feel monogamy (having only one sexual partner at a time and not being in any way sexual with anyone else) is what's universally ideal—or that it's the only acceptable way to do sexual and romantic relationships—and that without it, something is very wrong. Quite a lot of people also see anything that isn't exclusive as being cheating, even if everyone involved is being honest with each other and has mutually made sensitive, careful, and clear agreements with each other about nonmonogamy—ways of doing sexual or romantic relationships that are not exclusive, in any way or just some ways. Sometimes people in nonmonogamous relationships work harder to honor their agreements in their relationships than those in monogamous relationships often have to. In other kinds of relationships besides romantic or sexual ones, people typically accept and often celebrate people loving or being intimate with more than one person at a time, for example, having a handful of great friends, not just one; or being a parent who has three kids and who loves all of them. But many people learned or decided that romantic and sexual relationships are the total exception to that rule and that having more than one of those kinds of relationships concurrently, or wanting something besides monogamy, is not okay at all, let alone something to celebrate.

But really, monogamy and nonmonogamy are just options, one no universally better or worse than the other. How good—or not good—either or the many ways of doing them are relates mostly to what the people involved want, what works for them, and how much effort they're putting into making their relationships good ones.

When we first start dating someone, by default things always start off as open; they aren't closed or exclusive yet because no one has made any agreements in that area. Unless and until those agreements are mutually negotiated and made—don't just assume anything about a new relationship, especially because people's assumptions aren't always in harmony or don't mean the same thing such as with a given title, like boyfriend or girlfriend—you should instead assume a relationship is not exclusive. If you or someone else wants to change that, you've got to ask, you've got to talk, and you've got to come to clear agreements that work for each of you.

Some people want sexual or romantic exclusivity, others don't, or they do in one situation or at one time, but not another. Some want it but agree to go without it when the other person doesn't, and vice versa; some people don't want it but agree to it anyway, often because they feel like they really have no choice. (And when that happens, it is not good news.) But exclusivity, nonexclusivity, and everything in between are always a choice: we all get to decide, in general and in a given relationship at a given time, whether we will or won't be exclusive, and if so, how and in which ways.

Monogamy—being with one sexual partner only—can feel like a rule for romantic or sexual relationships, but it isn't written in stone; it's a preference and a choice. Monogamy works for a whole lot of people just fine and is what plenty of people want and need. But for others, it may not work so well, or they simply may not want that model; they may prefer an open relationship or polyamory (see page 153). No model is better or worse but

WHAT WORKS FOR *YOU?*

Here are some things to think about to create a relationship model that works for you and your partner:

- **Time together:** How much time, alone and with others, do you need from your partner? How much time do you have available to devote to the relationship? What sorts of time are you looking for: private, with family and friends, at school, on the phone, on the Net?

- **Time apart:** What do you both need in terms of having enough time to manage all the parts of your life *and* be sure you get plenty of time to be by yourself, whether that's working on your artwork or just hanging out listening to music? How do you feel about your partner just dropping by and about times that are good for phone calls, texts, or chats and such?

- **You, them, and everybody else:** How do you want a partner to fit into all of your other relationships with friends, family, the rest of your community? How much do each of you need in terms of family approval and inclusion? For instance, if you're queer, how do you both feel about being out or not with your family? What about disclosure to parents in terms of sex? How do you both feel about how much time you want to spend as a couple with all of your friends and with your own friends without your partner? Are there any friends or family who do or might create conflicts you need to talk about (such as an ex who has since become a platonic friend)?

- **Fenced in:** Almost every sexual and romantic relationship has an invisible fence of sorts around it that defines what we want to be for just us and our partners. What are your limits and boundaries in terms of sexual activities? Do you want monogamy—having each other as exclusive sexual/romantic partners—or a more open or fluid relationship? What level of openness is okay for you? Is flirting with outside persons okay? Sexting? Engaging in physical sexual activities with others? If so, what are your limits there, and how do you want to manage them? What are your partner's feelings: how do they define monogamy, an open relationship, or friends with benefits (FWB), and how does that mesh with your own needs and definitions?

- **Number one and number two:** What priority does a romantic or sexual relationship have for you? Do you and your partner or partners want or need it to come first, or after, or with the same level of priority as other parts of your life, including school, work, friends, family, sports, personal projects, and hobbies? What do each of you want when it comes to sex and what pri-

just a better fit—or not—for the people involved. What relationship models and specifics people choose, what's most likely to make choices go well is that they're what each person truly wants, for starters. And when that's followed up with clear, mutual agreements that feel like they'll really work for everyone, together and separately, honoring those agreements and discussions and adjustments as needed or wanted over time, any model of relationship is likely to go well.

What might you want? I suggest centering these types of decisions related to exclusivity more on *you* and what you know or think *you* want to do and limit than on what you think or know someone else wants or prefers. It's just too easy

---

ority does it have in your relationship? Are your wants and needs pretty similar or compatible?

■ **Grunt work:** How will you both shoulder shared responsibilities like birth control and safer sex, initiating and facilitating important discussions, managing limits and boundaries, and making joint plans with friends and family? Who pays for what when something costs? What joint responsibilities are both of you comfortable shouldering, now and in the near future?

■ **What's in a name:** What one calls a relationship or a partner can be a big deal to most of us (but not all of us). Is it important to you to be called the boyfriend or girlfriend, or not to be? Is your relationship what you and the other person or people would consider casual or more formal or committed? How do you want it to be? Some common relationship models have names like "friend with benefits," "boyfriend" and "partner," which are pretty darn vague and often don't mean the same thing to everyone. Do certain words or phrases carry special meaning or expectations for you, such as those (in)famous three little words: "I love you"?

■ **End goals:** Some people enter relationships with certain expectations: sex, cohabitation, marriage, or lifelong partnership. If you and your partner have end goals you're pursuing or want to pursue with each other, are you on the same page? If not, is there time and room for compromise, whether that means accepting that this isn't a permanent relationship, that one or both of you agree to adapt your end goals, or that you both are willing to see how it goes over time to find out what's really best for this particular relationship?

■ **Extra value:** How will you work practical issues related to values? For instance: if you or your partner doesn't believe in sex before marriage, how have you agreed to manage that? What ethics and values of yours are deal breakers for you? Are there gender or relationship roles you feel you need to have filled—or avoided—to make a relationship work for you? What expectations in terms of roles and values does your partner have of you? How do you manage and work out differences in values?

■ **Emergency!** Do you know each other's individual style of dealing with crisis? For instance, do you get quiet, withdrawn, or bottled up, while the other person is a yeller? How do you feel about privacy in crisis, in terms of what gets discussed with friends and what shouldn't? Communicating these things in advance and working to find methods of crisis management that you both feel good about can help you avoid a lot of misunderstandings and pain when you're already hurting or stressed out. ■■

to get all caught up in insecurity, jealousy, and even a desire for control or ownership of someone—all common responses to possibilities with exclusivity—and those feelings can wind up being what people consider most. That, of course, leaves out at least half of the whole picture: the half that's you. And if we don't know what we want for *ourselves*, we can't make *any* relationship choices well, including this one. It also might sometimes initially feel easier to just agree to what someone else says they want rather than taking the risk of telling them what *you* want, too, even though in the long run it's much more likely to be anything but easy and to leave you, that other person, or both, unhappy.

DID YOU KNOW? . . .

It should perhaps go without saying that how willing and able people are to practice safer sex and maintain sexual health should be a factor in the decision to close things up or keep them open. Anyone in sexually nonexclusive relationships who is sexually active with other partners exposes themselves and others to greater sexual health risks. The health risks increase exponentially with every additional partner, just like we're exposed to more viruses like colds or flus the more people we come into contact with. The only sound way to reduce those risks is by practicing safer sex, including the use of sexual barriers and getting tested regularly for sexually transmitted infections. Someone who isn't ready for that or who just doesn't want to take those precautions probably isn't someone ready for all the extra effort and care having more than one partner at a time requires.

So, start with yourself and what you would or wouldn't do. Do you want to be exclusive? If so, in which ways and how? In which ways don't you? Given you might have the opportunity to be romantic or sexual with more than one person at a time, how many people—if more than one—do you feel like you have time or emotional energy to be in relationships or sexual interactions with at once? Do you want to deal with being part of the interactions or relationships among those people, as is often part of the deal? How much time and energy do you want to put into creating agreements, checking in about them, and adjusting them as needed? If your answer is "not much," then a more closed relationship is likely what you want and will be able to handle. If you want something open or more open, for it to go well for everyone involved, you need more emotional bandwidth and time to do all the communicating involved with these options.

Now you can also look at those other parts: what does the other person or people want when you talk with them about this? What do they seem willing and ready to handle and manage? How do you feel about them being exclusive or not? If any of these choices or parts drum up insecurities or fears in you, can you deal with them, or are you not there yet? Do you *want* to? Can the other person or people deal with what you want when it comes to exclusivity or openness? Do *they* want to?

Put all this information together and you're ready to get talking with the other person or people so you can decide together what you are and aren't agreeing to and how you want to do monogamy or nonmonogamy together.

Healthy exclusivity agreements are about actions, not thoughts or feelings. People can soundly agree to, for instance, having genital sex only with each other and not anyone else, but they can't soundly agree to not experience attraction or sexual fantasy about others. Our actions are choices we usually have sovereign control over; our thoughts and feelings aren't. People are usually attracted to more than one person in the world, including when they're gladly with someone they think is more amazing than amazing itself. When people agree to any kind of exclusivity, it's not usually because a person they want to be exclusive with is the *only* person on earth they want to be with in those ways but because, of all the people they're attracted to and could explore a relationship with, that person is the one person at that time they want to be exclusive with.

It also isn't sound to ask someone to stop experiencing their solo sexuality or sex life (masturbation) that involves only themselves, not other people. And it is never, *ever* healthy or okay to ask someone else (or to be asked by someone else) to have close, emotionally intimate relationships or any kind of relationships with only *one* person. People need and benefit from a range of relationships with different people, including family, friends, teams or clubs, support networks, and—when it's what people want and agree to—romantic or sexual partners. If what you or someone else is after basically is total domination of another person's heart or sexuality, neither monogamy nor nonmonogamy can give you that, and that's a good thing. That kind of aim or behavior isn't the stuff of emotionally healthy relationships or interactions—it's control or abuse.

Polyamory

Polyamory means having more than one romantic or sexual partner at once—or being open to that idea even if the opportunity isn't currently available—and usually at least one of the partnerships is a committed one. Polyamory isn't "cheating," nor is it simply "dating" lots of people at one time. It's about making a conscious choice to have more than one ongoing partner, with full disclosure to and agreement from everyone involved. Open, polyamorous relationships may involve more casual secondary relationships or hookups, for some, sometimes even in the company of another partner. Polyamory also usually involves more than one partnership, and each involves some level of commitment: a dedicated intention, in feelings or actions, to each relationship and to any shared agreements that are part of that relationship.

DATING AND RELATIONSHIPS 3.0

It's a misperception that relationships can't begin, exist, or be sustained online or through mobile applications. But it's also a misperception that you can have the *same sort* of relationships or interactions exclusively through technology that you can have in person. Technology provides only one means of how and where you connect.

Let's lead with some pros, because they're often overlooked, especially by

HOW DO YOU FIND A FANTASTIC RELATIONSHIP, ANYWAY?

■ **Be open:** If you refuse to believe anyone else could like or love you as you are and you keep all your doors and windows firmly closed and locked, there's no way anyone else can get in in the first place. Intimacy—even just the pursuit of it—requires some vulnerability.

■ **Be prepared to be surprised:** The people you really click with, with whom you have a major love connection, may very well not look or act like your "type" or be anything like you idealized, expected, or imagined. Ideals we have about love and relationships early on are usually unrealistic and based on others' ideas—through media like movies or TV or what we pick up from family or friends—instead of being realistic and really about us as unique people. That surprise can be a bit confusing at first, but it's often part of the adventure!

■ **Be self-aware:** Learn who you are, what you want and need, and where you're going in life—with and without partners. Spend time with yourself so that you can do some real self-reflection to know all of that based on who you are, not who someone else is and who they want you to be. Self-awareness puts you in a much better place to know the good stuff when you see it rather than focusing on how others see you, who *they* are, and what they might want from you.

■ **Learn to love and accept yourself:** It sounds cheeseball, but if you don't earnestly care for yourself first, and love and accept who you are, nobody else is going to be able to do it very well either. And if we can't love ourselves, we can't do a very good job loving someone else. Bonus: if you're really being yourself all the time, when someone does fall for you, you don't have to wonder if it's really you they're into. You'll know it is.

■ **Trust your instincts:** When you feel in your guts that something just isn't right, chances are it's not. When your instincts tell you that something is really right? It probably is. By all means, temper those feelings with logic, but pay attention to your instincts—they're pretty smart.

■ **Stop looking so hard:** You're more likely to find quality relationships when you're living your life fully rather than spending every waking moment fixated on hooking up or finding a partner. Desperation isn't generally attractive to emotionally healthy people, and someone who will really love you for who you are is going to be attracted to you when you're following all of your dreams as an active participant in your own life, clearly able to drive the car of your life all by yourself. As strange as it may sound, although we've got to put what we want out there once we do get involved with someone, to get to that starting place, we often benefit more from living our lives without looking than we do from engaging in any sort of epic hunt for love.

■ **Take positive risks:** "Nothing ventured, nothing gained" is the order of the day. To get something started or kick things into high gear, someone has got to make a move at some point—asking someone on a date, getting a phone number, expressing love or care, even just saying hello.

■ **Know you're always worthy:** Everyone *is* deserving of love and affection. Everyone. That includes you. ■■

older people for whom online-anything isn't something that has been part of their sexual or romantic lives.

If you have social anxiety of any kind or otherwise have a hard time connecting with people face to face before you're comfortable with them, or you just find in-person dating superstressful, online opportunities can be everything. For those who live in very small or homogeneous communities or in places where who they are and who they want to date aren't accepted—such as if you're queer or gender nonconforming—online technologies can really diversify the dating pool and potentially provide safer opportunities to meet people for romantic or sexual relationships. And when people go about online dating smartly, it can, in fact, be safer than dating in person.

When people get very involved online, they often really work and hone their communication skills through all that communicating in writing and in words through e-mail, messengers, chat, or videoconferencing. It can be easier to communicate while NRE has got you in a whirl and when in-person chemistry and physicality aren't in the mix.

If your online dating or relationships are long distance, keeping sexual pacing slow is pretty much built in. If you want to avoid the impulsive decision making that can often be part and parcel of any new love, lust, or both, keeping things online can help with that, too: it's much harder to all of a sudden move in together after a month or two when you live in different cities.

For people who have a hard time really sticking to what they want in dating, online dating platforms can make it a lot easier to put out there who they are and what they want more clearly and confidently than they would in person. For people seeking more casual sex or what might be called "alternative" relationships, online options and apps can provide a more accepting environment with a bigger pool of potential partners than they'd find in their in-person communities. And for anyone having a hard time wrapping their brain around dating as being a kind of interpersonal shopping, online and mobile tools for dating or hooking up make that very tangibly obvious.

On the Other Hand . . .

All of the ways we can get to know someone in person include ways we can get to know each other online, but the opposite isn't true. How someone is online isn't always how they are in person, and how we feel about them online won't automatically be how we feel about them in person. So, if we are in something with the aim of moving it to an in-person relationship, we might be in for some tough surprises, such as discovering that we have no sexual chemistry whatsoever with our online partner when we thought we would because we liked their looks (would that chemistry was so simple!), that someone's in-person behavior isn't at all the way it is online, or that someone is not who they presented themselves online to be.

If you only knew your friend or partner in a classroom, would you know them the same way you do when you also see them at home, alone and with friends, with your family and theirs, at work and at play? Nope.

Often, when we're on the computer talking to someone, it's in our leisure time. We get to take as long as we like to say something, and we can even edit it as we go, something we can't do when we speak. Our writing skills may give the impression that the way we write is the way we are—when often that isn't the case. If we get involved with someone we haven't met in person, we may find that it feels easier to get closer to them without the static of physical attraction, face-to-face talking, having to see how a person meshes or doesn't with our friends and family. Overall, it can be really easy to sustain illusions about people in online relationships, easier than it is to get out of touch with reality in in-person relationships.

In-Person Big Plans: Made Best in Person

Try not to get too invested in online relationships, especially as maybe-in-person or maybe-long-term-big-serious relationships, before you meet the person and establish a relationship in the context of your entire life and theirs—not just a small online sliver of it. Starting to talk for real about moving, engagement, or marriage, for instance, before you've even met

BASIC ONLINE SAFETY

- Withhold very personal information for a while—not days a while, but weeks or months a while. Keep home addresses, school names, phone numbers, last names, private social media handles, and the like to yourself. If you use an e-mail address that identifies you clearly in any way—such as one that includes a school or college name or your full name—register an alternate e-mail address for yourself that's more generic to use for online dating. Once you've been talking to someone online for a few months, if you want to know them more, you may even want to set up a public meeting *before* you give out information that could result in stalking or other dangers. Often, we're able to get a better feel for who someone really is by being around them in person rather than online or even on the telephone. If someone really pushes you for personal information fast, that's a big-time red flag. You'll want to disconnect rather than connect more closely by giving them what they're asking for.
- The first few times, don't meet someone you know only online alone or in a private or unfamiliar place. Make sure you tell someone you can count on—a close friend, a family member—where you're going and at what time you expect to be back, or bring along someone you trust. This person doesn't have to sit right there with you; they can always sit a bench or table or two over and read a book. If you use a cell phone, make arrangements for someone to call you a half hour into a meeting to make sure everything is going okay and that you're safe. If a person you're meeting balks at the smart, cautious steps you're taking, that's often a big sign that their motives aren't safe. If you meet someone from online and pick up a weird vibe or feel unsafe in any way, trust your instincts and just get outta there.
- Be honest. If you're sixteen, don't say you're nineteen. If you're in a committed relationship

someone is unrealistic and pretty reckless. We may like to think that in-person physical attraction and chemistry are irrelevant, but more often than not, they're *very* relevant. The way we communicate together in person, the way the rhythms of our lives do or don't work together, and how a partner relates to our friends and family are all important, too.

It's ultimately best to consider online relationships and interactions as dating—not serious enough to build too much of your life around until you meet the other person and spend some real time with them and in their lives (and not just one meeting). If and when you take the step to in-person dating, mating, and relating, and that all goes well, then it's time to start getting more serious.

Another easy rule of thumb: figure that whatever context some kind of big deal may be happening in, most of our talking about it and agreeing to it should happen in that context, too. In other words, if the thing we're talking about or agreeing to is about something mostly offline and in-person, it's usually only going to be very sound to mostly talk about and agree to it offline and in-person. On the other hand, if the Big Thing you're talking about, like a commitment of some kind, is only really about online, then it's probably

with someone, even if it's on the outs, don't say you're single. There is a person you're communicating with on the other computer. Purposefully deceiving them—or them deceiving you—just isn't okay. Recognize that many people online are *not* honest, sometimes about very critical things like their age, motives, and relationship status. If you don't feel safe being honest because of something that makes you very vulnerable in the world—for example, if you're transgender—that's okay and understandable; holding back on sharing this information is not about deception but about personal and emotional safety. Rather than giving information that is not truthful, a better move can be to keep private anything about that item or to say that you aren't comfortable talking about it if someone asks about it. If someone feels like they absolutely need to know that thing or they don't want to keep talking or get more involved because of it, so be it.

■ Keep your radar up for questions that feel weird or inappropriate in any way to you. Unless you're expressly pursuing sexual hookups online, someone who asks you how you masturbate or if you're a virgin the first few times you talk to them probably isn't on the up-and-up. Someone asking for photos of your body or a blow-by-blow physical description of you is cruising (and if they're legally an adult and you're not, they may even be breaking child pornography laws and involving you in that crime) or looking for something to masturbate to rather than trying to get to know you. (That doesn't have to be a bad thing, but if it's not what you also want and feel safe with, it's obviously not going to be a good fit.) Someone who tries a sneaky way to get you to give them information you're keeping private—for instance, if you don't give them your phone number, but they then ask what school you go to, what street you live on, and if you have a private line—is not trustworthy and may in fact be predatory and dangerous.

Safety issues aside, the prime catchphrase with Net relationships is: *Walk, don't run.* ■■

all good. If someone's asking you to sign a five-year lease for an apartment, you're going to want to at least *see* that apartment and have an experience of being in it to even know what "it" is a big part of your decision. We can have ideas about or someone can tell us a whole lot of things about apartments or the neighborhood they're in that don't square with reality, and that's also true when it comes to people and relationships.

Safety Dance!

How safe things are online also varies and depends a lot on what we are or aren't doing to protect ourselves. Unfortunately, it is much easier—and much less risky for the perpetrator when it comes to getting caught—to stalk or harass someone online and to do so in much bigger, far-reaching ways than anyone could manage in person. So, we are always more vulnerable online, regardless of whether our relationships or dates or hookup interactions start online. Always do what you can to manage your risks wisely and to protect yourself.

When *Run, Don't Walk* Is the Catchphrase

If you're a legal minor, I'm going to go ahead and take one of the few Heather-gets-to-state-a-personal-opinion passes I afford myself and tell you something: I think your best bet is to hold off seeking casual sex via tech. Around sex and technology, the legal rights of minors are so bad and the legal and practical protections so poor, way too many people who aren't safe and who are looking to abuse or exploit young people know this all too well. Your stakes are also higher because peer or community sexual shaming about casual sex tends to go into overdrive when it comes to young people. Also, it's easier for people to invade your privacy or find out about your sex life when you're seeking it online than when you keep it more private.

On the other hand, if you do go there, when you use online or mobile technologies expressly to seek casual and immediate sex, "Walk, don't run" doesn't make a lot of sense because running is what you want to be doing. It also goes without saying that avoiding safety risks doesn't really fit with this context either; some risk is usually the point. That said, you really want to do all the things you can do to ensure your basic safety, and even to double down on some safety issues to make up for other areas where you're leaving yourself more exposed.

WITHOUT A MAP: RELATIONSHIPS OUTSIDE THE BOX

Some kinds of relationships—like being a heterosexual couple in a sexually exclusive relationship, to name an obvious one—have plenty of cultural support, representation in the media, and very visible in-person modeling. Even when people want to reconfigure or adapt relationships that are presented as the most normal, ideal, or best, there are a lot of examples they can use to contrast and compare, and usually there is still a lot of cultural and social support.

But a whole lot of relationships aren't as—or at all—normalized or visible, or they are considered dangerous or wrong. Really, when it comes to relationship models or kinds of sexual or romantic relationships, the "box" that defines what a lot of people think of as common, normal, ideal, or best is much, much smaller than the diverse range of relationships in reality.

Some kinds of relationships people may consider "alternative" are relationships like these:

- Those between or which include queer people—as well as relationships that are simply more queer in their structure, roles, or dynamics than heteronormative
- Interracial or cross-cultural relationships
- Casual, open, or friends-with-benefits relationships, or sexual relationships that aren't also romantic
- Romantic or sexual relationships among more than two people
- Relationships that encompass great differences in religious or spiritual beliefs or practices
- Asexual relationships or relationships in which one person is asexual and the other isn't
- Age-disparate relationships
- Online relationships
- Relationships with a strong sexual component, like domination and submission, that isn't just in play during or around sexual activity (see page 245)
- Relationships in which people are cohabitating or creating some version of family together (which may include children) without any desire or plan to ever get married

Some kinds of relationships, including some in the list above, can have big, built-in power inequities that make them

TECH TIP

Using the Internet or mobile technology for dating or hooking up? When people get into their twenties, they use these technological ways of dating or seeking sexual partners more commonly. A Pew Research report from 2013 found that nearly 40 percent of people between the ages of twenty-five and forty-four years are dating online (and around 10 percent of those between eighteen and twenty-four years are).

Really, the "rules" of tech dating are not so different from those of in-person dating: online or offline, there *aren't* rules at all, just what works for you and anyone you're dating, which should include not being a jerk. Otherwise, just keep in mind the usual dating—or trying to interact with people in a positive way—basics. (See page 150.) You'll want to build up trust and familiarity gradually, rather than all at once, and consider your personal and emotional safety.

Tech tools are just that: tools. They're just new vehicles or helpers to do a lot of the same things people have always done. The way people "do" dating or hooking up with tech tools is very similar to how people have done those things in the past without them.

That can be something you need to remind some much older people about, by the way, especially if you wind up listening to how unsafe or stupid it is to hook up, date, or get into a serious relationship that starts with tech tools. (Surprise: pretty much as safe or unsafe as in person.) People might also try to tell you how *no one* in anything good or real had it start online. (I am pretty sure the 5 percent of people in committed relationships or marriages that started online would beg to differ.)

more precarious. The power inequalities might be between the people in the relationship or originate from people or systems outside of the relationship that affect the relationship.

Relationships with big power or agency disparities, in which one person has rights or power—privilege—the other doesn't have or has considerably less of, can look like this:

- One person is still a minor while the other is a legal adult.
- One person has disability and the other doesn't.
- One person is poor and the other isn't.
- One person is undocumented as a citizen and the other is.
- One person is gender nonconforming while the other is cisgender.
- One person is taking social or economic risks by being in the relationship that the other person isn't.
- One person has a safe and supportive community while the other is unsafe or unsupported in theirs.

Heck, even in the most culturally normalized kind of relationship, between cisgender men and women, there are big inequities just based on gender alone. For example, the far greater burden to prevent possible reproduction falls on women, and that's also because the far, far greater burden falls on the person who can actually become and be pregnant. People in heterosexual, cisgender relationships often adopt unhealthy roles or dynamics that are considered normal or ideal rather than doing what they can to create healthier dynamics, in part by acknowledging, addressing, and working to balance out those power and privilege differences as best they can. Power inequities are not only part of less common or "alternative" relationships: they're prevalent in the most culturally sanctioned kinds of relationships there are.

Sometimes a relationship is not very visible or normalized *and* has some built-in power imbalances or inequities. Whether you're in or considering something in this category, here are some key helps:

Is it healthy? If a relationship is emotionally healthy (you can gauge this based on the information in this section of the book and in others that list hallmarks of healthy relationships), then everyone involved is probably already doing a great deal to manage any big (or smaller) inequities and is doing that well. In many situations, so long as everyone involved—*especially* the person with more power or agency than the other—does their best to understand and be aware of inequities, make adaptations and compromises, and share power so that the scales are more balanced, even relationships with some big divides can be healthy, safe, and beneficial to those involved.

Sometimes we develop a blindness to problematic dynamics in a relationship because we're so focused on the way the relationship is being seen or treated by outside people or systems. It's also pretty easy to hold even tighter to a relationship—even if it's not a good one—than we otherwise would because we feel like it's us and the other person against the whole world. A lot of outside drama or strife tends to take up tons of emotional real estate, sometimes leaving little to none for the relationship itself.

Every relationship has problems, especially if it lasts more than a few days, weeks, or months. And in marginalized relationships, or relationships involving marginalized people, although the marginalization itself, bias, and social stigma certainly cause a whole bunch of problems, they are rarely the *only* source of relationship struggles. Discrimination or social stigma are for real, and for real awful. But don't let knowing and feeling that blind you to other possible problems or big conflicts *in* the relationship. Marginalized people or groups are far more vulnerable to abuse than those who aren't marginalized, and most abuse happens *within* intimate relationships, not outside of or around them. So, be sure that if you're having a lot of conflict, you are looking within the relationship as much as outside of it to evaluate and work on (or leave) it. Hold the relationship to the same standards you would any other and have and only be in healthy, safe relationships.

Don't fly solo or blind: Educate yourself about the kind of relationship you're in. If you're in it, chances are good there are resources about it: books, websites, or online or offline support communities. Because something is less visible or normalized doesn't mean you have to do it without any kind of road map. Don't go it alone. Do what you can to find people in similar kinds of relationships and stay connected for support and perspective when you need it.

Bias check in aisle two: Bias and bigotry may well be things you deal with from people or systems outside your relationship. People are often unaware of their own biases—or they have convinced themselves or mistake a certain bias as genuine concern—so you may not only face bias but also face it from people who don't know that's what it is or just won't own up to it.

Bias is best unlearned by simple, slow exposure to whatever group or relationship the biased person has an issue with. If your family has an issue with your interracial relationship, avoiding family members altogether (unless that's the only safe option for you or your partner) or getting snarky about the issue isn't as productive as slowly and coolly letting them get to know your partner over time. That may also involve—if you're not independent from your family—accepting limits they put on your relationship or your participation in it; pushing back hard against them to try to change them fast won't help. Doing what you can to cope for the time being and taking baby steps to shift people's thinking or trust will.

Something some activists learned during the fight for marriage equality is that trying to move someone's position a lot all at once very rarely works. People just tend to dig in more when we push them too hard or ask them to somehow think very differently from the way they do. What works better is aiming for slow, incremental shifts, for gradual, even subtle movement, rather than radical change.

For change to happen, people have to be at least willing to start to make shifts.

Most people are or can get there, but some people are particularly stubborn in their biases. Talking about issues of bias outside the context of your relationship, such as in discussions of current events, can also be helpful, because those are less in-your-face. You might also find some extra help in support or activist groups that focus on tolerance.

You may have to face the fact that your relationship will never be accepted by your family or current circle of friends. You may even decide that, given a certain level of bias, you can't maintain the relationship in a way that's healthy or beneficial for everyone. As with many types of less-accepted relationships, patience is also key: sometimes, the mere test of time alone takes care of things. Or you may decide to distance yourself from those whose biases are putting up the roadblocks or to sever your relationships with them. That can be a very hard choice to make.

When it's not bias but is real care and sound concern: Sometimes resistance about your relationship isn't about bias even when the people being unaccepting *have* biases. Sometimes resistance is based in genuine, sound concern about a particular relationship or its context. A lack of support for you being in a relationship that's abusive or controlling, for instance, is about your relationship being unhealthy and you or a partner being unsafe in it, not about the age, race, gender, or religious belief system of the person being abusive or controlling. And if you have fewer rights or less power or agency in that relationship to boot, someone who suggests it's particularly unsafe and dangerous is right—it is. Someone being very wary about your specific friends-with-benefits situation that seems to leave you chronically unhappy isn't being wary of *all* those types of relationships but about your specific one and how it seems to be affecting you.

To figure out whether bias is or isn't a player in people's reactions, just pay close attention—attention to yourself and your relationship and attention to the other people or systems that are reacting poorly. You may need to check your own biases as well; it's easy to believe that discrimination is fair or right if we've been surrounded by and immersed in that bias ourselves. Honestly and openly bring the evaluations you make to the table, and communicate them clearly and with as much patience as you can muster to anyone else involved. Take the high road and do your best to keep your cool. The other person or people who are in your relationship need to do that, too.

Have and hold limits and boundaries: If you're facing intense pushback, set some limits and boundaries. You can ask that certain conversations be limited or ended. You can set a hard limit on anyone badmouthing you or your partner. You can ask anyone who wants to say a whole lot about your relationship to read up using a resource you recommend and to make sure they're listening as much as they're talking. Limits and boundaries should also be part of your relationship, and you may have some that are specific to dealing with outside strife and others for inside imbalances. For example, you can make boundaries around spending time with someone's friends or family who are unsupportive or emotionally abusive (that could include an agreement that you both will leave as a team if and when things get ugly) or set limits with a partner when it comes to things like them using (or not acknowledging) their power privilege. Limits and boundaries are part of every kind of healthy interaction and relationship, and when and if there are power inequities within or around the relationship, we often need more of them.

Trust your instincts: When there's less cultural or social support for something, fewer maps to look at, or some built-in inequities, it's often harder to suss out whether a relationship and what we're doing within it are right for us and others. Our instincts are always valuable and trustworthy, and when we have less information to work with, they are especially great and reliable resources. Pay attention to how you feel, and do what you can to align your head and heart. If all your own guideposts give a strong thumbs-up, you're probably good. If not, start thinking, talking, and considering solutions.

[THOSE THREE LITTLE WORDS]

Feeling and saying, *"I love you"* is no small thing for most of us. They're just three words, sure—but so much can be read into them and meant by them, it's dizzying. One person may say them very casually and freely, while to another the words are sacred and something they are more choosy about saying. Some people aren't comfortable speaking those words at all, because they feel they're so overused as to be meaningless, or they feel those words imply actions they're not comfortable with, or they're just plain scared to say them.

What's "real" love, anyway? Would that there was one answer to that question!

Overall, I think love means that you accept and respect someone for who they are, strengths and weaknesses *both,* not just for who you want them to be or what role you want them to play in your life. In many ways, more than anything else "real" love is about friendship, not sex or romance. Love usually means you care very deeply for someone, not because of *what* they are to you but for *who* they are to you, as is. Love usually comes without many conditions: the person we love doesn't have to look a certain way, be our boyfriend or girlfriend, or call us a certain number of times per week. This doesn't mean you shouldn't have boundaries but quite the opposite: when we love each other, healthy boundaries are both part of the mix and something we'll always want to support. Love involves support, even when giving that support creates a result that isn't so great for us, like encouraging a partner to attend their choice college even though it's two thousand miles away. It involves really caring for someone, not just when they're well but when they're sick; not just when they're happy but when they're upset, too. In many ways, love often feels like being **home**—a place we feel is safe for us, where we don't have to worry about impressing anyone or always saying exactly the right thing, where we can be ourselves. It's both parties giving as well as receiving. When someone loves *you, and you them,* it should involve all of these sorts of things.

It's sometimes easier to talk about what love isn't than what it is. Love isn't obsession, infatuation, or fixation. It isn't control, rescue, or ownership. It isn't validation of self-worth or self-image. It isn't a means to make someone stay with you or do something specific for you. It isn't a way to manipulate someone's emotions. It doesn't make us unbalanced or dizzy (that's how passion, new relationship energy, and being "in love" make us feel). Real love won't leave us feeling like half a person or like someone else is treating us like one.

It's normal to be nervous when you start to feel love bubbling up in you and growing. It may even make you want to withdraw a bit, because loving someone is big, scary stuff. If and when you want to say those three little words, the other person may not say them back or may be overwhelmed, shocked, or surprised that you've said them. They may not yet feel ready to say them, or they may even say "I love you, too" just because they don't want to hurt you, even if they aren't sure about their feelings yet. And you might react in these same ways to someone who says it to you first.

As with everything else that involves another person, all of that is okay; just try to talk it out honestly and with care. Partners don't always have to be in exactly the same place at the exact same time for our relationship to be healthy and beneficial. We both just need to feel okay about where we're both at. Talk about what those words mean to you and what you mean by them if and when you say them. You can even talk about why you don't like the L-word, about baggage you may have attached to it, about misuse of that word. Heck, you and yours can invent new words altogether for your feelings if you like. Everyone communicates differently, too, so words may not even be the best way to show the love you feel. When people say you "just know" that you love or are loved, most of what they're talking about is actions, not words.

You can't screw up by really loving someone. You can get your heart broken, a relationship may not go as you'd like, or you might be disappointed, but these are all inherent dangers when we live fully, not locked away in some small, sterile room by ourselves without ever taking any risks. Loving someone for real is pretty much always a good thing. Same goes for really being loved.

THE TEST OF TIME: LONG-TERM RELATIONSHIPS

Most couples therapists and relationship experts consider the first six months of a relationship to be the period in which two people are getting to know each other; what comes afterward is considered long term. These professionals usually work with older people, however; young-adult life tends to have a different pace and velocity. For teens and young adults, feelings are often more intense from the start, and attachments form more quickly. To account for that, I figure that if you're a younger person and you've been in a relationship for three or four months, you can consider yourself to be entering something potentially long term, according to your clock.

Here are some things to expect if you're going to try to go the distance.

What's Typical in Long-Term Relationships?

▶ **More vulnerability:** It's normal to start to feel more vulnerable, even more insecure, when a relationship has lasted a while. Your partner knows you better and you've likely shared a lot more with them than with someone you've only dated a short time.

▶ **Doubts about hanging in there:** There's nothing wrong with doubting or questioning a relationship. It's not a sign of disloyalty or betrayal; it's a sign of an active mind and is what people do who are trying to stay aware and keep evaluating their relationships as they go, which we always need to do. There's also nothing wrong with wondering if, maybe, you're missing out on other things because of a long-term relationship. Remember: there is no one type of relationship that is best for everyone, so if you start feeling that something long term and serious isn't right for you, it's okay to go with what works for you and switch gears.

What feels best to you is only up to you. Solid relationships where two people have mutual feelings for one another *are*

SOULMATES, THE ONES, AND FOREVER-AND-EVERS

It feels wonderful to be involved with someone who says they'll always love us, forever and ever—and who is saying that because they earnestly feel that way. Yet, most romantic relationships of our youth will not be the relationships we're in forty, twenty, or ten years—even one year—down the road. We're much more likely to find our longest partnerships when we're out of our teens and early twenties. The average span of a teen's first sexual or romantic relationship is usually less than six months. According to some studies, like the one from the National Longitudinal Study of Adolescent Health, it's most common for young people, especially teens, to be in romantic or sexual relationships that last a few to six months, not many—or even a few—years. That reality does not make your or someone else's *feelings* of big or eternal love any less important, nor do you need to be jaded about the whole works. But a little reality can go a long way in terms of protecting your heart and keeping your current relationship as excellent as it can be: when someone really feels like that, their feelings *are* real, those feelings just don't dictate how they will feel twenty years from now, next year, or even next week. Feelings can be fickle, even the big ones, and even when we don't want them to change.

Appreciate and honor those *feelings* of forever, but do most of your planning for right now and the not-too-distant future. Spend most of your time right here in the present. How we feel isn't a guarantee of what will happen, whether we're talking about romance, sex, or our desire to travel the globe. If you separate your feelings some from practical plans or expectations, not only can you have a relationship that's grounded but also you can be sure you don't miss all the great things going on today that often get taken for granted when you're too busy daydreaming about tomorrow.

hard to come by, and nurturing them does take a big investment of time, patience, and energy. Few people in healthy, happy relationships are going to be missing out on anything valuable, because little is more valuable. So, if you've got a really good thing, and you know you want something long term, don't take it for granted.

Obviously, if a long-term relationship is keeping you from achieving other goals, if it's causing conflict, if you just don't feel able to maintain it, or if you question it more than you actually enjoy it, it's worth considering terminating or changing the terms of the relationship. And if your friends and family are observing that this is the case with you, it's worth a listen. One aspect of long-term relationships is that, over time, a partner becomes more involved in your inner circle: your closest friends, your family. When they're a viable part of that core, you're both going to have to work with that integration and give it more cooperative care and attention than you did when you were more casually dating.

If you are in something long term and have family or friends who are skittish about it, or you are—talk it out. If they have specific concerns (such as your rushing into marriage, or relationship blind spots you seem to have), hear them out, tell your side, come to compromises if you can. Often cultural differences about dating and sexual relationships crop up between generations. For example, although you expect a parent or guardian to be totally on board with something ongoing and serious, in fact, their disapproval may surprise you because more casual or noncommittal dating was more normal for them. Even if you don't agree with what's being said—and you don't have to—just hearing it can alert you to issues to watch out for, and working with everyone can strengthen *all* your relationships.

▶ **Less sex or sex with a slightly different flavor than you might be used to:** It's common for the intensity of sexual feelings to fizzle a bit over time and for the frequency of sex to slow down. As people settle into a relationship, sexual activity can move away from the forefront, and that doesn't mean anything is terribly wrong. Partners may likely have sex less often over time, or their sexual activity may have peaks and valleys. But usually, in good relationships, although the frequency of sex may decrease, the *quality* of sex improves because you've had time to get to know one another; learn about each other's responses, likes and dislikes, wants and needs; and develop a level of sexual communication you couldn't have had right at the start.

For people who held off on any kind—or all kinds—of sex until they were in a long-term relationship, it may mean the beginning of sex for you, a whole new aspect of your relationship to get used to and work with.

If you and your long-term partner are still holding off on sexual activity, until marriage or just a far later date, you may find that waiting gets more challenging the longer you're together. If that's the case, revisit and reevaluate both your needs and wants. Make sure that celibacy is what you both still want, and if it isn't, talk about how to make your changing wants or values work between you. If you or your partner find that decreased sexual frequency or intensity is an issue for either or both of you, talk it out; reinvest yourself in the relationship and in the fun of refreshing its spark. Be creative: now you've got even more tools to do that, because you know one another even better.

▶ **Disagreements:** When you're just getting to know someone, it's normal to let a lot of things that bother you slide. You're still getting your feet wet, finding your comfort zones, and developing the trust and comfort to be able to really speak your mind. Also, often we are on our best behavior and at our most accommodating when things are new, so as a relationship goes on, more conflict can tend to crop up.

If you find that you and yours argue a bit more than before, there's no need to leap to the conclusion that all is lost. Certainly, if those arguments are ugly or become constant, or if you find you disagree on things that pose a very big problem—like birth control, life goals, or people near and dear to you—you've got a problem. But having a few more conflicts or arguments, ones that might not be resolved quite as easily with a cuddle or a cute emoji, is normal when two people stick around long enough to discover things they disagree on and have the confidence and comfort with each other to disagree.

▶ **Relationship shifts and tougher breakups:** At some point, you may be looking at a relationship model change or a breakup. It's pretty obvious that the longer you're with someone, the tougher a change or a breakup can be. When it takes longer to get to this point, it can take longer to get over. Inertia can be a huge factor in long-term relationships that aren't going so well. It may seem easier to learn to deal with a dysfunctional relationship than to go through a breakup, to be alone, to be dating again, to cultivate new relationships. It usually isn't. When something is over, it's best to let it be over. Seek out a new way for both of you to be happy apart, or in a new configuration, instead of going nuts trying to make a relationship that just isn't working or that has run out of gas keep going.

If something sudden and intense facilitates a breakup—like a partner's cheating, an accidental pregnancy, or a job or school transfer—you're probably going to need a good deal of time to grieve and plenty of support from friends and family. However, sometimes a longer relationship does reach a natural end in a way that's oddly pretty comfortable and easy.

Looking Toward the Future

It's most common for people in long-term intimate relationships to eventually want to create some version of family together, like by moving in together, getting engaged or married, or bringing children, pets, or other family members into the mix. Some of that is the stuff of decades or more, each a book—or fifty books!—in its own right. And for most of the readers of this book, that stuff, if and when it's wanted, is still pretty far off. But here are a few basics if you're considering making any major commitments.

For those of certain religions or cultural beliefs, living together before or without marriage isn't an option they want or feel safe choosing. Sometimes pregnancies people choose to carry to term aren't planned, so planning for a family isn't always something people do far in advance. But whenever possible, taking small steps with major commitments is the way to go.

Living on your own or with roommates, for instance, before living with a romantic partner is something most people can do. Take serious time to really talk through all the details and possible issues that cohabitation, marriage, kids, or all of the above can entail—with your partner and with other friends and family whose perspectives you value. Giving yourself and anyone else involved the necessary time before committing to something giant should always be okay. If it's not, moving forward probably isn't so wise.

This really should go double for things like marriage and parenting together, where on top of all the emotional and practical obligations and other big stuff major legal agreements—some of which tie you to someone in ways you or they may not always want—are at play. Talk about it with your partner in depth, with a keen eye toward *all* you'd be opting into—not just daily life and family stuff but also legal and financial issues. What do you and yours really feel about marriage, parenting, the legal aspects of any commitments (such as signing a lease), and any built-in gender or economic inequities? Are there ways that something might legally bind you that you or they feel uncomfortable with?

If it's kids you're thinking about, check out Chapter 12.

If you feel your mind changing at any point in the process of entering into major commitments, **say something.** Don't keep it inside for fear of hurting your partner or because *not* getting married or living together scares you (even though the idea of doing those things doesn't feel so awesome either). Part of major interpersonal commitments always involves honest and open communication, such as talking through concerns, doubts, fears, wants, and not-wants. There should be a lot of communication happening in the making of commitments. You also want to make sure that everyone making agreements knows what they're really agreeing to, wants to agree, and feels willing and able to honor their agreements. Be flexible with yourself and your partner. Throughout our lives, we grow and change all the time, so learning to be flexible in any situation is a major key to having healthy relationships.

[IN CONFLICT]

When people get close, conflict always happens eventually. That conflict can be large—like dealing with an unplanned pregnancy or someone wanting to shift a relationship to a long-distance one when that feels like it would be a terrible heartbreak for the other person—or small—like someone wanting to go out and party when the other just wants to stay home and cuddle or someone not calling back when the other is lonely. The longer any relationship we have goes on, the more we'll deal with conflict. More of it tends to come up, and as time goes on we also usually become more confident voicing conflict rather than trying to avoid it.

Some people suggest that good relationships don't involve conflict. For that to be true, everyone involved would basically have to (1) be the exact same people (and this is not even a guarantee because we're often in conflict with ourselves), (2) be sleeping their way through the whole of a relationship, and (3) never ever grow and change as people as we are wont to do. People are often in conflict from small ways to big ones. To more accurately gauge how okay and emotionally healthy we and our relationships are, we need not look at whether there is conflict so much as look at how we deal with it, alone and together.

Unfortunately, many people aren't schooled when it comes to resolving conflict. Whether we're talking about at home, through media, at school, or with peers, most of our models related to conflict are substandard, at best. So much of what we learn is usually a lot of avoidance or some backward idea about how not resolving conflict is noble. It's also common for us to learn to either explode or bottle up when conflict arises rather than to accept, deal with, and resolve it.

How many friendships have you seen or experienced that have been swiftly and suddenly destroyed or deeply damaged because of a conflict where someone—or everyone—utterly flipped out? Probably at least a few, especially if you attended middle or high school. Sometimes the only way people can resolve conflict between them *is* to part ways—some conflicts are just too great and otherwise unsolvable for people to stay together. But just as often, if not more so, a conflict *can* be resolved and a relationship not just salvaged but also strengthened. And even when people decide to separate, when they deal with conflict well, the separation is rarely the kind of nuclear end that so often happens otherwise.

Resolving conflict also delivers a nice self-esteem and personal growth bonus: handling conflict like a pro feels so much better than blowing up, teaches us good things about ourselves, and gives us tools to better relate to others as well as ourselves. It's something that can give us a real feeling of control and mastery over our lives and feelings. When so much of life as a young adult can feel out of control and it's so easy to feel clumsy or lost, that's a megabonus.

Conflict Resolution: A Crash Course

1. Take a minute (or even better, a few): If we're hurting or upset with someone, commonly we feel a strong urge to react to them or the situation immediately, like we just want to get those hard feelings *out* of us before we implode. Sometimes whether we react doesn't even feel within our control—but it is. Exploding isn't any better than imploding, especially when someone else is in our direct line of fire. When conflict arises and you're running hot, center yourself for a sec: take a few breaths, remind yourself of who you are and who you want to be at your best, and cool down your upset at least enough to really think and feel totally in control of your emotions and behavior. If you can slow it all down even just a little bit, you'll be able to start resolving the conflict instead of simply reacting to it, and that is more likely to make things better instead of worse.

2. In before out: To even get an idea of how we feel about something and the best way to deal with it so as to move forward to solving the conflict, we've got to talk to ourselves before we talk to anyone else. Sometimes, we have hours, days, or even weeks to process on our own; in other situations, the conflict happens right now, in our face. Whatever the circumstance, we want to do what we can to check in with our feelings as well as our thoughts, and check ourselves before we wreck ourselves or anyone else. We can always ask the other person to give us a minute and can even step outside or away for a little bit to get that space. If anyone refuses you time or space and tries to force you to stay in a hot conflict or stirs things up more, they aren't ready to resolve the conflict but only want to create or increase it. It's time to run, not walk, to get the space you need.

3. "I" statements: That phrase always sounds corny, but it's really important during conflicts to stick to *our* thoughts and *our* feelings and to own and express *our* experience of things rather than to focus totally on the other person or to assign them motives. So, for example, say, "I have a hard time feeling heard when you talk at the same time I do" instead of "You don't listen to me." Instead of "You make me feel so jealous," swap out for something like "I'm really struggling with jealousy over your friendship with her." Sometimes conflict is simply one person not getting the impact of their behavior on someone else, so now and then an "I" statement can solve the whole issue.

4. Where and when: Resolving conflict, especially the kind that's got someone really upset or scared, is difficult and takes real energy and focus from everyone involved. So, pick environments for working through conflict that make room for that fact. Trying to resolve a conflict through texting, with a bunch of other people around, when someone is in the middle of something else, or when you're really tired isn't the way to go. As much as you can, pick mediums where no one has to shortcut or be multitasking. (I said not in SMS messaging already, right? It's such a recipe for disaster, so let's just say it twice.) Set things up so everyone involved has the time, energy, and ability to pay very close attention to each other.

5. Patience, grasshopper: If both people are doing their best to resolve it and be cool with each other, a minor conflict can often be squared away in one talk, sometimes even within a couple minutes. The big or harder stuff, not so much. When a conflict is major, complex, or requires more negotiation or when someone involved is really struggling with managing it, resolution is often an ongoing process and project that we work on over time, with a series of talks and agreements, not just a chat, a hug, and a "No worries, we're cool." If even with a lot of time, resolution just feels impossible, then consider calling in reinforcements (like someone you both trust to help mediate or your favorite perspective-givers) or having a different kind of talk.

6. Accountability is magic: Just taking responsibility, clearly and earnestly, for our own stuff usually goes a very, very long way in resolving conflict. Acknowledging life history stuff that has nothing to do with the other person but that is bogging us down, ways we may have intentionally or carelessly created the conflict, or areas we know we're not good with conflict and need to work on is a type of accountability that can put you and someone else in a space where you're ready to solve the conflict. So often we just want to feel seen, heard, and respected, even when we don't agree or we really aren't happy with someone else. Even the outcome we usually want the least—not being able to resolve conflict and having to end or massively change the nature of a relationship—hurts a whole lot less when everyone involved clearly owns their own stuff instead of piling the blame on someone else.

[DYSFUNCTION JUNCTION: THE CRUMMY STUFF]

A lot of relationship problems aren't the end of the world and can be managed and repaired, sometimes without even having to work all that hard. The biggest part of the battle isn't fixing problems so much as it is recognizing that there *are* problems and being willing to address them and work a little to seek out healthier patterns of behavior. According to the Mediamark research (and plain old observation), more than half of all young adults report that their relationship causes them stress, and it's likely a lot of that stress could be alleviated just by recognizing dysfunction when it's in the mix and developing skills to manage it. Facing problems and working through them don't have to be awful. For many people, doing so strengthens their relationships with their partners and themselves.

The following isn't an all-inclusive list by many means—there are whole sections of bookstores with books on how to deal with relationship issues. Rather, these are just some of the more typical, key problems that teens and emerging adults report facing in relationships and ideas on how to handle them.

All by myself: We're often given the impression that it's better to be in a love relationship—any relationship—than not to be in one, and that just isn't so. Being single doesn't mean a person is undesirable or unattractive. In many cases, a single person simply isn't interested in relationships at a given time or is waiting to meet someone whose needs and wants really work with their own.

Entering into or staying in romantic or sexual relationships primarily to avoid being alone is a really bad idea. Not only is it hard to have good judgment when you're so freaking scared of being alone or sick of your own company, it usually means you're using the other person, in a way, to try to fix feelings that you need to work on by and for yourself. It's also all too easy, when you're in a relationship and deathly afraid of being alone, to become dependent and clingy, which can tank even a good relationship. A study done by the Department of Psychology at Macquarie University in Australia found that, in relationships, both partners were equally dissatisfied when either partner suffered anxiety over abandonment or fear of being alone. Too, some experts have linked fear of abandonment with abusive behaviors: a partner afraid of being alone may be more inclined to try to control their partner to ensure that they stick around.

For relationship's sake: Feeling funny because you're twenty and have never been kissed and can't wait another second? Sexually frustrated? Does it seem like all your friends are in relationships right now, and you'd better get one, too? Are you with someone just because they're interested in you even though you're not as interested in them? Feel the need to prove to parents, friends, or yourself that you're mature enough or attractive enough to have a relationship, no matter with whom? Just plain bored with your life?

Entering into or staying in a relationship because you are primarily concerned with "having a relationship" is a really good way to ensure that at least one of you, and likely both, will feel like crap in pretty short order. Looking for and accepting just any relationship with anyone at all who'll have you is a lot like putting just anything into your mouth when you feel hungry: sure, sometimes you might get a lovely piece of cake, but other times you're going to wind up with a mouth full of dirt.

The good stuff is worth waiting for. If you feel the need to have some things in the interim, you can, and you can get them in ways that are fair and healthy. You can date more casually. If you feel sexually frustrated, you can masturbate. If you're lonely, you can make friendships and community connections based on interests other than love and sex.

The Great Escape

Some kinds of escapism—a kind of diversion that gets a person mentally away from their usual realities or routines or from parts of their life that are challenging or just plain awful—with like, love, and lust aren't a bad thing. Without at least some escapism some of the time, we'd all lose our damn minds. Getting away from our stresses, strains, conflicts, and frustrations sometimes and in some ways is actually healthy and helps us manage stress and stretch our imagination, which is always a good thing. And when things are or have been truly awful for us, it can very much be a way to survive.

The keyword there is *some:* escapism is something we want to make sure to keep in balance in our lives. We also want to keep an eye on where we're looking for it and how. Make sure that your relationships aren't based in escapism to the point that no one is actually dealing with—or even acknowledging or seeing—the for-real realities. Also, be sure you and any relationship partners aren't being escapist in ways that are truly dangerous and unsafe—emotionally or otherwise—for anyone.

Romantic or sexual relationships, especially when they're new or new to us, are often so engaging and intense that it's pretty easy to get totally sucked in and to wind up losing ourselves. Being intimate with someone else gives you opportunities to explore who you *want* to be. That is just fine, and sometimes that's also who, it turns out, you *are.* But other times, it's full-on, full-time role-play, which doesn't make for mutually healthy interactions for long.

We can know we've taken a bad turn with escapism in our relationships when we're trying to run away from ourselves or things we just have to deal with or we create connections or relationships that just aren't honest and real. Sometimes escapism in relationships becomes downright dangerous and destructive, like when people engage in shared substance abuse or other self-harm.

Healthy escapes can be great, including those with someone else, such as getting lost in the fun of a festival weekend, going to the movies pretending you're famous critics, playing in the park like little kids, or losing an hour to some deeply awesome sex. If at any time, though, you ever find yourself feeling—even if this is how you want to feel—like you're having a hard time getting back in touch with yourself or knowing who that is, reach for a lifeline. If a self-check doesn't get you right, ask for help from someone you trust.

Liar, liar, pants on fire: Lies and important omissions cause big problems in relationships, whether you're not being fully honest about your feelings, seeing someone else when you're supposed to be monogamous, saying you feel sexually ready when you really aren't, or staying in a relationship that is itself based in some way on lies.

Sometimes, you may have to or want to wait a little before you disclose to a partner major things that make you vulnerable; for instance, sexual abuse or domestic violence survivors often take a while to feel comfortable sharing their history, and someone who doesn't ever want kids can take some time before they say so to someone who might. But you do need to share important information. So, if you're waiting, be sure you're doing what you can to get to the point of disclosure before you or the other person gets too invested and involved.

Between partners, even when it's hard to tell the truth—when it may mean hurting a partner's feelings or putting the relationship at risk—you should always be working toward the truth by just spitting out the tough stuff or by taking small steps to move to being fully honest in time. This can even mean telling a partner you have something important to share but haven't yet built the trust and comfort you need to do that just yet. If you have some sense of what you need to feel safe and sound to be honest, you can share that with the other person so that, if there's something they can do to co-create and build that sense of safety and trust, they can get started.

Drama major: A lot of people confuse drama with love, affection, or real connection. The higher the level of drama gets—friends or parents disliking a partner, promises of marriage, a profound age difference, even emotional or physical abuse—the more we might assume a feeling of love or passion exists because the emotional stakes are raised. That's understandable; after all, writers have been using that exact same device to elevate their readers' emotions for thousands of years. What so many people learn romance is or should be more often involves conflict than accord. But.

Often, people are simply reacting to those escalated circumstances or unhealthy ideals, and the drama can keep young couples together like glue but also stands in the way of real love, intimacy, and healthy emotional bonding. So, if the drama kicks in, try to recognize it and remember that then, more than ever, is *not* the time to leap in blindly but to step back and really look at what's going on.

Traffic patterns: One partner may want to move things along—things like sex, commitment, going public as a couple—a lot faster or slower than the other. Sometimes the general pace of a relationship flows pretty organically and with ease and great mutual timing, but other times you wind up with stalls, speeders, or bottlenecking, and you may need to direct your relationship traffic with more effort and intention. Either partner has the right and the ability to turn on a green, yellow, or red light at any time. If you find you're feeling rushed or stalled or that the pace of your relationship just isn't in your control, stop where you are and evaluate. Talk to your partner about how you're feeling and what pace is more comfortable for you and why.

You might want to be sexually active with a partner but feel emotionally unprepared for it or know you can't afford birth control or sexual health care. A partner may want to be monogamous but may be worried about doing exclusivity too soon and then feeling fenced in instead of enjoying it. Outside factors may also affect pace, such as parents having rules or restrictions that don't allow for serious dating or sex yet. Relationships don't exist in a vacuum, and as young adults, all our choices don't get to be fully our own yet, so we sometimes have to manage and accept limitations and disruptions to our ideal relationship speed limit.

Tug-of-war: Feel like you have to try to earn a partner's time, attention, or love? Are you making a partner work pretty hard for things you should be giving easily? Don't feel fully worthy, or feel someone you're seeing isn't? Do things just feel unbalanced?

Everyone who gives love, care, respect, and affection is worthy and deserving of love, care, respect, and affection. No one has to earn it. If you're having to work your buns off to get attention or time from your partner, if you often feel you're begging or pleading with them for the things you need, or if, on the other hand, you feel really reluctant to give very basic things to a partner, that inequity needs to be repaired or it's time for that relationship to be over.

A relationship is a lot like a seesaw: if one person isn't carrying their weight and is making the other do all the work, somebody's going to stay stuck on the ground and the other person will be stuck dangling in midair. To make the seesaw worth riding, both people need to be doing the give-and-take evenly.

(Not enough) space case: Of course, when we really connect with someone sexually, romantically, or both, we want to be together. But just like a fire goes out if you suffocate it, so it goes with relationships: everyone needs some real room to breathe and space and time away from a partner to *keep* wanting to be together. This is often a challenge with relationships when we're young. The intensity that's so common when people are new to all this and, often, when they have more free time than they will later in life, tends to result in a total immersion with each other when possible (and is probably a big part of why young relationships tend to burn out about as fast as they flared up).

For all the great things technology has given us and the ways it can benefit our relationships, it's also added extra challenges in this department. After all, in the past when people weren't in the same space, they most often were truly apart. But not now; now not being in the same space in person often just means a shift to texting, chatting, emailing, and social media, including some people watching what the other is doing even when they are not directly interacting.

Be sure you're mutually unplugging on a regular basis. It's fine to keep in touch these other ways, but not if it means you're never apart, never alone, never really spending time with the other people in your life where they get your whole attention. You can even set times of the day or days of the week when you agree you both get some real radio silence. Take good care to maintain the other relationships and parts of your life rather than letting them all go or pushing them away in favor of a romantic or sexual relationship. Relationships and intimacy need as much room to breathe as they need closeness.

[ADVENTURES IN SPLITSVILLE: BREAKUPS AND HOW TO DEAL]

Even when a breakup is the best way to go—or all the choices feel like crap, and it just seems the least crap of them—breaking up is rarely fun or easy. It usually hurts in one way or another if not in all ways. It is safe to say that everyone is going to have to deal with at least one breakup in their lifetime. There are ways to do a little damage control to take care of yourself and your ex or soon-to-be ex.

When Is It Time?

Have you gone round and round with a given issue or set of issues, tried everything—including healthy conflict resolution or adjusting agreements—to make it work, all to no long-term avail? Or have you (one or both of you) just given up? Is your relationship clearly not mutual or balanced? Do you spend more time arguing, fighting, or in uncomfortable silences than feeling good and enjoying each other? After you spend time together, do you feel drained, sad, or hopeless instead of energized, happy, and supported? Do you or your partner simply feel done with the relationship? Do certain aspects of it just no longer feel "there"—for example, the sexual attraction has diminished greatly, the romantic feelings have fizzled, your friendship has gone kablooie? If so, your breakup train is pulling into the station. And if a relationship has become physically, sexually, or emotionally abusive or manipulative, it is absolutely time to head for the door and close it behind you.

Often, with well-balanced people we really care for and with whom we have been open, a "breakup" isn't so much a dramatic split—one person coming out of nowhere and announcing it's over—as a rearrangement and a mutual agreement about that rearrangement, like agreeing to create and go about a nonsexual friendship instead or to just part ways, wishing each other well. With a little time, patience, and communication, someone who doesn't work out as a lover or partner can become one of our most cherished close friends. Most of the time, breaking up, when it's the right thing for someone, isn't the sign of a weak or uncaring person or of people just blowing each other off; in fact, it's generally a pretty clear sign of real caring, self-awareness, and respect, including respect for the relationship.

How Do You Do It?

When a breakup is looming on the horizon or you have started to consider making a break, ideally you want to talk about it together. That may mean saying something like, "I know we [or you or I] have been working on *<insert big thing here>*, but I'm starting to feel like we should talk about the option of splitting up, too." That way, you can both have some time to consider that choice and then share what

HEALTHY/UNHEALTHY

What's in a healthy relationship? According to Access Excellence, a national education program affiliated with former US Surgeon General C. Everett Koop, in a healthy, beneficial relationship, both of you are:

- Able to find healthy ways to work through disagreements together
- Able to make decisions together
- Able to share honest feelings freely and to trust each other
- Able to understand yourself more, not just your partner
- Able to respect one another's feelings and opinions, even if you disagree
- Able to feel comfortable, respected, loved, supported, safe, and secure

What's expressly unhealthy?

- My partner or I set or would like to set all or most of the rules for our relationship.
- My partner is or I am often jealous or possessive.
- My partner follows me around, checks up on me a lot, or insists I check in constantly, even when it's difficult or impossible for me to do; or I do any of these things to them.
- My partner is very concerned with how I look, what I wear, who I spend time with (friends, family, coworkers), and how much time I spend with others; or I have these strong urges to control my partner in these respects. My partner or I may okay some friends or family, but only those who have a blind loyalty to my partner or me, or friends and family who are loyal to only one of us.
- I hide things that I think would upset or anger my partner (phone numbers, letters, photos); or they feel the need to do so with me.
- Either my partner or I don't talk about parents' or friends' objections to or worries about our relationship, or we are afraid to disagree with each other—even about the small stuff—or talk about problems in the relationship.
- My partner yells, calls me names, puts me down, accuses me of things I have not done, or seems to always have something negative to say about me, my family, or friends; or I do so to them.

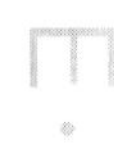

you're thinking and feeling as you go, making the whole process more gradual rather than sudden.

It's normal to take some time to think through a potential breakup by yourself or with your support system of friends before bringing up the possibility to a partner. But once you *are* considering it in earnest, don't hold off too long before telling your boyfriend or girlfriend. There's a difference between a breakup and a trip to the dumps. Ideally, breakups should happen jointly and be a process because they affect both people, so both get to make choices.

There are some exceptions to that ideal: If your partner is very dependent, codependent, emotionally unstable, or abusive, you may find that a gradual, cooperative approach to breakup doesn't work. If, for instance, you've tried to talk about a split

- I feel as if no matter what I do, it isn't enough to earn my partner's attention, approval, support, or love; or my partner feels that way about me.
- I am or my partner is afraid to say no to sex in general, to refuse sexual activities one of us likes but the other does not, or to ask for things that one of us likes, wants, or needs sexually.
- I or my partner refuses to use birth control or safer sex practices.
- My partner threatens me or has threatened me, my property, pets, friends, or family; or I have done so to my partner.
- My partner has, or I have, a bad temper and/or major mood swings.
- My partner hits, throws, or breaks things when angry and/or has pushed, hit, grabbed, restrained, or otherwise physically hurt me; or I have done such to them.
- I feel that my partner's anger is my fault and/or feel that, if I change or behave a certain way, they will behave differently; or my partner feels this way about me.
- I have or my partner has an exit plan for when it gets "really bad."

The behaviors above are often parts of a dangerous or abusive relationship; if you find you nodded a "yes" to at least a couple of them—and certainly if you found even more—you have sound reasons to be concerned or to start getting concerned if you aren't already. Control and abuse most often escalates and becomes constant. Even if, for example, emotional or verbal abuse does not escalate to physical or sexual abuse, those abuses are still harmful and unhealthy and are still abuses, not healthy behaviors that are parts of a healthy relationship. But in most cases, emotional or verbal abuse does escalate to physical or sexual abuse. So, even if you're thinking, "Well, they at least aren't hitting me," or "They haven't raped me. They just call me names and pressure me," know that, sadly, in time those things commonly will happen with someone who is in any way abusive.

For more information on identifying, responding to, and dealing with the impacts of abuse, see Chapter 11.

with a partner again and again and they just won't hear you or they beg and plead and simply refuse to let you end the relationship, you may just have to handle it on your own. Make clear you're done—this isn't the time for pussyfooting about; you need to be very, very clear—and ignore phone calls for some time, or call on friends or family to help mediate.

It may not be safe for you alone to discuss a breakup with or make a split from an abusive or volatile partner. If you at all think that they may harm or try to harm you in any way if you discuss a breakup or even tell them it's happening instead of keeping quiet until you can get out of there, trust your instincts. If your safety is at risk, the usual rules do not apply. You may need to make the split with little fanfare or warning, with safeguards in place. For example, break up in public and let your family know not to let this person in your house later, or tell school or job authorities your intentions to make a break.

The Mourning After

There's no one way to process a breakup. A breakup is a loss, even when it's a wanted or accepted loss, and grieving with a breakup is as personal and individual as with any other kind of loss. Even people who were together for years and who had loads in common will often process a breakup differently, and of course, it also depends on how a specific relationship and breakup went. Some people need lots of time alone; others need extra time with family or friends. Usually, after a breakup, we're whacked with a bevy of mixed feelings. You may find you miss your ex and are happy they're gone at the same time, that you're sad and sappy and pissed off all at once. Honoring and accepting those feelings—all of them, recognizing that none of them are right or wrong, they just are what they are—in constructive ways is important. If you need to cry for a few days solid, do it. If you need to sit with friends and kvetch about every stinky thing your ex ever did, that's just fine. Expressing yourself and your feelings in ways that work for you—via creative writing or playing music, for example—is a great help. Try throwing yourself into things you usually enjoy and find satisfaction in, such as sports, research, work, chores, and hobbies. Putting our feelings into some kind of tangible form and using them to fuel us in some way helps keep them from eating us alive or getting us stuck in them.

Trying to push all of your feelings away or deny them is not dealing. Certainly, you can't be processing all of the time; other aspects of your life need your time and attention, and they may be a needed comfort or distraction. But make sure you're taking at least *some* time to work through what you need to and to just feel how you feel, without having to pretend you're happy or okay all the time. It's okay not to be okay.

Sometimes, breakups come after a very long time of knowing things are over or heading that way. So, when they finally do happen, you may already have processed your upset, or you may just feel relieved. If you had emotional investment in a relationship, but feel you have *zero* processing to do, it may just come later. But overall, there's no rule that, postbreakup, everyone has to be seriously depressed or upset.

After a breakup, it's also common for friends or family to express that they're not sure about your feelings or how you're managing them. They may think you should move on more quickly, stop crying at a certain point, or even be more upset than you are. Sometimes, people will butt in that way because it just hurts to see you, someone they care about, suffering. But they may also be projecting, assuming you should feel how they have felt or wish they did after a breakup. Sometimes, even when you've been in a relationship for only a very short time, a

POSTBREAKUP BEHAVIOR THAT JUST ISN'T HEALTHY

- You show up at their house, dorm, locker, or on their social media, even if they've made clear they aren't comfortable with that and want you to leave them alone. You keep texting or calling when they've asked you to stop or are obviously setting you on ignore. You use technology or other ways to keep an eye on them and not let them separate from you. These are all forms of harassment and stalking.

- You threaten suicide or harm to yourself or them, their friends, family, or property. That is a form of emotional abuse.

- You cannot, even a couple of weeks later, keep it together to do any of the things you normally enjoy or to cope with your normal daily life and responsibilities.

- You engage in forms of self-harm, such as self-mutilation, drug or alcohol abuse, or knowingly dangerous sexual behavior. You truly do not feel that you can go on, weeks after the breakup, and are sincerely worried about your survival.

- You try to sabotage their friendships, dates, or other current relationships, or you deliberately spread lies or half-truths about them to make them look bad. That is emotional abuse and harassment.

- You would take them back in two seconds, on *any* terms at all, or no matter how badly they've treated you.

- You lie or manipulate them to try to get them to come back, or to keep them from breaking up with you, by feigning illness or pregnancy, for example, or threatening self-destructive behavior, using blackmail, making promises you know you can't keep, or agreeing to things that don't work for you (like agreeing to an FWB, when you really only want a serious relationship).

If any of this sounds like you or someone you have just had a breakup with, reach out to a friend, trusted adult, or family member (*not* your ex—you two are done); be honest, and ask for help. If all else fails, and you or an ex are just completely off the map in terms of healthy behavior, call in serious reinforcements; parents and school counselors can be of great help in these sorts of situations. If feelings of shame are keeping you from asking for that kind of help when you need it, do your very best to just ask anyway, even while you're feeling like that, so that you can get safe, and then resolve those feelings later when your safety is no longer at risk. ■■

breakup feels as huge as one of a much longer and deeper relationship, and that can be tough for others to understand. Set clear limits and boundaries with others if you need to.

Of course, you'll probably want to tell most advice like this to stuff it if you've just had a breakup. That's normal, too. You can always come back to it later.

CLOSE THE GATE WHEN YOU LEAVE

Closure is important when something comes to an end. So, it's normal for exes, either after a breakup or in the midst of one, to want to talk out all of their feelings as they tie things up. That may include making plans and room for a friendship during or after or saying things that were left unsaid. Or, sometime after a breakup, you may just want to write a letter or have coffee with an ex and talk about things you've figured out or residual issues you feel bad about or want to understand better. Often, especially when the timing for that feels right for everyone involved (rather than, for example, when people are trying to get that when everyone is still angry or upset with one another), those can be really productive conversations, sometimes even leading to quality, long-term friendships. But in some situations, especially with really bad breakups, you may not be able to, or want to, get resolution with a partner; that's something you may need to do for yourself or with the help of friends, family, or a counselor.

["JUST" FRIENDS?]

In most cases, if you want to be friends with your ex and have that friendship be a good thing for all of you, it's going to take a little time. It's normal for people to need a few weeks or months—sometimes even years—to themselves, sometimes with little or no contact, to process a breakup, let alone start forging a new kind of relationship. If a breakup was very amicable and during your romantic or sexual relationship you also were or grew to be excellent friends, a shift to a friendship that doesn't include sex, romance, or both can be almost instant and really easy. But having the kinds of relationships in which all that is going on and we're really doing breakups well often takes time to learn, and often there are extra circumstances to deal with—such as anyone starting to date someone new immediately after a breakup, and someone right in your social circle, no less. So, chances are it's going to be at least a little more—sometimes a lot more—challenging to shift to friendship.

After some time has passed, as far as developing a friendship goes, you have to feel and work this stuff out together, and it's normal for it to be touch and go for a while or for certain subjects or places to be off limits (their new boyfriend or girlfriend or places associated with sexual or romantic experiences you had together). You may hit snags now and then, like you can with any friend where your stuff together is big or has a lot of history. Some issues that were problematic in your romantic relationship may also continue to be issues in your friendship, and you may or may not be able to work them out any better than you did as partners. Sometimes shifting to a platonic friendship turns out to be exactly the kind of relationship you are great together in; sometimes no kind of relationship is a good one.

A lot of people say or decide they want to be "just" friends, often as a consolation prize, as if a romantic or sexual relationship were automatically better than platonic friendship. Really, it's not, even if our culture presents it that way (and it most often does). All relationships are different, and what type they are doesn't dictate their quality. People who weren't very good together as lovers can turn out to have a far better relationship as friends. If you've known the person you were with for a while, you probably already *do* have a friendship as part of your existing, albeit changing, relationship.

The cornerstone and hallmark of *any* kind of healthy, rich, and enduring relationship *is* friendship, so if anyone tells you that's not important or that friendships aren't as big a deal or as intimate, know they either sadly haven't had important friendships in their lives yet or particularly rich romantic or sexual relationships or they're just not seeing through the fog of some of our world's most idiotic ways of presenting and talking about people and our most important values. Above all else, learning to cultivate friendship and how to be and have a friend—even with exes, regardless of whether they end up as your best friends and family or as casual, friendly acquaintances—are beyond valuable.

8

To Be, or Not to Be . . . Sexually Active

What we're talking about over the next few chapters is **sex with other people and how to figure out and make your own best choices if and when you're going to be sexual with someone else.** Because the definition of what sex even *is* can be so confusing, let's make this one clear: ***sex with a partner is consensually engaging in sexual activities with someone else.***

Consensual means *everyone* involved wants, is asking for, and is giving a glad hells-yes to any sexual activities, without pressure, obligation, or ambivalence—and with a pretty good idea of what they're getting into. Sexual, in the way I'm using it here, simply means something a person is actively and intentionally engaging in with someone else with the aim of expressing and exploring their sexuality.

A potential or current partner might be someone you call your girlfriend or boyfriend, but they also could be your best friend, an acquaintance, a spouse, a fiancé, or a casual hookup.

Consensual sex with partners is about everyone involved **freely and willingly engaging in close contact with each other, often (but not always) including genital contact, usually with the shared aim of experiencing pleasure or expressing or exploring sexuality.** That can be a make-out session, fingering or a hand job, sharing a sexual fantasy, oral sex, vaginal intercourse, anal play (or even just showing someone your naked butt), mutual masturbation, massage, or tech sex. Some of those, none of those, or all of those—and things not even in that very short list—may or may not have great importance or relevance to you. They may or may not be a "rite of passage" for you and yours the first time you do them or the 267th time you do.

From a healthcare and harm-reduction standpoint, sex is any of the activities that often is sexual and also poses known physical or mental health risks. When we're talking about sexual health, it really doesn't matter whether someone experienced something as sexual or not or calls something sexual or not. In a medical context, it just matters whether something *can* be sexual, or often is sexual, and *also* has a healthcare component or possible health impact.

Only you can assign a given value or importance to what you do and who you do it with. You can define *sex* for yourself, and only you can even really come up with your own lived-experience, just-your-own-self definition of what being sexual is for you. Only we can define, for ourselves, what is or isn't an expression of our sexuality, over time and in general or at any one specific time. That's why we can't tell someone else what is or isn't an expression of *their* sexuality; just because something is an expression of our sexuality or something we feel is a superbig deal doesn't mean it is for someone else. That's all very individual.

But those bigger umbrella definitions of sex and sexual activity all include things that, if we're going to be part of them, we should give real thought to (and not just when we're young!). We must do the best we can to make informed choices that are most likely to be good for us and everyone involved.

We automatically do this kind of intentional and careful decision making about other things, like driving a car, for example. Driving can be fun and go just fine, but it also could be bad news in any number of ways and even do a considerable amount of harm, especially if we aren't all thoughtful, careful, and wise. Most people think that's a no-brainer. Thinking about sex like this should be, too. You (might) want to take a ride with someone, but you probably don't want it to end by running into a tree.

Let's face it: many people don't give their sexual choices enough thought. It's more common for people to give a lot of

Later on in the book (Chapter 11), we'll talk a lot more about how any kind of sexual abuse or assault might be (or might not be) sex for the person doing the abusing or assaulting. For the person or people being abused or assaulted, it's rarely sex. Just like how someone whose backpack was stolen isn't likely to consider themselves as having participated in gift-giving but instead considers themselves as having been robbed, the same goes here. So, if you are reading this and are a survivor of sexual abuse or assault—as so many of us are—figure that unless you yourself want to call and consider any of that sex for you, sexual abuse or assault isn't what we're talking about here. This is about sex that's consensual and wanted by everyone involved.

"It"

What is "it" all about? "It" is often common cultural shorthand for whatever sexual activity we've decided (or our peers, partners, culture, or community has decided) is *the* rite of sexual passage or *the* activity that means, to us or others, that we have become or are being sexually active. Often, "doing it" is assumed to mean penis-in-vagina intercourse, and the first time we do "it" is almost always supposed to be a profound rite of passage and a Very, Very Big Deal.

But. (And it's a really big one.) Not everyone is heterosexual or has sexual partners for which those two sets of parts are at play, whether the people involved have those parts or not. Not everyone is interested in having intercourse—for some people, not right now or not today; for others, not ever. And for plenty of people, a sexual activity or experience they felt was *their* rite of passage may not have been intercourse, or there may not have been one Big Partnered Sex Thing at all. There may have been several "its," and there may be more to come: in a sexual life someone can really enjoy, explore, and grow with, there really should be.

Some people later realize that their big sexual rites of passage didn't even happen in their teens—even if they were sexually active then. Some adults, even those who have been sexually active for years, are still *waiting* for a One Big Thing. Some feel that there really isn't one important or cornerstone partnered activity at all but that their sexual rites of passage were the first time they had an orgasm with masturbation; how they felt about sex or their sexual selves; a relationship they were or are in; or doing things to sexually empower themselves, such as their first sexual healthcare exam, the first time they laid out all of their limits or boundaries confidently and held all of their own lines, or the first time they were honest with a partner about what they really wanted sexually.

With anything this hazy and loaded, it often pays to redefine things as much as we can, to try to think about things in new ways, and to define them for ourselves. That's especially helpful with something as incredibly individual and personal as sex.

For now, let's not make a big deal out of "it."

thought to their "first time" but far less to many of their sexual choices before *or* after. That's hardly ideal. Also, it's not the way to create or build a healthy, safe, and satisfying sex life. Given the level of sexual dissatisfaction, lack of communication, ignorance, and all-around screwed-up-ness running amok when it comes to sex, it's pretty clear that that *common* approach just isn't working very well. Almost all of us could use a renovation in terms of the way we think about our sexual choices and how we make them, no matter our age or level of experience.

For sure, the first few sexual choices we make *are* often very important and worth taking time to consider. And, yes, here's hoping your first few times with any sexual activity will be great. But *all* the sexual choices we make are important and worth taking time to consider, and *all* of our sexual experiences can be great (the fact is, over time, they usually are more often, not the other way around) and watershed in any number of ways. That's important, not just to protect you and others from trauma or other serious undesired outcomes but to enable you to have a sexual life that's much better and that has more layers than "not bad," or "not risky," or "not painful"—that's as *excellent as it can be*. After all, if the very best we could hope for from sex with partners was that it didn't suck or mess up our whole lives, it would be pretty bonkers to be part of it at all. Especially because sex is something completely optional and not having it causes no harm to anyone.

Sex shouldn't just be about avoiding bad sex or harm but should ideally also *be good and beneficial.*

When you decide to start being sexually active—what's called your "sexual debut" in public health and sex education—*is* a pretty big decision, because stepping onto that path does dictate some things you may need to be responsible for, have as part of your life, or manage from that point on, such as preventative sexual health care, including contraception and safer sex practices and supplies, and managing sexual relationships, by themselves and with the rest of your life. You can always choose to have any kind of sex with a partner once and never again—with them or period. You can even engage in sexual partnerships for a while and then never have another sexual partner again, ever. So, although some things only come into play if you become and stay sexually active, others are factors ever after, with more sex or not.

When you are at the point where you're making choices about sex with partners, start with the Sexual Readiness Checklist (page 186). If just looking at that list makes you dizzy or freaked out, that's a feeling to pay attention to: if you feel that way when faced with the simple realities of being sexual with others, now's probably a bad time to become sexually active. If you find yourself rationalizing why you don't need half the stuff on that list, or why it's unimportant, you're probably rushing or in some big denial about what healthy and happy partnered sex requires. If you flipped right past it and feel you have no need to look at it at all, you are seriously kidding yourself, even if you already *are* sexually active. If, in going through the list, you find you already have most of those things in hand or in mind, then you're probably in really good shape in terms of readiness.

We're not going to miss out on a good sexual opportunity if it's not actually a good sexual opportunity. In other words, if all or most of the things that make sex likely to be good aren't there, what we're probably missing out on if we don't take that opportunity is a crummy or so-so experience, not a great one. Sex that people experience as good and sex that we all feel good about usually tend to happen only when we're in the right headspace for it, when we have the things we need, when we don't feel pressured or rushed to make a choice too quickly, when whatever sort of relationship we're in supports sound sexual and emotional health and well-being, and when our wants and needs align pretty closely with our partner's.

Text continues on page 188

THE SEXUAL READINESS CHECKLIST

Material Stuff

■ I have a safer sex kit (see page 298), including several up-to-date, quality condoms and/or other safer sex barriers, lubricant, and any other basic safety items for the activity or activities I want to engage in, and my partner or partners and I each know how to use them and are comfortable using them.

■ For any activity with possible pregnancy risks, I have a single or combined method of birth control (which can include condoms) if my partner or I want to prevent pregnancy (see Chapter 12).

■ I know where to find and how to contact a local sexual health clinic or my existing sexual or general healthcare provider.

■ I have at least some money I can access easily and use at any time (ideally "some" is a couple hundred bucks, but you have what you have), and I have funds for a "sex budget" of at least $50 a month to take care of birth control, safer sex items, and annual testing and sexual health care, including having to treat or manage a potential sexually transmitted infection (STI) or pregnancy. If I don't have that, I *do* have free or cheaper ways to access all of these things; I am covered under a healthcare plan or service that can cover (if applicable) pregnancy, neonatal care, gynecological visits, STI testing, and birth control via public health care or clinic care; or I have the funds or means to pay for these services, even when I need them very quickly.

Body and Health

■ I am ready to soon begin, or have already begun, any needed annual sexual and general health care and exams and disease and infection screenings (see Chapter 10). The same is true of my partner.

■ I understand and am familiar with my own anatomy and my partner's basic anatomy (see Chapter 2) as well as the basics of the sexual activity I want to participate in, STIs, and human reproduction (if applicable).

■ I can tell when I'm feeling sexual desire and when I'm sexually aroused and when I'm not; I have some idea about what I need to feel desire and be aroused, and I can comfortably communicate when I am not wanting something or am not aroused. I feel my partner can say the same.

■ I can relax and feel comfortable during sexual activities without a level of fear, anxiety, or shame that I don't feel I can manage.

■ I feel confident that my partner and I clearly understand the possible risks of any sexual activities we may choose to take part in and that we know how to minimize them and are ready to take care of ourselves by reducing the risks that we can.

Relationship Requirements

■ My partner and I understand what consent is (see pages 192–199), and I feel confident that we are each able to give full informed consent to the activity or activities we're going to engage in. I am able, and gladly willing, to engage in mutual, active, and meaningful consenting with my partners (see pages 192–199).

■ I am able to set limits (to say no or even just "not that way but this way") when I want to and hold those lines for myself with someone else; I can trust my partner to easily respect them at all times, and vice versa (see page 191).

■ I can assess what I want for myself and separate it from what my partner, friends, or family want, and I feel my partner can do the same.

■ I trust my partner, and I know myself to be trustworthy.

■ I feel I can tell my partner what I want and need sexually and emotionally and when I do and do not like something, and I feel able to hear and respect them when they do the same.

■ I can talk to my partner about sex, in or out of bed, and can be honest and clear when I do, and I feel they can do the same with me.

■ I have basic respect for my partner: I care about my partner's health, emotions, and general well-being, and I behave accordingly; I know that my partner cares about mine and shows that care in their actions and sexual behavior.

■ My partner and I have already discussed most of these issues together, in advance of sexual activity.

Emotional Items

■ If my partner or I have any strong religious, cultural, ethical, political, or family beliefs or convictions that pose serious conflicts to any kind of sexual activity, we have evaluated, discussed, and resolved them (see page 200).

■ I can and will take responsibility for my own emotions, expectations, and actions, and I know my partner can and will do the same, even when that is difficult, makes me feel embarrassed, or creates conflict.

■ I can handle being disappointed, confused, or upset about sex, and I am prepared to handle a partner's disappointment, confusion, or upset well (see page 204).

■ I have some people I trust and can count on with whom I can talk about sex, and I can go to them for emotional support and for help when I am in a jam, and I know that my partner also has a support system like that.

■ I understand that sex and love aren't the same thing, and I do not seek to have sex to use it to manipulate or harm myself, my partner, or anyone else. I feel my partner's sexual motives are sound, safe, and realistic as well.

■ The partner I am considering being sexual with does not abuse me, and I do not abuse them (see Chapter 11).

■ I feel confident neither of us is entering into a sexual situation that is likely to be emotionally unsafe or harmful for either of us or more than either of us can probably handle (see Chapter 11).

■ I feel my partner and I both understand that sexual activity may change our relationship in any number of ways (ways that are great or ways that suck), and we feel we can handle and accept whatever may (or may not) happen.

■ I feel I can emotionally handle a possible pregnancy, disease or infection, or rejection from my partner, and I feel my partner can handle these things as well. ■■

[**GREAT SEXPECTATIONS**]

A day rarely passes when we're not exposed to at least one—often limited or oversimplified—message about what sex is, what it's supposed to be, how great it is (or not), how important it is (or not), or how big a part of our lives it should be (or not). Those messages are often biased, strongly flavored by the person doling them out, intentionally or not. A friend going on about her sex life can exaggerate or report enjoyment that wasn't really there to make herself or her partner look good or feel better—or, if it wasn't great, to signal she's worried something is wrong with her. Someone preaching about the apocalyptic dangers of sex may be inflating or misrepresenting the risks based on their own moral agenda or their own experiences of sex. A film may show us totally unrealistic sex or sexual relationships just because it suits the plot.

Our fantasies about and expectations of sex or our sexual lives are often far from our realities or realistic possibilities. (They also sometimes aren't even healthy, such as romanticizing having no say or jealous rage.) Expecting sex to be like what we see in the movies or popular culture is unrealistic, and thinking it's made of magic is an error. In real life, it's quite a good deal different. In the movies, for instance, rarely do we see a couple taking care of their sexual health with regular exams and testing, which a sexually active person has to do to keep themselves and their partners physically and emotionally well. In the movies, rarely do we see "quiet" orgasms or sex that's neither awful nor earth shattering. In the movies and in popular literature, rarely do we see the full spectrum of anyone's sex life or sexual relationships and all the many, many issues that must be dealt with. Rarely do we see boring, unhappy endings to sexual conflicts or see them without someone involved being

NEW PERSPECTIVES

When you're thinking about becoming sexually active, it can be helpful to talk to people you trust and respect who became sexually active around the same age you are or in the same sort of environment or set of circumstances as yours. Although their experiences may not be identical, listening to others' feelings about their early sexual experiences and choices is often helpful when making your own decisions: you can be reminded of some possible positive and negative outcomes, including some you may not have thought about, and get a sense of how you feel about them.

Young people and older people often have a big disconnect when talking about this stuff. Often, neither party actually listens very well to the other. But nobody has to agree; we just need to listen and to be heard. Parents, guardians, or other adults can be good people to talk with about sex. They have valuable perspectives, just like you do, and potentially good help to offer. They're people, too, who often went through the same things and who have some hindsight you don't yet, even if you don't feel the same way or draw the same conclusions. For more on talking to parents and other potentially supportive adults, see pages 380–381.

made out to be a jerk just by virtue of merely being human. Rarely do we see couples taking a long, slow time, and with reasonable conversation and kindness, to wade through issues—instead, we usually see colossal fights, huge dramas, or stormy, wailing breakups, all within the span of an hour or two max. Rarely do we see average-looking people with average-looking bodies, people who have emotional needs (as people do) and who communicate realistically—which often includes a lot of awkwardness and unsexy talk—about sex. So, if you base your expectations on things like movies, books, porn, or friends' accounts of their relationships, you're bound to end up feeling confused, lost, or disappointed, and you will likely find it hard to stay grounded in your very real relationships and sexuality and deal with them appropriately.

It's not uncommon for our expectations of partnered sex to end up having little or no resemblance to what we actually experience. Those surprises can run the gamut: there will probably be things we expected to be better, and things we enjoyed more than we expected to. You may even find that what happens *does* meet your expectations to the letter. We're all unique, our expectations are all unique, and so is the sex we have.

Get Real: Unrealistic Expectations and Scenarios

Although sex with others potentially has a lot to offer, sex can't do some things:

- Sex with someone cannot give us enduring self-worth, self-esteem, or long-term positive body image.
- Partnered sex cannot substitute for our own exploration or understanding of our bodies.
- Engaging in sex, by itself, cannot give us reliable information about sex outside our own unique experiences or about sexual health.
- Sex in and of itself cannot provide love or emotional affection, friendship, support, relationship commitment, or security.
- Sex cannot substitute for other kinds of communication.
- Sex is not the magic key to being thought of or considered an adult or mature; it cannot magically beam anyone out of adolescence and into adulthood (sorry).
- Sex doesn't have to be painful or scary, a first time or any time after.

You might find it helpful to make a list of your expectations—it's easier to find out what they are when we take them out of our head and let them see the light of day. Jot down some things you expect: sexually, physically, emotionally, in terms of your relationship, in terms of your whole life. Let yourself write the whole range of your expectations, from the stuff you feel is pretty realistic to your ultimate ideals and worst nightmares, and even the stuff you think or know is just silly. Just get it all out there so you can have a good look and be self-aware. A list like that can also help you bring those expectations to the table when you and your partner talk about being sexually active. No need to show up on a date with the whole thing printed out and a dotted line for them to sign on—having the general gist in your head will do just fine.

A good deal of what we expect includes some of our basic wants and needs. For instance, if you expect to spend time together after sex, snuggling and talking, you can figure out how important that is to you: Is it essential, or would it be okay if that didn't happen? Is it something you need to tell a potential partner that you need? If you expect a certain pace or certain activities, are those wants or needs? Once you've got that list, you can go through it and get a pretty good handle on your basic wants and needs even if when it all happens you find you don't need all the things you thought you would or that you want things you didn't expect to.

REGRETS, WE'VE HAD A FEW.

A big worry many young people have about becoming sexually active is that it will be the wrong choice, with the wrong person, or at the wrong time. There are lots of people who regret their early sexual choices. (There are also lots of people who don't.) There are many reasons why regret might come into play, from the obvious (something unwanted, unexpected, or traumatic happened) to the not-so-obvious (they feel regret simply because they assume another choice could have been better). Sometimes, those worries are based on age (*Is this too young? Is that too old?*). Although age can be part of the equation, often it, too, is really an issue of expectations. Some studies have found that the younger a person is, the more unrealistic their sexual expectations are likely to be. If your expectations of sex are really inflated or unrealistic, don't be too surprised when you do have it that it doesn't measure up. And given that the sex we have later is often better than our first experiences with sex, it's also not surprising that many people feel the sex they had later "should" have been the sex they had first.

Do know that a whole life lived without *any* regret is awfully unlikely. As you may know from that time someone's grandpa showed up at karaoke, Frank Sinatra had a few regrets, but what he felt was important was that (more, much more than this) he did it his way. The best any of us can ever do is make the best choices we can, and in this area of life, like any other, when those choices are about what really feels like our own rightest way at the time, based on our own circumstances—like we're living our lives *our* way. If we do that, like Frank, we'll probably only have a few, too.

MYTH BUSTING

Mindfulness and intuition are your pals in the choice of when to start having sex. Learn to listen to yourself and trust your own authority and sense of self. If your head or your gut says "not just yet," pay attention. If you feel that you have to hurry up and make a choice, remember that if you don't feel "Yes!" instead of "Er . . . I guess so," the best decision is usually to wait and give it some real thought. But if it all feels really right right now—including all the stuff on your checklist, not just the stuff in your heart or between your legs—it probably is time. When you're doing a good job of listening to them, you really can trust yourself and your gut feelings whether you like what they're telling you or not.

No Harm, No Foul: Limits and Boundaries

Your wants and needs determine many of your limits and boundaries. This can be a tricky area to navigate when you're new to sexual partnership, because it's common to have a better handle on all this stuff when you've been sexually active for some time. It's hard to know all of the limits and boundaries we want or need when we haven't had a lot of—or any—experience to find out. Plenty of people don't figure out good limits and boundaries for themselves for decades. For obvious reasons, setting boundaries and limits can be especially difficult for anyone raised in a way where they've gotten the idea they're not allowed to have them, such as people raised as girls and women and people who grew up living with abuse. So, in terms of having certain areas of your body touched or engaging in certain activities, you may find that you just don't know all of your general limits and boundaries yet and that your feelings change as you go—often they vary from day to day, partner to partner, and life phase to life phase.

Many limits and boundaries tend to shift and adapt as we grow and change. Different issues and different relationships and interactions prompt different limits and boundaries to come up. Because communication is the order of the day in sexual partnership, so long as we all keep talking and keep those windows of opportunity open, we can keep our partners in the loop, even if all we're saying is, "I'm not sure how I feel about doing this right now for some reason, but I'll keep you posted when I've thought about it more," or "I don't know if I'll be okay with that kind of sex or not, but I want to try and see, and will let you know how it is for me once we try it."

We can know and establish some limits and boundaries in advance. You probably, for instance, have a good idea of how "far" you want to go in terms of the sexual activities with someone and the risks you're willing to take in regard to safer sex or contraception. Those are limits. There may be lines you won't or don't want to

WANT. NEED. HUH?

The difference between a want and a need is that a need is usually nonnegotiable. Going without what we just *want* can sure suck and be disappointing, but it's not likely to be traumatic. Going without what we *need* can be traumatic, especially in situations like partnered sex, where we're very vulnerable and the risks can run high.

Divide and conquer. Figure out which is which. Try not to make exceptions with your needs; it's almost never worth it. Talk about them and your wants with your partner, and listen to their wants and needs. When it comes to needs, make sure everyone's can be met. If they really can't, and they are very much needs, try to get a sense of whether they might be met with someone else later (and until then, you put a hold on doing anything where those needs can't be met) or whether with a given partner or situation it is really unlikely those needs will ever be met, now or later. It sucks, but if your needs—again, not *wants* but *needs,* as in nonnegotiable—can't be met, you may have to change a relationship or nix sex with someone.

cross, such as having sex in public, having penis-in-vagina intercourse without birth control, or having certain parts of your anatomy looked at with a magnifying glass and a flashlight during sex. Those are boundaries. Again, as time goes on, you can adapt, erase, or add to those as need be, and you probably will. But you'll always want to keep both in mind and express both when you're making or negotiating sexual choices.

[CONSENTING]

If you're going to be sexual with another person, you have many variables to consider, but there's one thing everyone has to be on board with **no matter what:** active, meaningful, and mutual consenting.

Active, meaningful, and mutual consenting is about always asking or checking in with each other, not just doing sexual things to each other and then seeing how the other person reacts. Just doing something to someone first and only *then*—if then!—checking in is like taking someone's phone, making a bunch of calls, and only then asking, "Is it okay if I use your phone?" That wouldn't even be okay with a phone, let alone someone's body.

Consent is about reaching and being in agreement about which things we want to do or explore with others sexually and *how* we want to do or explore those things. It's also about what we don't want to do and how we don't want to do something. Those things may be physical activities such as kissing, manual sex, or intercourse or may be things such as sending or sharing sexual texts, using (or not using) safer sex methods or contraception, or whether we're okay with the words someone wants to use for our body parts.

It's about our limits and boundaries—our no's or not-that-way's—as well as our wants and desires—our yesses and our I-can-haz-more-of-that-oh-pretty-pleases. It's about *everyone* involved in any given sexual interaction or potential sexual interaction—about everyone, not just one person.

Consent isn't something we negotiate or give only once; it's something we're doing throughout sexual activity. If someone consents to one thing, that doesn't mean they're consenting to anything else, just to that one thing, at that one time, in that one way or context. Consent is *always* something we or others can revoke. Everyone always has the absolute right to change their mind, at any time, including after they've already said yes.

Also, consent is only meaningful (including from a legal standpoint) when we and others can truly give it freely. We can't consent sometimes, such as when we are asleep, intoxicated, in severe physical or emotional distress, feel we may be harmed if we don't (duress), or don't even understand what someone else is asking us to do with them in the first place.

Active consenting is a shared responsibility of *everyone* engaging in or who wants to engage in any kind of sexual interaction. And consent is only meaningful if it isn't coerced. Coercion is when someone says yes or otherwise gives consent to go along with something not because they want to but because they are talked or otherwise pushed into it or they have been made to feel that they don't have a right to say no. Coercion is not consent.

With meaningful, enthusiastic consent, we can all make and voice any choice without feeling forced, manipulated, intentionally misled, or pressured. It means we're in an interpersonal environment where what we want is mutually valued. It means we are in a situation where the other person does not have radically more power than we have and is not using any power they do have to influence or guide our sexual choices. It means we and our partners feel and truly are safe for each other. It means we feel able to say and accept yes, no, or maybe without fear and that our limits and boundaries are completely respected. Feeling free and able to say yes and to say no isn't only important to keep from getting hurt or hurting others; it's also important because a big part of a satisfying, healthy sex life and sexuality is grounded in free choice. Meaningful, enthusiastic consent makes any kind of sex much more likely to only ever be something we really, really want: we don't tend to enjoy things much, if at all, that we're made or choose to be part of when we don't want to.

If you want one word to define what consent is, whether we're giving it or getting it, **it's YES.** Consent is yes a million times over, for the love of all things sparkly, awesome, and delicious, and not a minute longer if you want to do it too, please, **YES.** Everyone's yes doesn't always look or sound the same, of course, but there are often common threads. A yes with words is a lot easier to understand and recognize than some other kinds of yes. But there isn't always a question, exactly, to say yes to. Sometimes it's just saying what we want. Sometimes yes is inviting someone else to do something with us. Sometimes yes is using hands to pull someone closer or voicing an excited squeal or moan.

It's potentially all those things, for *all* the people. When it's really not, for anyone, then we're not involved in consensual sex anymore; we're either part of abuse or on the very slippery slope to it.

Consenting might seem like a big duh; if it does to you, know it unfortunately isn't so obvious to everyone. A lot of people have had experiences when someone hasn't first asked them about doing something to or that involves them before doing it—like giving a hug, moving a piece of hair out of their face, or making plans for them without checking in with them. Many also have had experiences when they haven't felt free or allowed to answer as they'd like when people have asked something of them. As children, a lot of our lives involved people doing things to us without asking or against our will, whether it was Grandma Marge kissing us on the lips when we really didn't want her to or someone making decisions that are about us without asking for our input, like switching us to a different school without giving us any say. Too, we have a whole lot of historical precedent of situations that didn't recognize a need for consent or that set the standards for consent so low as to allow a great amount of sexual abuse and assault to be unrecognized, disbelieved, or dismissed.

So, it's not surprising that when it comes to sex and consent, more people seem to have trouble understanding, accepting, feeling a right to, or having

What Are Some Clues Someone Doesn't Care About Consent?

When someone doesn't care about consent, they may act like they're in a big hurry. They may act like you or others owe them sex or they owe you sex. They're not asking how you're feeling or what you want; they seem only or mostly focused on themselves or they are *only* focused on you and seem to have none of their own desires or limits. They can act like you, as a whole person separate from them, aren't actually there. They're ignoring or trying to change some of your stop signs, such as pushing them away, not wanting to get naked, saying you're not sure, or saying no. You may feel unsafe or worried, are unable to speak up or say no, or worry they're unsafe or can't speak up. They can react with anger, resentment, or self-injury when you don't immediately say yes to sex. They don't seem to have personal boundaries or care about yours.

If any of those things are going on, do yourself a favor and just get away from that person or situation pronto. If you were wrong, it's okay —no one is done any harm by *not* getting laid.

any idea how to actively do meaningful, mutual consenting. Legal and social definitions of what constitutes meaningful consent and what constitutes abuse or assault have been changing in a good way: more people and social systems are recognizing that a lack of a no isn't a yes and that real-deal consent is a must for people to have an emotionally and interpersonally healthy and truly satisfying sexual life.

[A (NOT SO) BASIC CONSENT HOW-TO]

Consent works best centered in communication using words, in whatever language everyone involved can communicate with and understand. There are other ways to express and affirm consent, but they're way trickier, and when those ways work well, it's usually because the people involved already use and have used words with consent and have established good, solid patterns of communication with words.

Explicit Consent: Using Words

This Kind of Consent Is a Must With:

- First-time sexual partners
- New relationships or partners
- Someone who is new to sex in general
- Taking the least risk of getting your lines crossed or crossing someone else's lines
- A rekindled sexual relationship, when it's been a while since you were sexual with someone but are again now
- When you know or suspect you have a hard time reading nonverbal cues or that your own nonverbal cues may be tricky for someone else to interpret
- Someone healing from sexual abuse or assault, especially if it was recent

Consent with words is using language to make clear what we want and don't want, what our desires are and are not, and what we do and don't feel ready for and to ask these things of others. Sometimes it's about one person asking for something and the other replying; sometimes it happens in unison.

When we say or express an "I want," we're voicing desire. Desire can be a strong feeling, so we might not always voice it delicately. The way we voice sexual desire matters when it comes to consent, though: we need to be mindful of how our words express what we want while still leaving room for others to express what they want, especially because we won't always want the same things or want them at the same times.

There are ways to voice desires and seek consent that support consent and good sexual communication. And there are ways to voice desires and seek consent that can stifle mutual consent and communication, making it hard for someone to freely consider and voice their own choices in response.

Some Ways to Explicitly Ask for or About and Ensure Consent Is Given Are Questions Like These

- May I [do whatever sexual thing]?
- I'd like to [do whatever sexual thing]. Would you? If not, what would you like to do?
- How do you feel about doing [whatever sexual thing]?
- Are there things you know you don't want to do? What are they? Mine are [whatever they are].
- Is there anything you need to feel comfortable or safe when we do [whatever sexual thing]?

But That's Not Sexy

I'm not going to try to hard-sell anyone on consent, because if consensual sex—not abuse or assault—is what we want, it's a requirement, not an option. I'm also not going to argue with anyone about what they do or don't find sexy. It's not my place, and it's also supertiresome for everyone involved (including me).

Instead, I'll say this: communicating a lot about a thing we are super-into (aka: geeking out) tends to be something people *like* doing and find amplifies how they like and enjoy a thing. As in, "OH MY FREAKING GAWD, this cupcake is *EVERYTHING*. I want to MARRY this cupcake. NOM NOM NOM."

This is also often how it goes with explicit consenting and other clear sexual communication: when people are into what they're doing or want to do together, talking about it only tends to get them more turned on, not less. "But that's not sexy" is a thing more often said about consenting when a sexual experience itself probably isn't going to be all that sexy in the first place. Expressing ourselves with and during sex is part of what makes it clear no one is having sex with a corpse.

If being sexual together is a turn-on, talking about it together probably is, too. If not . . . ***well.*** People also often are reluctant to ask because that gives the other person a bigger opportunity and ability to say no. **It should.** I think we can all agree that, although definitions of sexy may vary, what is never, ever sexy is doing something to or with someone sexually that they do not want to do and that you don't give them a real chance to opt out of or stop.

- I want to do [whatever sexual thing] with you, and it feels like the right time for me. Do you want to do that and does the timing feel right to you?
- I'd like to have sex tonight. Would you? Anything you want to do or try? If you want to have sex, should I also order a pizza now so it can be here for postsex munchies? What kind?

None of this has to be superformal, and no one has to learn to do all of this, for everything sexual under the sun, all at once. Like anything else when it comes to your sexual life, you get to—and should—go at a pace that matches what you are and anyone else involved is ready for.

Just like initial asks, check-ins don't have to be formal or interrupt anything we're enjoying. We can also use moments to check in that may already have presented a pause, such as someone having to pee, the phone ringing, falling off the bed, switching up a position, or a big laugh we're trying to catch our breath from.

Consent check-ins can sound like, *Does this feel good? Still into this? Are you comfortable? Anything you need or want right now? You seem quiet: are you okay? Anything I should stop doing or do that I'm not doing? I feel good: are you feeling good, too?*

Columbia University Health Service's Sexual Violence Prevention and Response Program provides one of my favorite basic ways of thinking about and doing consenting well:

Signs You Should Stop

- You or a partner are too intoxicated to gauge or give consent.
- Your partner is asleep or passed out.
- You hope your partner will say nothing and go with the flow.
- You intend to have sex by any means necessary.

Signs You Should Pause and Talk

- You are not sure what the other person wants.
- You feel like you are getting mixed signals.
- You have not talked about what you want to do.
- You assume that you will do the same thing as before.
- Your partner stops or is not responsive.

Keep Communicating

- Partners come to a mutual decision about how far they want to go.
- Partners clearly express their comfort with the situation.
- You feel comfortable and safe stopping at any time.
- Partners are excited!

Nonexplicit Consent

Over time, people who build trust and become intimate usually feel comfortable using fewer or less frequent consent-in-words and more nonverbal cues or ways of doing consent that aren't explicit. That's generally okay so long as it feels okay to everyone involved, but this way of seeking and trying to suss out consent is a lot trickier. Most words have very clearly defined and pretty universally understood meanings. Body language? Not so much. It's easy to "read" body language and other possible cues wrong and to cross each other's lines because we did.

What Can ***CONSENT*** Sound Like?	What Can ***NONCONSENT*** Sound Like?
Yes	No
I'm sure	I'm not sure
I know I want that	I don't know
I'm so excited	I'm so scared
Don't stop	Stop
WOOHOO!	[total silence]
More!	No more
I want to . . .	I want to, but . . .
I'm not worried	I feel worried about . . .
I want you/it/that	I don't want you/it/that
Can you please do [insert thing to please do here]	Can you please not do [whatever]
I still want to . . .	I thought I wanted to, but . . .
That feels good	That hurts
Mmmmmmmmm	Maybe
HELL YEAH	I love this, but . . .
I love this	I want to do this, but not right now
I want to do this right now	I don't know how I feel about this
I feel good about this	I'm not ready
I'm ready	I'm not sure if I'm ready
I want to keep doing this	I don't want to do this anymore
[Insert praise to your deity of choice here]	This feels wrong
This feels right	

A recent study from the Havens Sexual Assault Referral Centres (*Where Is Your Line? Survey Summary Report*) of more than a thousand people ages eighteen to twenty-five found that fewer than half of young adults interpreted someone pushing them away as a no, and over 60 percent did not assume crying meant nonconsent. That same study found that more than one in five people expect intercourse after other kinds of touching and that 25 percent of women have been silent when a partner did something sexual to them that they did not want.

That's a good example of how unreliable nonverbal "signs" or "signals" of consent can be. Because it's so easy to muck up this way of ascertaining consent, we all need to be cautious about ditching or reducing consent in words and make sure that, before we do, we've established good communication overall and have it as a pattern and precedent we know we can fall back on any time we or a partner is not 100 percent sure we are interpreting or can interpret nonverbal consent correctly. We also want to be sure to still do check-ins with partners during less-talky sex time. And before moving on to this kind of consent, you should be very sure it's really the right situation and relationship to ditch a lot of talking, for you and for a partner: go figure, you decide that by talking together, with words.

This Kind of Consent, Paired with Consent-in-Words, Is Best Saved For

- Longtime sexual partners
- When everyone involved has already had a good deal of sexual experience
- When you and a partner understand that you are taking greater risks of overstepping boundaries and limits, are each okay with that, and are each willing to take good care of each other if signals get crossed
- When you and a partner already communicate nonverbally well in other situations
- When you and a partner each feel *very* confident you can read each other's more subtle cues
- When you have used verbal consent to establish that you're going to start using more nonverbal consent

Some people ask how they can tell by looking when someone is aroused, in part to try to establish nonverbal consent. The trouble is, physical signs of arousal are lousy nonverbal signals of consent. Why? Because even when those things are happening because someone is aroused—and just as often, they're happening for other reasons—someone being aroused doesn't mean someone wants to be sexual or be sexual in the ways someone else does. It really is that simple.

What Can Signal Consent Without Words?

- Direct eye contact
- Initiating sexual activity
- Pulling someone closer
- Actively touching someone
- Nodding yes
- Comfort with nudity
- Laughter and/or smiling (upturned mouth)
- "Open" body language, such as relaxed, loose, and open arms and legs, relaxed facial expressions, turning toward someone
- Sounds of joy, like a satisfied hum or enthusiastic moan
- An active body

What Can Signal *Non*consent Without Words?

- Avoiding eye contact
- Not initiating any sexual activity
- Pushing someone away
- Avoiding touch
- Shaking head no
- Discomfort with nudity
- Crying and/or looking sad or fearful (clenched or downturned mouth)
- "Closed" body language, like tense, stiff, or closed arms and legs, tight or tense facial expressions, turning away from someone

- Silence or sounds of fear or sadness, like whimpering or a trembling voice
- "Just lying there"

The golden rule when it comes to trying to do consenting that isn't in words? If you don't feel about 200 percent sure, switch back to words. It really is that simple.

[ACCEPTING AND RESPECTING NONCONSENT]

Part of being ready for sex related to consenting isn't just about being ready to say yes or no or asking for what we want but also about being ready and willing to hear answers, limits, and boundaries from others we're bummed about.

Everyone knows it can suck when we want something with or from someone else that they don't want to share or give, most certainly including with sex. Sometimes it's just a momentary bummer, and other times it can feel like a real heartbreaker.

But when someone is not clearly giving, sharing, or continuing consent or is nonconsenting, there's only one sound way we should all respond: to absolutely accept and respect their response or their lack of agreement and participation and to immediately stop the action (if something physical was going on) or not move forward. Although we are allowed to *have* whatever feelings we have, it's really important we manage and express our own feelings appropriately, avoiding things like voicing anger, sulking, or emotionally withdrawing, which puts sexual pressure on someone else.

We may need or want to work through our feelings and theirs (they can be bummed out, too!). That might be sensitively—not manipulatively—asking for some time to ourselves to clear our heads and cool down our heart rate, and then calling each other later to check in and assure each other it's all okay. Maybe we'll need to have the other person affirm that they still like us. You can ask if they want to do something to share some comfort or to get close in other ways, such as having a cuddle, holding hands, or doing something else entirely, like taking a walk together, catching a movie, or hitting some karaoke to have a laugh.

It's worth noting that sometimes a nix to sex can result in us doing something else equally—or even more—exciting and fun. It's always possible that what starts out seeming like a bummer can turn into something really great. Not having the sex we want blows, but if it means we wind up having an ad hoc roof party, a moonlight swim together, or a really deep talk that brings us closer than having sex would have, it can be a blessing in disguise.

If someone's no isn't about sex, full stop, it's okay to ask if there's something else they'd like to do sexually. It's also okay to ask why someone doesn't want to do something sexual at all or anymore—but make it clear that question isn't about you trying to convince them, change their mind, or suggest they need to justify their no. You want to be sure you're asking that at the right time, too: if they seem upset or stressed—or you are—it's probably not a good time and is probably best to talk about it a few days down the road when everyone is feeling less vulnerable. You can open a conversation like this with something like, "I was totally okay with you not wanting to do [whatever it was] anymore yesterday, but if you're up for talking about it, I'd like to hear about why so I can better understand you and also do my best to help us create a sex life together that's best for us both."

Long story superduper short? We all have to ask before we do sexual things, even though there are different ways of asking. We all need to hold off on doing sexual things with someone else until and unless they make it clear to us they want to do them, too. We always need to ask how, because there are a lot of ways of doing any given sexual thing, and a yes to the whole thing isn't a yes to any particular

DID YOU KNOW? . . .

When you get a big no, only ask the once. If you ask someone to do something with you sexually and they tell you no or otherwise give you the clear message that not only do they not want to do that thing now but also they don't want to do that thing, period, or anytime soon, do **not** ask again the next hour, day, or week.

With that first no, you can tell them that it is something you'd really like to do, so if they ever feel differently, you'd like it if they brought it to the table and let you know. That's okay. You can also just leave it; when someone asks us to do something sexual we don't want, we can generally assume that if we change our minds, it'd be okay for us to ask them to do it. So, if we ask someone for something we want and they don't, we can pretty much count on them asking us to do it if they ever change their minds. They already know we're interested because we already told them that by asking.

way we can do it. We also need to make sure we're someone a partner always feels comfortable saying no to, not just yes to, and that we keep consent ever ongoing.

And we've just got to remember that no does *not* ever mean yes. Maybe does not mean yes, either. Yes means yes. And saying yes should always feel just as awesome as hearing it. If it doesn't, yes probably isn't what we or someone else really wants to be saying.

CONSIDERING YOUR ETHICS, BELIEFS, CULTURE, AND VALUES

Your own system of personal beliefs, ethics, and values—including any religious or spiritual beliefs or traditions—is a big part of who you are. Ignoring or disrespecting it, or allowing others to, is usually a recipe for disaster. Whatever your cultural background or community—and however you feel about it—that's also often another big part of who you are as a person. Both of these things also play big parts in our sexual choices and lives and how we feel about them.

Some people find it easy to experience sexuality and create sexual lives with themselves and others in alignment with all of those things. But not many. More people have some areas where it's not that challenging, and others where it is. And to some, it can *all* feel like one big conflict, even when they are not even having any kind of sex with partners but are just thinking about it or experiencing their own sexuality by themselves.

Some cultures or systems of ethics, values, or beliefs are in direct conflict with what we know to be true based on science or people's actual lived experiences. Some put forth a lot about tolerance and acceptance but are not tolerant or accepting at all in some ways. Some fit many people's sexualities and sexual choices well but are a terrible fit with the sexual lives and choices of others; some fit hardly anyone's sexuality or sexual choices. Some even stand counter to what we know to be vital for anyone to have sexual lives that are emotionally or otherwise healthy for everyone, like those that endorse or enable sexual or domestic violence, nonconsent, or sexual or gender inequities. And how we feel about any of these systems isn't always the same as how we feel about any of the flaws in them. Someone can, for instance, absolutely abhor the suggestion that women owe men sex as a duty but feel very attached to a system or larger tradition that endorses that idea.

To alleviate some of the giant load that all this usually puts on us, it might be helpful to apply this question to your sexual choices: *"What would my best self do?"* Who is your best self? The person you aspire to be, want to be seen as, and feel really, really good about being. That's really what all of these things ultimately are about, so just cutting to the core can help reduce some of the emotionally loaded static of things like cultural traditions and religions but still get you to the heart of things.

Conflicted? You're so not alone. You've probably got two big learning processes going on at once here: learning how to make your own best sexual choices, including in this regard, and learning who exactly you are in the first place, including what you, yourself, believe and who you want you to be. It'd be hard not to be conflicted. Plus, you might have other issues at the root of or piggybacking on conflicts with these things and your sexual choices, such as having low self-esteem, having grown up in abuse, or having internalized and self-inflicted homophobia or biphobia.

See if you can't find someone or more than one someone you suspect or know to be in a similar place as you are. The Internet can be an amazing place for finding people who are rethinking certain systems, cultures, or ways of considering ethics and talking about it in group forums or on blogs and for reading posts from people who have had these struggles so you can get some ideas based on their choices and feelings. It can also be a good place to seek alternatives. There are so many variations on these themes and systems that finding something that you never knew about before but that turns out to feel like a right fit for you is pretty easy.

Just talking it through with someone else who gets it, even if what they chose or choose to do isn't the same as what you are or will, can go a long way, especially when so many of these issues are so linked to our sense of community.

It's always fine to leave anything, including a system—be it something internal, like your own frameworks, or external, like a culture or religion—that does you any kind of harm, including emotionally, or that just doesn't feel like a right place for you to be. That's what some people do. Sometimes that's not an option, or not one yet. In that case, what people do varies. Some kind of suck it up and go through the motions until they can leave systems outside of them or adjust their own systems for the better. Others do what they want to with their sexual or love lives and figure they'll let the resistance, judgment, or other crumminess come and try not to let it get to them. You may be thinking that all this is easy to *say* rather than *do,* but knowing you have options can help. This is one of those things where only you can figure out how you'll deal and what you'll do.

There's another option: if you're feeling a great love in your heart for a certain system of beliefs, ethics, values, or traditions but have some big conflict or trouble with some part of it, you can try to accept that conflict and let it be in conflict until you can figure out what you want to do to work it out (which could even be nothing).

Wise words from Walt Whitman here (the only person in this book with the distinction of being quoted more than once, I'll have you know): *"Do I contradict myself? Very well, then I contradict myself, I am large, I contain multitudes."* Sometimes, we feel one way while literally feeling utterly differently at the same time. No matter what it happens with, it can be seriously confusing, but it is very much for real. You may need to just allow yourself some real time—days, weeks, months, even years; whatever you need—to try to sort this all through. In the meantime, that may mean holding off on making all or certain sexual choices until you do feel at least clear or resolved enough to be sure that you can live with whatever decisions you make. If it does, that's okay. **Remember:** whatever the issue, including when there are no issues at all, everyone gets to wait, hold off on, or table for now any kind of sex, with anyone, ever, that doesn't feel right for them in any way.

If you are currently living within a system where the conflicts it has with your sexuality or sexual life put you in real danger or subject you to abuse, my best advice is to always do whatever you need to do to be safe or get yourself safe before you do anything else. So, for example, if having sex before marriage would result in big external and internal suffering for you, or if getting caught with a partner of your same gender could mean getting kicked out or abused, do what you can to save those things for when they can happen in contexts in which you are safe and not in danger physically and emotionally. They'll be so much better when you don't have to risk your life or well-being for them, I promise. It's terrible to have to live under or within any kind of oppression or enforced sexual repression, but if you want to get to the other side, where you can get out from under this, you've got to survive it first.

You may not discover what some of your sex ethics, limits, or boundaries are until after you cross those lines; that happens to nearly everyone at some point. But even when you're just starting out with partnered sex, you likely have plenty you *are* aware of, so be mindful. If you're not sure about them, deal with them the same way you'd cross a busy street: be cautious and slow instead of running out into heavy traffic. And talk to your partner to see how your ethics, values, limits, and boundaries mesh with theirs to be sure you can be mindful of one another.

[WHAT'S THE RIGHT AGE FOR SEX?]

Age in years is certainly a factor when it comes to the legal aspects of sexual partnership, and sometimes when it comes to certain sexual health services. But in many ways, age in years isn't a helpful way of determining sexual readiness. Mostly that's because we aren't all the same maturity at the same age, nor does everyone of a given age want or need the same things or exist in the exact same circumstances. Sex—of whatever kind, in any given situation—may feel and be right as rain for one person who's fifteen but wronger-than-wrong for another fifteen-year-old.

Some health risks or negative outcomes are attached to having certain kinds of sex—especially and particularly genital intercourse but also oral sex—when people are in their teens, especially their young teens, including higher risks of dating abuse and of some kinds of sexually transmitted illnesses. But when it comes to being *ready,* nothing magical happens the day a person turns fourteen, sixteen, eighteen, or twenty-one. Not physically, not emotionally, not sexually. The right age for you to have sex is when you can deal with all the things on the Sexual Readiness Checklist (page 186) and when it feels like it's right for you and yours—to *both* of you. Readiness for this isn't about how old someone is; it's about whether they're at a point in their lives and in the right situations to feel and be ready.

[TO PLAN OR NOT TO PLAN, THAT'S THE QUESTION]

Being as prepared as we can for sex is smart. Talking about becoming sexually active with the intent of getting there, having safer sex tools and birth control ready in advance, getting STI screenings done, finding spaces and times that are safe and private are all part of it.

Planning special times for sex—especially when you've got something pretty unique cooking—is also fine and fun. But spontaneity is an important part of sex, too. Being spontaneous or flexible is important, especially once people move out of the honeymoon phase of a relationship, because one partner will probably want to have sex or engage in a certain sexual activity at times when the other partner doesn't want to. So, we all need to be able to make allowances for that, and have those allowances made for us.

Too much planning or sexual plans writ in stone like some kind of binding contract make it easy for people to feel obligated to have sex and to start a pattern of having sex when they really don't want to, and that's never good. So, seek a balance: enough planning to be smart and not too much to make sex feel like a dentist appointment looming or like something someone has to do just because a plan was made.

[LIGHTS, CAMERA, ACTION!]

A lot of people are concerned with looking and acting "the part" during partnered sex. Worries about shaving or not shaving, about the size and shape or taste and smell of body parts are common. Wondering when we should be moaning and when we shouldn't, if laughing or being silly is okay, if there are "right" things to say during sex, when eye contact should or shouldn't be made, and even what our

Many young people assume that the majority of their peers are sexually active or having intercourse, even when statistical data show that's not so. Many studies have shown that a scary percentage of people in the world—of all ages but especially young people—lie to friends and partners about their sexual experience. It's a vicious cycle: if everyone assumes everyone else is already sexually active, a whole lot of people start exaggerating or lying about their level of sexual activity or taking part in sex they don't really even want just so they don't feel left behind, left out, or like a weirdo.

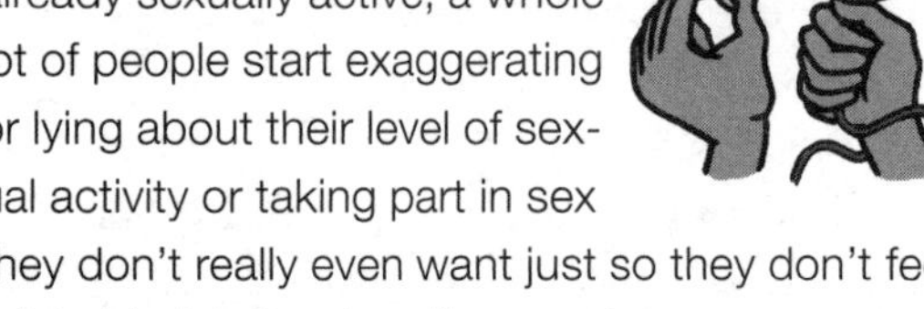

Currently, in the United States, the average age at which teens report they start having genital intercourse is seventeen years. For the last couple of decades, the age at which people first have this kind of sex has been increasing, not decreasing. In other words, your parents were probably younger—not older—than you are or will be if and when you have sex with a partner.

face should look like aren't atypical concerns. A lot of folks stress about doing something the "wrong" way.

The only person you should be when you're having sex with someone is yourself. For serious. (And, yep, even if you're role-playing, you're still you.) If you usually shave or wax, fine. If you don't, that's cool, too. If you taste and smell like a person, not candy or a rose garden, that's to be expected: you *are* one. If sex with you and yours isn't like sex in the movies, that's a given—this is real life, not the movies. Sex in the movies is as accurately depicted as, say, someone having a piano dropped on their head in a cartoon. If you don't look like a supermodel or an action figure, congrats! Welcome to being part of at least 95 percent of the population. Sex with a partner shouldn't be a performance or a beauty contest; it should be a place and an experience in which you're able to enjoy being yourself intimately with someone you know wants to be with exactly you.

[WORST-CASE SCENARIOS]

Some young people who first become sexually active together never have sex together again, and for plenty of people, sex may change a relationship in negative and unexpected ways. Often, one partner won't reach orgasm easily or at all or will feel sexually dissatisfied in some way. Sometimes, things happen during sex that we're embarrassed about or ashamed of: bleeding, loss of erection, farting, or a moan that sounds like a dying moose.

With both STIs and unintended pregnancies being highest for people between the ages of fifteen and twenty-five, it's pretty obvious that plenty of people get very unwelcome surprises from partnered sex. Some people discover during sex with a partner that they may be an entirely different sexual orientation than they thought or that they have sexual desires they didn't know they had and aren't at all comfortable with. For some, becoming sexually active all by itself creates big problems with friends or family.

When something that can feel so wonderful, that's supposed to be so wonderful, nets such bad results, it can be hard to handle. Being ready for some bad stuff is smart. Remember, sex *does* carry risks, physical and emotional. Keep in mind what those risks are. Be sure in advance that you think you can at least handle them—even if it won't be easy.

[BUT WAIT—]

If you want to save some or all sexual activity until a later time (like when you're older), a different situation (like when you don't live at home anymore), or special event (like getting married), that's A-OK. Just like not waiting for some or all of it is A-OK.

The same is true with engaging in some kind of sex once, and then not wanting to do it again.

One of the cardinal rules of consensual sex is that you *always* can change your mind. You can like an activity one day and not want to do it the next, or you can be sexually active and later opt out, or you can be sexually inactive and opt in. It's completely okay to get your mind set on a given sexual choice for a while, and to stick to it, and then to find that it doesn't fit you or serve you well; adapt as needed. That's what you're supposed to do.

[BEING A PRUDE (AND OTHER REALLY CRAPPY NAMES FOR CHOOSING NOT TO BE SEXUALLY ACTIVE)]

If you choose to let sex with partners or dating sit on the shelf, just like people who choose *to* have sex often have to deal with, you might experience negative messages or unsupportive behavior from your peers, culture, and even your parents. Just as people throw shade at sexually active people, the same can happen to people who choose not to be or who feel the sexual opportunities they have had so far just aren't good enough to go for it. Prude, slut; stud, loser; good girl, bad girl: same crappy coin, two different sides of it.

When sex isn't something you want or doesn't feel right, you get to opt out, and it's smart to opt out. Being part of sex you don't want or that doesn't feel right tends to result in unhealthy, dysfunctional, or plain-old-crummy relationships, a sexual life you probably won't feel good about or enjoy, and feeling in conflict or out of touch with yourself. A big part of being at peace with and enjoying our sexuality and sexual lives is making choices that feel in alignment with our wants and needs, our ethics and values, things we want to explore, our abilities, and our limits and boundaries. When it's not what we want, "no" or "not now" is not only something we can say, it's usually the best thing to say.

Is anyone—including your own mind—suggesting that because you're nixing sex for now, you're a prude and are sexually shackled or repressed?

Concepts of "sexual repression" and "sexual liberation" are not universally defined but are very (oh, so very) arbitrary and personal. These aren't labels we can simply assign to people or things that we can know anything about just based on whether someone does or doesn't want to have sex. Much like words for sexual orientation and gender, these are words best and most accurately expressed only by someone about *themselves* on the basis of their feelings, experiences, and introspection.

I think being as clear and strong about a sexual no as a yes is strong evidence someone is sexually liberated and empowered, not repressed. People who do not (yet!) feel sexually empowered feel they can't say no. Someone who feels empowered sexually is usually someone who's good at advocating for themselves in what they want and don't and at setting whatever limits and boundaries they have. Someone who feels sexually empowered tends to take real ownership of their own sexual wants, don't-wants, needs, and choices.

Liberation, of any kind, is centered in freedom, and freedom is centered in people having the power, ability, and right to make their *own* choices. Empowerment is about a real feeling of power and agency in our own, unique lives based on our own unique personalities and circumstances. So, if and when you want to opt out of sex or a sexual relationship, know that holding to that limit, regardless of what someone else wants from you, is something that supports liberation and empowerment, not something that opposes it.

By the way, some people choose to reclaim and use the word *prude* to express part of who they are without feeling crummy about it, just like some people do with *slut*. The origin of the word *prude* goes back around four centuries, when it originally meant a "woman who affects or upholds modesty in a degree considered excessive." Considered excessive by *whom*? Clearly not *that* "woman," or she wouldn't be making the choices she is. This may feel familiar: just like the word *slut,* it's a term usually based on *other* people's standards, ideas, and wants about people as a whole and their sexuality—what they consider too much or too little for someone *else*. It's not just about someone's own ideas about and standards for themselves, which are what we support if we want people's sexual lives to be healthy and beneficial. You may find it's powerful for you to reclaim a term like "prude," swapping it from being something people use to try to control your sexuality to something you feel represents the sexuality you want. Who knows, maybe Super-Prude is exactly the kind of identity that will help you flip the bird at people who don't respect you for making your own choices. It might feel like just the word to support you in sticking to what you want.

[INTIMACY: BONDING BASICS]

Therapists generally define intimacy as an emotional space in which two people can be free to be themselves without reservation, both accepting and supporting one another. Sometimes, emotional intimacy (becoming close via feelings or emotions) and physical intimacy (becoming close through touch, sexual or platonic) are differentiated. When people talk about intimacy in a sexual context, they're either talking solely about physical intimacy ("intimacy" and phrases like "we were intimate" are sometimes used as delicate ways to refer to sex) or about emotional intimacy, which can occur during sex as well.

Studies like "Greater Expectations: Adolescents' Positive Motivations for Sex" show that a desire for intimacy—for just plain being close to someone, whatever that means to us—is often one of the biggest motivations young adults have in choosing to become sexually active. It's important to bear in mind that partnered sex cannot, all by itself, cement or deepen a relationship or create emotional intimacy that isn't there already, but many aspects of partnered sex *can* enable *greater* intimacy. When we share our sexual selves with another person, we are potentially taking physical risks and risking rejection, disappointment, or deeper feelings and attachment. So, much of the time, we're engaging in sexual activities or relations with people we already feel some degree of intimacy with or want more intimacy with (even if it's only for an evening).

Are You *Mental?* Yes!

Often, sex with someone we already have an emotional bond and intimacy with can elevate our feelings, both during and after sex. Whereas saying that one specific sort of sexual relationship or another is "better" or "worse" is biased and inaccurate, we *can* say that sex with greater levels of intimacy is most often experienced differently, physically and emotionally, than sex with less intimacy.

No sex is *just* physical. **None.** Because sex is a whole-body process that utilizes the brain more than any other body part, and because it involves all of our senses, including our sense memory, partnered sex always includes emotional aspects. (Even though they can feel like they're coming from your heart, emotions actually come from your brain and your endocrine system, not your circulatory system.) That doesn't mean sex must be or always is *romantic* or that love, of any kind, is required for enjoyable, healthy sex. It doesn't mean that one can't have sexual partners outside romantic relationships primarily or purely for sex alone.

But it does mean that even very casual sexual partnerships, like hookups or FWB scenarios, do have some emotional aspects—such as seeking out companionship or company, wanting to explore various feelings through sex—and do involve varying levels and kinds of intimacy, just like romantic or longer-term relationships.

No one relationship model or type of sex automatically equals more or less physical or emotional intimacy than any other. Physically, someone may feel most connected to another person during vaginal or anal intercourse, while another may feel most intimate kissing deeply. Someone in a romantic, close relationship may sometimes feel distanced or unable to communicate freely during sex, while someone else having casual sex may have an emotional epiphany and feel incredibly close to the other person, able to be sexually freer because of the anonymity or the sudden connection. Or vice versa.

Our levels of intimacy within relationships and during various kinds of sexual activities all vary based on who we are, whom we're with, what we both want and need, what the relationships are like, where we're at in life, what social conditioning and life experiences we've had, how we're feeling on a given day, and how we nurture and protect that intimacy.

[VIRGINITY: PAST AND PRESENT]

When people talk about a "virgin," they're usually talking about someone who has not had penis-in-vagina intercourse. Well, sometimes. Actually, it's hard to say—this is one of the most vague, arbitrary cultural terms there is.

But the common concept of a virgin as someone who hasn't had penis-in-vagina intercourse leaves a lot of people out in the cold. Defining sexual partnership as only that kind of intercourse would make someone who has had more than one partner, but no penis-in-vagina (or penis-anything) intercourse, a virgin. The most standard definition of virginity—which is almost always more about and more impactful on women than on men—also suggests that a woman is not a fully sexual being or doesn't have a sexuality at all until or unless she has had intercourse with a man and that couples who engage in sexual activities other than intercourse, or who don't even want to or can't have intercourse, are somehow not having "real" sex. On a similar note, the emphasis put on intercourse can cause people to engage in sexual activities they don't really like because they want physical intimacy but are ashamed or afraid of having intercourse. People who have been sexually assaulted—who have in no way participated in consensual sex, or really even sex at all—are often thought to have "lost their virginity."

The usual concept of virginity also makes sex a commodity: a passive thing that someone gives and someone takes. But consensual sex everyone wants isn't a thing; it's an action. It isn't passive; consensual sex doesn't just happen. No one just trips and falls on someone else with their penis or vagina and then—ohmygosh, they're having sex! Consensual sex is something people do, and if they're not doing it, it's not happening. And consensual sex—especially consensual sex people also happen to really enjoy—isn't about anyone giving or taking something. It's about sharing, co-creating, and actively doing together.

So, Who's a Virgin and Who Isn't?

What it means to be a virgin—if virginity is a construct you want to work with—really can be defined only by you, and it has to do with how *you* define sex. Someone else can't do it for you, and you shouldn't allow anyone else to do so. (If abstinence or virginity is being asked of you by your church or parents, ask them to define it, explicitly, because what they think it means and what you think it means may be very different things. Ask questions. If you're going to agree to something, you should be sure you understand and can live with all the information.) Virginity shouldn't be a standard by which you judge others or by which you allow yourself, when it's in your control, to be judged. It shouldn't be a symbol of status or a lack thereof. Sex—or a lack of it—isn't something that should be used to value or devalue anyone or as a bargaining chip for anything or to manipulate anyone.

As out there as it may seem, you might give some thought to abandoning the concept of virginity altogether. However nicely or in different contexts some present it now, it is an idea that throughout history has been sexist, heterosexist, classist, and oppressive. Virginity as an ideal has actually done the opposite of what many would think it aspires to do: it has *de*valued sexuality and intimacy—and women—rather than making them more valuable.

DOORMATS AREN'T PARTICULARLY INTIMATE

Limits and boundaries don't inhibit intimacy: **they increase it.** We open up a lot more to someone emotionally by having and setting limits and boundaries than by going without or keeping silent about them. Being open doesn't mean being open all night like a mini-mart. Being open is being honest about your feelings, wants, and needs, even when they don't align with your partner's. Part of getting close to someone else means increasing your compassion and empathy with them, and theirs with you. Some limits and boundaries may be temporary (like, say, waiting to have intercourse until you've been together a certain amount of time) and some not so temporary (like not engaging in anal sex, ever). But we've all got them, and they're part of who we are.

Limits and boundaries aren't just a big *no.* They are the support systems that give us the trust, safety, and freedom to be able to say a big ***yes*** to the things we do want, need, and feel ready for.

You can't "give" someone your genitals, and someone else can't "give" your sexuality to you. Both of those things, and all the rest of you, are all yours and are still all yours even if and when you're sharing them. Your value as a person and as a partner is not and should not be merely or primarily sexual. It's about the whole person you are, no matter your previous sexual experience or your lack of previous sexual experience. What makes something special isn't not having done it before; it's bringing your whole awesome self to the table whenever you *do* do it.

BE A BLABBERMOUTH! COMMUNICATING WITH PARTNERS ABOUT SEX

You can read everything from the *Kama Sutra* to *The Joy of Sex,* have a ton of sexual experience, or psychically channel Mata Hari, but if you don't know how to communicate with your partner, chances are good neither of you is going to have very emotionally healthy, beneficial, and satisfying sexual experiences, especially over time.

Communicating clearly and well about sex and relationship issues before you become sexually active with someone—the whole works, not just when whispering sweet or X-rated nothings into a lover's ear—not only puts you in a place where you can have satisfying sexual relationships, short and long term, but also helps keep everyone safe and sound both physically and emotionally.

If you have a car, you know that you've got to keep a pretty good eye on the oil in the engine; if you run out, your car's not going to keep working, even if it's in great shape—it may well explode in your face. Communication is the oil that keeps the engine of your sexual relationships running smoothly.

How to Talk About Sex

Talking with your partner about sex isn't just about asking what one person has or hasn't done before, wants to do, or gets hot just thinking about. Talking about sex with a partner also involves discussing the pace you're comfortable with; your sexual

THE (NOT REALLY) MYSTERIOUS HYMEN

For centuries, people believed that the most obvious proof of virginity is found at the vaginal opening with the presence of a hymen, or *corona*, and that virginity is only about people with those body parts. The lack of a hymen or a hymen that is not intact has long been considered indisputable evidence that a woman has been sexually active. Although this belief is still widespread, it is normal, as you know, for the hymen to become less visible over time as a result of any number of things that aren't intercourse or sexual. The hymen is less like a seal and more like a collar: even when "fully intact," it doesn't close the vaginal opening like a manhole cover. Some people are born with easily indiscernible hymens, and some with hymenal openings so large that their intact hymen doesn't look any different from one that isn't there at all. It's stretchy, too, and even after it has mostly worn away—from hormonal changes, menses and vaginal fluids, general activity, and solo or partnered sexual activity—small folds of it remain around the vaginal opening for the rest of a person's life. A "broken" or unbroken hymen is no reliable "test" of virginity. (For more on the hymen, see page 29.)

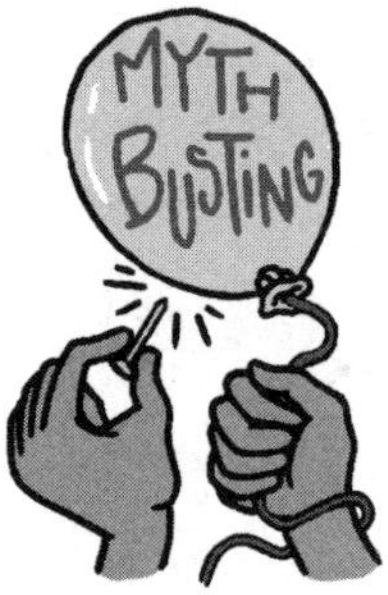

Neither is bleeding during first intercourse a piece of "evidence" typically used to "prove" virginity. Although some people do experience bleeding, plenty of others do not; there isn't a lot of study on this, but research mostly reflects that with consensual first-time intercourse, more people do not bleed than do. Another myth is the idea that the difference between someone who is and isn't a virgin can be felt, physically, by their partner. A virgin is "supposed" to be "tight." (For more on this, see Chapter 2.) Someone having first intercourse very well may feel tight (to a partner or themselves), but that is more often the result of nervousness, fear, and anxiety than it is a sign of whether or not they've had partnered sex before. It's also typical to think that first intercourse *must* be painful, and if it's not, then clearly the person with the vagina has had sex before. But for plenty of first-timers—those who are relaxed and aroused, who are as lubricated as they need to be, who have gentle partners, or whose hymens may have already worn away a good deal or are very flexible—intercourse isn't painful. It may not feel all that amazing, because, like anything else, practice makes perfect, but it isn't painful.

It's worth a look at the root of these beliefs and their cultural contexts before you decide whether to sign on with them. Idealizing things like sexual pain and bleeding, putting a monetary or moral value on the appearance of the body or someone's sexual history—let alone only for only one group of people, while the other group is exempt save for the power and privilege that that inequity gives them—or putting anyone through embarrassing and shaming virginity "tests" is serious sexism.

Even defining "real" sex as only one act that isn't enjoyable all by itself for millions of people is pretty bizarre when you think about it.

health and your partner's; what you want or need to be comfortable engaging in a given sexual activity; how you masturbate; how you feel about your body; what feels good and what really doesn't; safer sex and birth control; your sexual ethics and beliefs; the relationship model that works for you both—the works. Good sexual communication means you are creating and maintaining an environment in which you and your partner or partners can really talk openly about sex, in and out of bed, even when what you have to say isn't very sexy or isn't what the other person might want to hear. It means being able to say no and having no be accepted and easily respected without pressure to say yes; it means being able to say yes knowing that it doesn't mean you, or they, have to say yes every time.

It's no big shocker that talking about sex openly and intimately isn't very easy. Many adults in long-term sexual partnerships don't have the hang of it, and plenty prefer to avoid sexual discussions rather than practice them. A rare few of us grew up in households where sex was discussed healthily and openly. Good sexual communication generally requires more than single-word responses. For a lot of people of all ages, honest and open sexual communication is brand-new terrain.

Before you become sexually active with a partner, take a look at how you communicate with them about other things. Are you able to talk openly and freely about your feelings for each other, relationship models, time management, previous romantic/sexual relationships, peer and family relationships, and dealing with crises? If not, it's wise to pause and evaluate whether that partner is a smart sex partner for you yet; after all, if you don't feel comfortable talking about needing a little more time together or what's going on with your family, it's going to be a serious challenge to talk about wanting to be touched more here or there or about having a yeast infection. If daily communication, especially about things that are very close to your heart, doesn't feel pretty easy just yet, work on that first, or consider that this person may not be an ideal partner for you. Look at your own existing sexual communication in other parts of your life. Are you able to discuss sexual issues with your friends or your physician with a decent level of comfort and honesty (even if things sometimes feel a bit awkward)?

If you're already at that point, then you've got a good foundation for sexual communication. You can lay it down from the outset just by saying something as simple as (but likely less formal than), "Before we get sexually involved, I want us to be able to talk about sex together honestly and freely." Just making your intentions clear like that opens the door, allowing both you and your partner permission to talk and to be honest when you do.

If it feels to you as if you and a partner cannot discuss sexual issues—either because you don't feel ready or because you think talking about them will bring on anger, upset, jealousy, or massive insecurity—then you might want to wait to have partnered sex with that person until you both do feel able to talk more comfortably. You can also get more practice talking outside of bed because any conversation between the sheets tends to be a lot more loaded.

Once you have some simple, solid communication dynamics down, it's pretty much a matter of basic care and feeding: if and when you do start having sex with someone else, you'll keep talking to one another, all the time, and it should become second nature to always be communicating and sharing ideas, feelings, and experiences without trying too hard. It's not unusual, when you first start having sex with others, to go without superheavy verbal communication for a while because it's new, because you're caught up in all the things that feel good, or because things that aren't as you like them, yet, will just take time. Communication is important, but the sex you're having also doesn't need to feel like a lecture series.

It usually takes a few tries—and often more than that—to meet someone whose needs and wants are compatible with ours and who we can partner with to find middle ground that works for both of us. Because of that, it's tempting to let things go unsaid when we really need to be talking about them—things like limits and boundaries that aren't being communicated or respected, wants or needs that aren't being met, relationship models we know we can't deal with, or sexual velocity that is just going too fast. Resist that temptation if it happens. You don't want to set patterns or precedents for things that aren't okay with you or that aren't working for you because that makes it even harder to iron them out in the long run. Put your limits and boundaries on the table as soon as they come up. Even if that feels difficult, awkward, or risky to do, it is a lot easier to set limits earlier rather than later.

Speaking Your Own Language

Part of sexually communicating well involves using terms that both of you know the meaning of and are comfortable with. So, you and yours may hit roadblocks to productive sexual communication if, say, you're talking about "tea bagging" or "fingering" and your partner has no idea what you're referring to, or if your partner calls your genitals a "pussy" or a "prick" and those terms are offensive to you. Be sure that when you are talking about sex, you do so without making too many assumptions, and think about the language you are using to express yourself. Be open to making changes or clarifying to better the communication. Ask what words work for your partner; tell them what words and language feel best to you.

On a related note, everyone has different levels of comfort when it comes to "pillow talk"—talking about sex during sex for the effect of heightening arousal. Some people may like a partner to "talk dirty" during sex, but their partner may not be comfortable with that, or not yet. Again, these tend to be matters of compatibility, and by discussing them, even partners with some divergence of opinion can often find middle ground that suits both of them.

[BODY OF EVIDENCE: LEGAL ISSUES AND YOUR SEX LIFE]

When we're making sexual choices, we also sometimes have to concern ourselves with our larger community, including the legal policies of our cities, counties, states, provinces, and countries. Knowing what legal risks you or your partner may be taking and what legal consequences can be involved is important in making sexual choices.

For instance, a legal adult who is sexual with a minor may be breaking laws that can land them with criminal charges and lifelong sex offender status, and it can make a giant mess for the minor as well. Sending a naked photo online or with a cell phone, asking for one of someone else, or passing along one someone else sent to you, if anyone involved is a minor, most often this is considered child pornography, about as serious a crime as it gets. It's something to think seriously about before you snap, click, or share.

Laws vary a great deal internationally. Listing all the specific sex laws of every area around the globe would be not only beyond the scope of this book but also beyond the scope of a law library. This section is brief, but it focuses only on legal policies common in most areas of the Western world.

The good news is that all laws are available for you to research easily online. Hooray, Interwebs! To discover which laws apply to you, all you have to do is a little online legwork. Open up a search engine: the bigger, the better, when it comes to this kind of searching. Next, type in the kind of legal policy you want to find out about—for example, age of consent, pornography, sexual assault—and the name of your nation, province, or state. That should get you started. Ideally, you want to look for at least some institutional websites, which usually have domains like .gov or .edu. If you'd like to look through a law library instead, just add "law library" to that search string, and you'll see the big ones come up. Some laws around sex are national, and others are local, specific to provinces, states, counties, or cities; sometimes you'll be dealing with both national and local laws. But if you start broad, with national law, and look at credible sources of legal information, those sources often note when local policies apply instead or in addition.

If doing all that leaves you unclear, or you want backup with what you've read, you can try calling your local legal aid service with questions. If you have a college or university nearby, it may have a law library you can use. Law librarians, like most librarians, are awesomely helpful.

Here are some of the most common laws related to sex and sexuality, what the terms mean, and how those laws may apply to you:

Age of consent (AOC): The AOC is the age established by a county, state, or nation at which a person can legally give meaningful consent to sex with another person. Age of consent laws—which were initially sex trafficking policies designed to keep parents or other adults from putting children into prostitution—differ among states and countries. The youngest age of consent worldwide is currently twelve (in several countries, including Chile, Panama, and the Netherlands), and the oldest, eighteen, is the AOC of several states in the United States, including California. On average worldwide, the age of consent is usually around sixteen, but what's relevant to you is what it is in *your* specific area. Many areas or nations have an age of consent that isn't the same for men and women, and when that's the case, the lower age is usually for young men,

Text continues on page 216

TOP TEN REALLY CRAPPY REASONS TO HAVE (ANY SORT OF) SEX WITH SOMEONE ELSE

1. To try to keep them from leaving or having sex with someone else

Sex just to try to keep someone around is manipulative and controlling. It also rarely works.

2. To prove your maturity or independence

If you really need it, the best "proof" of maturity and independence is making choices on the basis of what's best for you and what you really want and need—choices that also aren't harmful or hurtful to you or others—no matter what anyone else may think of them or whatever they are. If that process and those choices involve maturity and independence, the proof will be in that pudding, all by itself.

3. As a substitute for exploring your own body

Nobody can or will ever know your body as intimately as you can. Some people report that they "just can't get into" or enjoy masturbation, and that's fine. Or they complain that it just doesn't feel the same as sex with a partner—and that's not surprising because they are different things, and they generally won't feel the same. Masturbation doesn't have to be your favorite thing. But do at least find your own clitoris or prostate by yourself first rather than asking a partner to seek it out for you and be your sex-ed teacher. Get to know your favorite places or your ick zones by yourself as well as with a partner. Learn the names of your own anatomy and where everything is rather than going for a road trip without a map.

4. To make your parents mad or get their attention

The trouble with this one is that most people don't even realize it's what they've done until ten years later, and then they have to suck it up and feel pretty stupid when it's clear this is exactly what they did. It's not fun, and it rarely produces the desired result. You may be putting yourself at risk for no good reason, using others or hurting their feelings, and ripping yourself off of the experience of having sex in an environment where it can actually be pleasurable and make you feel good about yourself. And you probably also don't want the kind of attention this'll get you, either.

5. Because someone else did it

I know you know what some old person or another would say about this, so I don't need to talk about cliff jumping here. To sum up: someone else isn't you. The best choices for you are the ones you make *for* you, based on your needs, wants, and abilities, not someone else's. Blaze your own trail: do it **your** way.

6. To fit in with friends or gain status with people

Sex for this reason is often a double-edged sword. Although it might net you status with some, it'll decrease your status or reputation with others. People who are your friends accept you as you are, and they like you for who you are, including your values and choices, even if they aren't the same as theirs.

7. Because your partner wants it, even though you really don't

Having any sort of sex because of feelings of obligation or pressure tends to leave a really nasty taste in your mouth for quite some time, and it doesn't do a lot for your self-image. If your partner wants to do something you don't, you can communicate that with a simple, "I'm sorry, but I'm not interested in/ready for/willing to do that. If and when I am, I'll let you know. How about we do this instead?" Any partner worth even considering, let alone having, isn't going to argue that point. If what's being suggested is a really big deal to them and just not workable for you, now or ever, you may have to deal with sexual compatibility issues at some point (see page 259). But even the least desired outcome of that is going to be easier to live with than participating in activities you really don't want to.

8. To just get it over with

That's an understandable thing to want to do with a job interview, taking out the trash, or getting rid of an ingrown toenail. But sex is supposed to be enjoyable and satisfying, and, like most good things in life, it being enjoyable and satisfying requires the right set of circumstances, the right timing, and being in a good place, all around. Partnered sex doesn't have an expiration date like a carton of milk, nor is it a requirement to fulfill at any given age or time.

9. Because you're bored or restless

Get a hobby. Volunteer for something valuable and important. Go hang out with friends. Read a book, see a movie, go biking or skating. Research the history of the most obscure thing you dork out about. Put silly hats on your cat. Write a novel. Clean your room, binge-watch a television season, give your dog a bath. Heck, masturbate. Sex with a partner has a lot of emotional and physical risks for everyone involved. If someone told you that they decided to climb Mount Everest or learned to swallow knives because they were kinda bored, you'd think they were a little whack, and the same goes with sex because of boredom.

10. To spite someone, even if that's just yourself

Maybe you want to make an ex jealous. Maybe you want to prove to someone who questioned your readiness, attractiveness, or orientation that they're wrong. Maybe you want to sting your best friend for dating someone you also liked. Maybe you cheated on a current partner and are so mad at yourself you feel that sleeping with four more people at a party is a justifiable self-punishment.

You don't want your sex or love life to resemble trash TV. You have to live with yourself and the effects of your actions for your whole life—you can't just change the channel. Make sexual choices you feel pretty confident you can live with and want to.

and the higher age for young women. Several areas also have a different age of consent for same-sex partners than for opposite-sex partners, and those policies usually set the age of consent higher for same-sex partners.

Some AOC laws allow for those who are not legal adults but who are older than the age of consent to legally engage in sex with someone younger than the AOC. Some AOC policies allow for some or all kinds of sex between legal minors and legal adults in specific circumstances. Legal policies that allow for sex between partners when one is younger than the age of consent and the other older tend to have specific windows: for example, it may be completely lawful for partners two or three years apart in age, a misdemeanor for those over five years apart in age, and a felony for anyone ten or more years older or when the minor is particularly young. Legal exceptions and grace periods that allow for reasonable age difference—usually a very small one—are called "Romeo and Juliet" policies; these policies might be in place because it is recognized that the age of consent policies in that area may unintentionally penalize peers, like a couple where one person is six months older than the age of consent and the other is six months younger than it. Areas in which AOC laws allow for some age difference do, however, usually stipulate that those exceptions aren't in play when the older person is in a position of additional power or influence over the younger, such as someone who is a teacher, religious leader, or coach.

What "sex" is in terms of AOC laws also varies: in some areas, it's limited to intercourse and oral sex; in others, something like fondling may be included. "Sex" in these laws and policies is usually very clearly and specifically defined. However, simply dating—without any sex of any kind in the mix—is never part of these policies. Nonsexual relationships with age difference are not a legal issue so long as those relationships aren't abusive (in which case, we'd still be talking crimes, regardless of age, but any kind of abuse of a minor by an adult often adds additional weight to those crimes).

Although you may have questions about the fairness or "legitimacy" of AOC laws or how they are sometimes applied (me too), the intent behind them *is* to protect people who are vulnerable, however flawed aspects or applications of those laws may be. Someone who has the full rights afforded to an adult always has more power and agency than someone who isn't yet afforded those rights. When used as a protection, as they were designed to be, these laws *can* help protect youth or help youth seek justice when they didn't or couldn't give meaningful, informed consent or were coerced into sex by someone with greater power and agency than they have. They also can make predatory adults less likely to seek out minors as sexual partners.

AOC laws are often misunderstood as legal policies that make sex between minors and adults criminal for everyone involved. But the partner younger than the age of consent is not breaking the law; the partner older than the age of consent is.

Statutory rape: The crime of a legal adult or person older than the legal age of consent engaging in sexual activity with a minor or person younger than the legal age of consent. Depending on the age of the minor and other circumstances, this may instead be treated as child molestation or be paired with other charges, like forcible rape, kidnapping, or corruption of a minor. But generally, when a teen is involved and they feel they consented to the sexual activity, it falls under statutory rape. Sometimes, statutory rape or similar charges can occur if a person is older than the age of consent but is still a legal minor and has had sex with a legal adult.

Statutory rape used to be something of an empty charge, but in the United States it's possible for a statutory rape charge to translate into registered sex offender status for a person's whole life. A state law known as Megan's Law requires communities to be informed when someone charged as a sex offender moves into their neighborhood. The person convicted may even be required to go door to door to tell neighbors who they are and what they have done. Being a registered sex offender can have a heavy impact on availability of jobs, places to live, custody agreements and parenting—the works. More often than not, people with registered sex offender status have committed serious sexual crimes. But sometimes it happens when no one intended or experienced any abuse or when someone is being discriminated against in some way, like because they're gay or of color.

Even when sex offender status is not applied, having a statutory rape charge on your record can mean not getting into college, not being considered for a job, or not being considered for leases because you've got a criminal record.

How could someone get charged? By a parent, teacher, friend, doctor, or neighbor reporting the known or suspected sexual activity. By someone younger than the AOC who originally said yes but who realized in retrospect that they really were not able to give full consent or were coerced.

The younger party in cases like these isn't the one who has broken the law, but that doesn't mean they don't suffer. This kind of thing can really turn your whole world inside out and upside down. Gender is a nonissue here: both men and women can be and have been charged with statutory rape.

Indecent exposure: This is the term for public acts of nudity, masturbation, or partnered sex. A lot of people participate in indecent exposure without even knowing it because what they consider public and what is *legally* public are two different things. For instance, having any kind of sex in a car in a public garage or parked out on public property, like on the street or in a park, is public rather than private sex, and thus indecent exposure. "Public nudity" generally applies to exposure of body parts deemed sexual, such as genitals and breasts.

Solicitation: In the most basic sense, sexual solicitation occurs when some form of sex is offered, accepted, or suggested in exchange for something else, such as money, higher job status, or a place to stay. Prostitution and other forms of sex work are a form of solicitation, and survival sex—such as exchanging sex for needed food or shelter—is not exempt from these laws. This can include online activity. On a related note, it's important to know that sex work is not legal for minors in the United States. And unlike the way some other sex laws are enforced, a minor can be charged, punished, or incarcerated for solicitation.

Child pornography: Creating, seeking out, or sharing explicit sexual material that involves legal minors. Developmentally speaking, not all people younger than the age of majority in the United States are children, but legally speaking, anyone younger than the age of majority is a child. The most common way these laws have come into play for young people involve digital sexual media, such as images made and shared that contain nudity or things that can otherwise be construed, by community standards, as explicitly or overtly sexual. In other words, if someone sixteen years old creates a digital image of themselves having some kind of genital sex with a partner or of themselves naked, or someone fifteen years old shares media like that with someone else, legally they often are considered to have engaged in child pornography, which is a felony crime that can carry very serious lifelong legal and social ramifications.

It's very important to remember that in most legal systems, **ignorance of or disagreement with the law is not a defense**. So, the fact that you don't see yourself or a partner as a child (you meant to make pornography, but certainly not child pornography, because you don't define yourself as a child) or that you didn't know something like this was criminal won't put you or anyone else involved in the clear.

Legal discrimination

Legal discrimination: Terribly, some legal actions or punishments are informed by bias and are applied with the intent to discriminate. For instance, we know from research that the reason we have more men of color than white men in the prison system in the United States is primarily because of racial (and economic) bias and that sex workers are much less assisted in the justice system in reporting and pressing charges related to sexual violence than are victims of violence who are not sex workers. The more vulnerable someone is and the less power they've been afforded in the world—like legal minors and members of other oppressed groups—the fewer rights they usually have and the more likely discrimination is to occur. Discrimination can happen to people charged with crimes and to people who are victims of crimes.

If you know or suspect any kind of legal discrimination is happening to you, ask for a lawyer, immediately, if you are in any situation in which you are being detained or visited by police. When you can, seek legal representation via legal aid or another kind of advocacy from individuals or organizations that act as advocates.

Sodomy: Sodomy laws criminalize any act of oral or anal sex, even between consenting adults. These laws have almost exclusively been applied to homosexuals and bisexuals.

Starting in the sixties, states began to repeal these laws, often with the help of the American Civil Liberties Union and other legal advocacy groups. At this point, fewer than twenty states in the United States still have sodomy laws on the books, and most sodomy cases are tossed out of court or repealed. In *Lawrence v. Texas,* 539 US 558, a landmark decision in 2003 by the US Supreme Court, two gay men sued over state sodomy laws—and won. This case essentially made even sodomy statutes that still exist basically unenforceable.

Sexual assault (rape): Sexual assault is when someone forces or coerces someone else into a sexual activity without their explicit consent or knowledge, often with the use of physical force or some form of emotional coercion. If a person consents to sex under duress, such as threats to harm friends or family, or if the victim has been given drugs or alcohol to produce consent, that is also rape or sexual assault. In some areas, rape and sexual assault don't mean the same thing legally; in others, they do. But in nearly any legal system, either term is used to describe sexual activity someone did to, on, or inside someone else without meaningful consent.

Rape, as a term, often has subcategories. "Forcible rape" generally implies physical violence. "Date rape" or "acquaintance rape" applies to a sexual assault committed by someone known to the rape victim. "Spousal rape" refers to a married person who has raped their spouse. "Gang rape" is a term for sexual assault in which more than one person assaults a victim. "Attempted rape" and "assault with intent to rape" are terms used to describe an instance in which rape did not take place but was intended or attempted.

Although very few people are confused about what physically violent or forcible rape is, many people are in denial about or don't know how to identify other types of rape and sexual assault. Coercion—pushing and pressuring a partner to have sex until they give in—is also sexual assault. Pursuing sex with someone who is clearly inebriated, under the influence of drugs, or distressed is also rape or sexual assault in the letter of most laws.

The majority of people who are sexually assaulted are women, and the vast majority of people who rape people of any gender—women, men, people who don't identify as either—are men. However, rape and other kinds of sexual violence aren't things that happen just to women by men: about one out of every eight rape victims is a boy or man, according to the National Crime Victimization Survey in the United States. For more on rape and sexual assault, see Chapter 11. And women both can and do also commit sexual assault, and their victims are also of any and every gender.

Unfortunately, sexual assault can happen to anyone and is something no one is immune from doing to someone else just by virtue of being a certain gender, race, age, or member of any other group. Who doesn't commit sexual assault is the person who chooses not to assault anyone; the good news there is that that, too, isn't about gender or other classifications. It's just about someone choosing ***never* to assault anyone sexually** and instead choosing to prevent assault and ensure they're only engaging someone in sex while doing the things we all need to do to ensure the sex is consensual.

Sexual harassment: Unwelcome and uninvited sexual advances, requests for sexual favors—even in the form of jokes—or other sexually loaded and unwanted verbal or physical conduct are considered sexual harassment when accepting or rejecting the behavior or advances could affect a person's employment, interfere with a person's performance, or create an intimidating, hostile, or offensive environment. Although the term is most often applied in job environments, sexual harassment can also occur in schools, community centers, and other areas. Catcalling—or street harassment—is another form of sexual harassment, as is slut shaming or "revenge porn," the malicious sharing of any sexual media made by someone that was intended to remain between sexual partners (or that was made without both people's knowledge or consent in the first place).

A charge of sexual harassment has the power and impact it has for the same reason it's so rarely reported: in a culture where sex is often seen as shameful—especially for certain groups—it's very easy to shame someone into silence when sex is concerned. Our culture also has a tendency to blame the victim of a sexual crime, especially when that victim belongs to a sexual or general minority. Victim blaming and shaming are so pervasive that whenever someone is the victim of any kind of sexual crime, be that harassment or assault, they'll often be more inclined to think and believe it's their fault than the fault of the person who actually did the harassing or assaulting. Sexual harassment isn't sexual assault (though it often is a prequel to it), so a lot of people being harassed figure their hard feelings around it aren't valid and that they'll just have to suck it up and hope it'll go away. A lot of people also think it's funny or harmless—it is neither.

"Bullying" is another word for harassment. So, if someone is bullying someone with, about, or around something sexual—like their sexual orientation, or like slut shaming, or by being very verbally sexual with them when that's not what's wanted—we're talking about sexual harassment.

Loitering: Loitering—being "in a place at a time or in a manner not usual for law-abiding individuals" and arousing "suspicion" among others or from the property owner—isn't a sex crime, per se, but it can be treated like one. Again, loitering laws are most often used against groups (such as gays and lesbians or teens) whose sexual activity isn't socially acceptable in a given area. Loitering laws can also be used to discriminate against vulnerable groups by being applied, for instance, when a transgender person uses what someone considers to be the "wrong" bathroom. Trying to evade or argue with security or law officers in any situation where you're on private property that isn't yours (which includes malls, stores, schools), even if you are in the right, is a bad idea and likely to result in a charge. So, if loitering is being suggested and clearly used as discrimination that you want to counteract, your best bet is to leave the situation, comply with the officer, and then later report it to another officer or talk to a lawyer or legal aid group.

Be careful and aware when it comes to the law. Certainly, some laws and the ways they're applied aren't at all fair or just, and certainly, it's a bit strange to have to consider the courts when making sexual choices for yourself. But legal issues exist all the same, and unless you're willing to go to jail to protest them, it's a really good idea to obey the law as best you can. And if you're going to take a risk, seriously consider not just the emotional or physical consequences but also the possible legal ramifications.

However, take comfort in the fact that if you're making sound sexual choices based on criteria such as in the Sexual Readiness Checklist (page 186), sex laws are not likely to be a big issue for you, so there's no need to freak out or obsess.

How to Work the System So It Doesn't Work You

You may at some point find yourself involved with the justice system as a victim, witness, or someone thought or known to have perpetrated a crime. Unfortunately, justice systems—and their related agencies—are often not fair or kind to young people. If you're a member of an oppressed group (or are both a young person *and* a member of one or more oppressed groups), like if you're queer or gender nonconforming, of color, poor, disabled, or undocumented, the same goes double. Ideally, laws are supposed to protect the most vulnerable people, but it just doesn't always play out that way. Many legal policies—more often based in bias or bigotry rather than malice—can be applied to do the opposite.

If you ever do find yourself involved with the law or the justice system as a victim, a witness, or someone reported for or charged with a crime, here are some of the most important and basic things to know so that you can do your best to advocate for and protect yourself and make the legal system work for you rather than against you.

1. Know your rights, ideally in advance. To the best of your ability, do your homework about your rights ahead of time so that you can consider them in your decisions. Again, ignorance of the law is not a legal defense: we're responsible for abiding by laws whether we know about them or not. So, it pays to do what you can to learn about the law and take it into account with your choices before you make them. It's also a lot harder to get run over by a legal system or other related agencies when you know your rights well enough to know when they are or are not being respected, and you feel confident enough in that knowledge to advocate for yourself.

2. Create an on-call crisis team. Pick at least one trusted adult (minors have little to no power in justice systems, so having someone with adult rights is important), you know, an in person, who could get to you and who'd have your back no matter what. Pick an advocate or advocacy organization you can reach by phone. Who's an advocate in specific situations? A particular person or agency—like a lawyer, legal aid group, or an advocacy group that provides in-person help for any special needs you have or for a vulnerable group you are the member of, such as a transgender rights advocate or a youth rights group. That advocate or advocacy organization doesn't have to be local, but they need to be able to be local or connect you with a local advocate. Parents can be advocates (or your trusted adult), but if your parents or guardians aren't people you know you can trust to advocate for you, choose someone else. Include contact information for your local police in this list, because, as a young person, it is more likely you will be the victim of a crime rather than someone charged with a crime. If you are a member of a group you know is highly discriminated against by your police, you can pick the number for your fire department or ambulance squad instead. Save phone numbers for your three choices in a mobile device if you have and use one, and write them down on a small card you can fit into your wallet, purse, or pocket. Try to always keep this information with you or memorize some of it. Sometimes a cell phone may get lost or taken from you, so it is wise to have a backup list.

3. Listen instead of talking. Listen to what law enforcement officers and people from any other related agencies say to you very carefully; that way you can know what is going on and be sure not to miss anything important. Do your best to keep quiet or say very little until you have a lawyer or other advocate there who's just for you. If you say anything at all, let it be to ask for that person. After they arrive, then is when it's in your better interest to talk.

4. Ask for legal representation. No matter what, let this be your mantra: "I want a lawyer." Or, in the event that your parents or guardians hired a lawyer for you and you do not want that one or a lawyer assigned to you, say, *"I want my own lawyer."* You have a right to a lawyer, and your own lawyer. Say it as many times as you need to until you get one.

5. Always assume that you have rights, power, and agency, and always ask for them. Sometimes you won't have some rights, power, or agency, and sometimes when you ask for any of these things you will be declined. But operate from a place of assuming you have all the rights, and gently but firmly insist on them.

BE PATIENT. Impatience is not a virtue and also can seriously mess you up in any part of the legal system. It's much harder to be patient when we're scared, defensive, falsely accused, or we're the victim of a crime who wants help and justice without having to wait or go through steps that, unfortunately, can feel terrible. But when we get impatient, we tend to get more reactive, more irritable, less careful; most often we tend to start behaving more and more badly. This isn't about judging anyone in such a spot. Unfortunately, behaving badly ends up hurting only ourselves. Feeling angry, upset, or just plain sick and tired of anything to do with the justice system or a crime is certainly understandable, but you want to do your best to try to stay (or at least act) patient. Muster the best behavior you can so that you don't get yourself in more hot water and can get all the help and protection you need.

9

Popular Mechanics: The Ins and Outs of Sex with Partners

Nobody needs—or could honestly give—a complete step-by-step instruction manual for sexual activities, which is why this chapter isn't one.

It's often assumed there's one "right" way to perform any sexual activity or one "right" order in which to engage in sexual activities. A lot of people also think that there are universals when it comes to being "good" or "bad" in bed. Sure, more people kiss before oral sex or intercourse than not. And, yes, a majority of people like some things that a minority of people don't. But sexual activities aren't simply a matter of a progression that builds up to penis-vagina intercourse or anal sex for everyone, and the order that feels right for a given person, or with a given partner, can vary a lot. Whereas any one sexual activity can be performed by itself, for most people a combination of activities is what's most satisfying. Sexual activities also aren't some kind of set menu everyone has to eat from with no substitutions, nor are they a list of requirements everyone must fulfill.

In case you haven't picked up on this from everything you've read here so far, human sexuality is as diverse as human beings are: what anyone likes and doesn't, wants and doesn't, and likes to do things vary widely not just from person to person but even for just one person—they can vary a whole lot from partner to partner, from one time of life to another, and even just from day to day.

What is essential is feeling able to communicate with your partner, to do what comes naturally, to be creative and spontaneous, and to learn what each of you enjoys by experimenting and communicating. If you don't worry too much or overthink it; if you're talking, listening, and attentive to your partner's nonverbal cues (when they smile, moan, turn a body part to you or push it closer, or pull away slightly), and if you are giving cues and responding truthfully and authentically, it's pretty impossible to do any sort of sex "wrong." It's common to get all hung up on doing things "right" and forget that it usually does come pretty naturally if you let it and just stay connected with what you want and what's okay—or not—with other people. **There aren't universal rights and wrongs** when you're paying attention to and respecting your partner, and they you. Sex is also like just about anything else in life: it's both something with a big learning curve—a new one for every single partner, with whom you're really starting from scratch, save knowing what you know about yourself sexually in some general ways—and something, as we learn and explore, with some parts that rock, some that are fumbles and lackluster, and a lot that is somewhere in between.

Much of sexual pleasure is psychological and emotional, about your brain, more than anything else. That doesn't mean what goes on with the rest of your body is irrelevant or unimportant—it's very important—but if you're feeling emotionally good about what you're doing; if you're both emotionally and practically prepared; if you feel safe, trusting and trustworthy, and relaxed with your partner and are simply enjoying being close to them and they with you, then most things are going to feel good without trying too hard. If you're communicating well with each other about what you want and don't, like and don't, need and don't and being honest in that communication, you're probably going to find out what feels great for *you* in no time. The only person who could make a sex manual for how to please your specific partner *is* that specific partner; the only person who could make one for you is you.

The sexual activities listed below are ordered in terms of increasing intimate contact, STI and pregnancy risks, and how common they are. The list here isn't divided by gender or orientation, because that would be silliness. Some heterosex-

Sexual activity

Just about anything in this section can be sexual or not. We might kiss our family members, and that's usually about affection, not sex. Someone's hands and our genitals are involved in sexual health care. And if someone is sexually assaulting someone else, although something might be sexual for the person doing the assaulting, it rarely is for the person being assaulted. So, what makes a sexual activity a kind of sex and not something else? When it's something everyone involved is consensually doing together because they want to explore, express, or share sexual desires, feelings, curiosities, and overall sexuality.

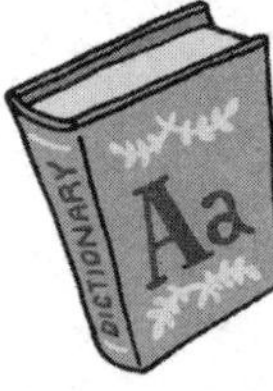

ual men engage in receptive anal sex with their girlfriends, and some lesbian women participate in blow jobs or vaginal intercourse using dildos or hands; the idea that there are "straight" sexual activities and queer ones is utterly busted. Any combination of partners can do just about any form of nearly any sexual activity, and what activities people do and don't do usually isn't just about—and sometimes isn't about at all—orientation or gender.

ABOUT THE PREGNANCY AND STI RISK ASSESSMENTS

You'll see that after each activity, the level of risk for pregnancy and STIs is noted. **These assessments are for the possible level of risk when birth control and safer sex practices are *not* used.** So, for example, vaginal intercourse is listed as high risk for pregnancy and STIs, but those risks can be massively reduced with a reliable birth control method and safer sex practices. How much risks are reduced depends on which methods were used for safer sex, contraception, or both, and how well and often they are used. (For specific information on birth control methods and their effectiveness rates, see Chapter 12, and for specific information on reducing STI risks, see Chapter 10.)

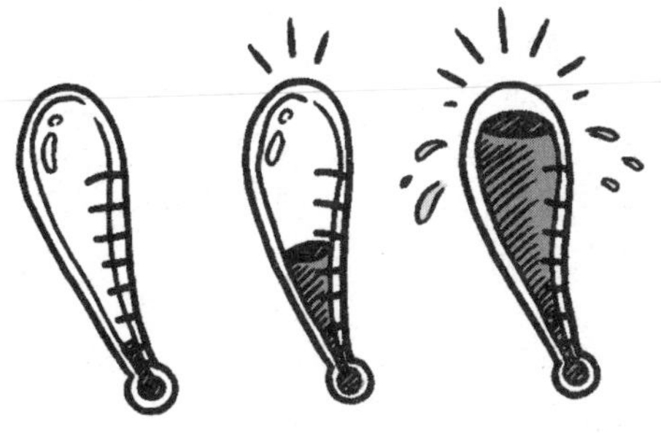

low risk medium risk high risk

KISSING

AKA: Making out, macking down, sucking face, smooching, snogging, pecking, French kissing.

What is it, and how do you do it? You know this one. Kissing is when two people press their lips together all smoochy-like or enjoy exploring one another's mouths or any other part of the body with their lips, teeth, and/or tongues.

Most folks know how to deliver a closed-mouthed kiss, but with a sexual partner, you shouldn't want to grimace or hold your lips supertight for fear of too much slobber from Uncle Joe or Aunt Gladys: you are opening yourself up to your partner through your mouth.

Some partners test the waters by kissing a partner on the cheek first. For a lip lock, you just lean forward and press your lips gently to theirs, tilting your head a bit to get noses out of the way. You can have a session of closed-mouth kissing for quite some time, just by repeating the kisses for as long as you'd like, and kissing whatever parts you and your partner choose.

Openmouthed, or "French," kissing means just what it says: your mouths are open in some way. That may mean using your tongue to explore your partner's tongue or lips and slight nibbles on the lips or tongue with the teeth. Kissing is a lot like dancing: both partners are taking steps by paying attention to each other's lead and rhythm. So, it's good to pay attention to the subtleties of what your partner is doing, and go slowly until you get in the groove together.

Kissing isn't just reserved for mouths: you or your partners can kiss any part of the body. Many people find kissing and outercourse (like petting, cuddling, and "dry sex") to be some of the most enjoyable and intimate sexual activity there is.

You might also want to be aware, because kissing (especially deep or extended kissing) does feel so intimate, that it may be something you and/or your partner is hesitant about or that you or a partner may be comfortable with other sexual activities before kissing, and that's okay. In that regard, it's also probably safe to say that if you really, really don't feel comfortable kissing someone (assuming you like other things and just don't like kissing, period), or if they're continuously hesitant to kiss you, that can be a sound cue that either you or they aren't feeling ready for sexual intimacy yet or that you may not be a good fit as sexual partners altogether, for any number of reasons.

STI risk: No risk to low risk. (No risk for dry or closed-mouth kissing; low risk for wet or openmouthed kissing, although if there is a cold (herpes) sore, other mouth sore, or injury present in either partner, there is a greater risk.)

Pregnancy risk: No risk.

[PETTING/MASSAGE]

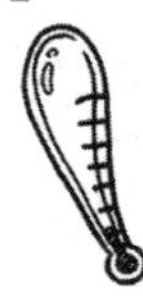

AKA: Feeling up, rubbing, necking, petting, touching up, outercourse.

What is it, and how do you do it? It's exploring and seeking pleasure with one another's whole bodies and the hands. For some people, the major draw is parts of a partner's body they think of as sexual or those that aren't touched in common, platonic contact: the neck or back, breasts or chest, stomach, hips, thighs, buttocks, genitals.

> Unless you or someone else wants it that way, there's no sexual activity that has to be done exclusively, when no one is doing anything else at the same time. What we know from studies about sexual satisfaction is that more people enjoy doing more than one thing at a time—like intercourse, when people are also using their hands to touch each other, or dry humping, when there's also kissing going on—than only one thing at a time. So, unless you or someone else doesn't want to or has a hard time focusing on more than one thing at a time, know any one activity on this list is more like one song in a mix than the whole mix.

Petting and massage can be anything from heated to really mellow and relaxed. You may even just be giving your partner a backrub because they're tense or sore, or because it feels nice, and it may or may not become sexual.

How someone likes to be touched differs from person to person and area to area. For example, someone may like their breasts or nipples squeezed, and another may just like light, feathery stroking. Sometimes partners limit touch to one area, as a way of focusing on that area or as an extended "tease." As with all intimate contact, communication is a good thing, and many people figure it out as they go just by asking, "Does this feel good?" or "More gently or more rough?" Feedback like, "I love it when you touch me like that there," or "You can do that a little harder if you want," keeps communication open.

During petting, massage, or cuddling, you can rub, stroke, knead, or pull your partner's skin with your hands and fingers, varying in intensity from very light, almost tickly touching to very deep kneading or massage. Sometimes you might add your mouth to the mix, licking, sucking, or kissing parts of the body.

People tend to forget (or don't know in the first place) that our genitals aren't the only sensitive or sexual parts of our bodies, not by a serious long shot. Our mouths, hands, and feet also have a ton of sensory nerve endings like the genitals do, and touching the whole of the body, instead of just the genitals, can increase intimacy and arousal. Plus, it feels good! Some people can even reach orgasm due to intense petting or massage or from touch to parts that aren't genitals: the breasts, neck, thighs.

When you're with a new partner, it's always a good idea to start by setting any limits of your own clearly and checking with your partner about their limits. You or your partner may have certain body parts you don't want or don't feel ready to touch or have touched. There may be parts of your body you still feel awkward with, and you can let a partner know about that. If you want to stay fully or partially clothed, communicate that, and encourage your partner to communicate their own needs and preferences. Activities like this can be a great place to set a solid foundation for active, clear consenting with these and other activities in the future.

STI risk: No risk, so long as no body fluids are shared.

Pregnancy risk: No risk.

Premature ejaculation

Young people who've got penises tend to reach orgasm and ejaculate very soon after any given sexual activity begins. According to studies, on average, someone with a penis—of any age—tends to reach orgasm, ejaculate, or both within just a couple minutes of intercourse.

The term *premature ejaculation* is an iffy one. It assumes there is one universally "right" length of time or minimum time that is acceptable for erection, and that's just not true. It's not "premature" for someone to orgasm or ejaculate within a few minutes; it's average. However, it can often be considered too soon or too fast if someone's partner needs much more time than that to get off themselves—as is usually the case for people who've got vulvas instead—and anyone involved has the idea that for the other person to get there, both people have to "last" with a certain sexual activity or keep an erection until everyone has had an orgasm or otherwise feels finished. Should one partner reach orgasm when the other still wants more sexual activity, that's very easily achieved with any of the sexual activities that don't require an erection.

If you've got a penis and feel like you're reaching orgasm or ejaculation in such a short time that *you* don't feel satisfied, or if you want to try to extend the length of time of erection for other reasons, you can also try masturbating before partnered sex; taking pauses of a few minutes from sexual activity when you feel close to orgasm; or making sure that the sex you're having is more full-body than just genital. An added bonus of condom use is that the ring of the condom applies pressure to the base of the penis, which can help maintain erection.

[MUTUAL MASTURBATION]

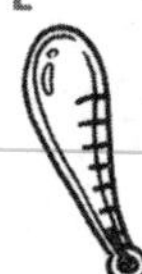

AKA: Circle jerking/jilling, flop-whacking, wankwatching (okay, so I made the last two up).

What is it, and how do you do it? When partners masturbate in each other's presence, instead of alone, it's called mutual masturbation. (Sometimes, *mutual masturbation* is also the term used to describe partners giving each other manual sex at the same time, but that's not what we're talking about here.) During mutual masturbation, there is no genital contact between partners; it is *self-contact* with a partner present. Both partners may be masturbating at the same time, one after the other, or only one person may be masturbating with a partner looking on.

It's common to have mutually masturbated with friends during childhood, puberty, or adolescence, by the way: plenty of people do or have done that, no matter their gender or sexual orientation. It's also not unusual to feel a little weird about mutual masturbation, especially at first or with a new partner. Usually, when we masturbate, we're alone and often feel freer with our bodies without the self-consciousness we may experience in the company of even a partner. Some people feel funny about it because they feel like someone else touching their genitals is acceptable, but masturbation is shameful and something to pretend you don't do or like: hopefully you know better than that by now. You or a partner might feel that if either of you "needs" to masturbate during partnered sex, it's because you aren't good enough at pleasing each other. Not so! Try to remember that none of partnered sex is a "need" scenario—any of us may just *want* to do different things at different times. And masturbating with a partner isn't a replacement for partnered sex, it *is* a form of partnered sex, one that can be a pretty great way to learn about things you and your partner like, such as the kinds of genital touch and sensation you enjoy.

STI risk level: No risk.

Pregnancy risk level: No risk.

[FROTTAGE OR "DRY SEX"]

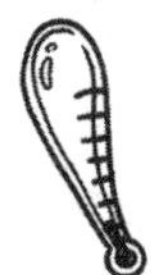

AKA: Dry sex, dry humping, grinding, freaking, body rubbing, tribadism (or tribbing), outercourse.

What is it, and how do you do it? It's when two people grind their genitals together (or grind their genitals against a partner) but while dressed (thus the "dry" part) and without any direct genital-to-genital contact or entry.

In any position where there is (covered) genital-to-body or genital-to-genital contact, both partners simply move their hips around to stimulate the genitals via pressure and friction. Some couples also enjoy dry sex by pressing the penis from behind into the buttocks; some couples position themselves to use each other's thighs or genitals for simultaneous stimulation that way. Because genitals are sensitive, you can get quite a bit of sensation from the warmth and motion of another's body, and because partners are often face to face and are usually engaged in full-body contact, it can be very emotionally intimate.

If one of you is nude or wearing garments that don't really cover your genitals or won't stay put to keep them covered (like a G-string), a latex barrier (a condom or dental dam) is a good idea to prevent accidental fluid contact (for more on barriers and how to use them, see Chapter 12). If everyone's naked, then we're talking about tribadism—scissoring or grinding *with* direct genital contact—which carries risks dry humping doesn't.

STI risk: No (if people are dressed) to low (if people aren't dressed) risk.

Pregnancy risk: No (if people are dressed) to low (if people aren't dressed) risk.

[MANUAL SEX]

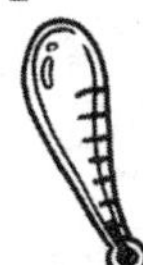

AKA: Hand job, fingering, finger-fucking, whacking off, wanking, jacking off, jilling off.

What is it, and how do you do it? Manual sex is when one partner is engaging a partner's genitals with their fingers or hands.

Manual sex can mean stimulation of the penis, testicles, perineum, anus, and surrounding areas; the vulva, including the mons, inner and outer labia, clitoris and vagina, and/or the perineum, anus, or surrounding areas.

"Fingering" is often assumed to mean vaginal entry only, when, in fact, more people enjoy either clitoral stimulation or pairing clitoral stimulation or stimulation of any other parts of the vulva with vaginal entry.

Bear in mind that the vaginal canal and rectum are curved, not straight. So, if you are going to engage in manual sex with those body parts, putting a rigid finger or three in there as if pushing an elevator button isn't likely to feel so hot. Instead, try to keep your fingers curved in a little, as if you were holding a ball, and feel out the body part you're going inside very gradually with your fingers, as it feels good for your partner. Like with any kind of sex, checking in with someone as you're exploring tends to go a lot better than just going at it like there isn't a person—a person who can give you information their body parts can't about what feels good—attached to the body part you're touching or are inside of.

If you are going to enter the vagina or anus with fingers, lubricant is advised for comfort and pleasure, and latex or non-latex gloves can also be used. Like gloves, handwashing also reduces STI risks just as well, but gloves can also make manual sex *feel* better, protecting the genitals from scrapes and abrasions from calluses on the hands, hangnails, or fingernails. Lubrication (what's lube? See page 294) is **really important,** as is starting slowly and gradually.

If you're not in a position to look at your partner's genitals and you want help finding any part of them to explore, like the external portions of the clitoris, just ask. So long as they know their own body well, it's pretty easy for someone to place your fingers where you and they are wanting them to be. Experiment with different levels of pressure, depth, and speed and with what part of the genitals you're touching. How direct or indirect someone might want contact with parts of the genitals that can be supersensitive—like around the ridge of the head of the penis, with the foreskin, the opening of the rectum, or the clitoral glans—varies a lot, so per usual, be sure to ask, check in, listen, and be responsive to the feedback a partner gives you.

An erection—either of the penis or of the parts of the vulva—isn't required for manual sex, so you don't need to wait for erection unless you or your partner has a preference.

Because genitals are *sensitive,* using lubricant—and saliva is a substandard lubricant, for the record, as well as a possible infection risk—for manual sex is a good idea. (You'll notice this is a reoccurring theme. Lube is always good news, while a lack of it rarely is.) That's especially important when you're going inside someone's body in some way, but it's something that often increases pleasure from manual sex when you're working with the penis, the vulva, or other external bits, too.

If you're engaging in anal manual sex, make sure to switch gloves or wash hands between anal and other genital contact to reduce bacterial infection risks. Before partnered anal play, experimenting alone and gently with the anus first is wise, both to understand how delicate the area can be and to be prepared for how intense the sensations can be from anal play.

STI risk level: Low risk.

Pregnancy risk level: No risk.

Deeper manual sex

More involved, as it were, manual sex is colloquially called *fisting,* but that's not because you make a fist and try to put it into a vagina or anus, which is unlikely to be anything but painful, if not impossible. Rather, this kind of manual sex involves starting with one or two gloved fingers (and lube, added as you go) and slowly working up to more, as it is—and only if it is—pleasurable for the receptive partner. If a whole hand is wanted by both partners, and four fingers feel good, the performing partner can then tuck his or her thumb into their palm or inside the fingers to make the whole hand as slim as possible, and then slide upward. Once it's all inside, that partner can then turn the hand back and forth, slowly open the fingers up gently and rhythmically, or go up and down, as is comfortable for their partner.

Fisting isn't that common, and the more fingers we're talking about, the less common it becomes. Fewer people will likely be interested in it, especially at the beginning of their sex lives, and more people are generally interested in vaginal fisting than anal fisting. While both canals really *can* make room for that much inside, and it can feel good, this can be hard to imagine if we're still getting used to the idea of single fingers, a penis, or a dildo inside the vagina or anus. As with any sort of entry to the vagina or anus, if the idea of deep manual sex makes you very nervous, it's smarter to opt out, because being scared or nervous not only inhibits arousal but also keeps the muscles of both canals from relaxing enough for deeper entry to be comfortable and pleasurable.

Very deep manual sex carries higher STI risks than less intrusive manual sex does.

[ORAL SEX: CUNNILINGUS]

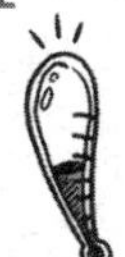

AKA: Eating out, licking out, going down on, going south, giving head, tipping the velvet.

What is it, and how do I do it? Stimulating the vulva externally (inner labia, clitoris, vaginal opening, perineum) and/or internally (the vagina) with lips, tongue, and/or teeth.

Although for many people the clitoral glans is the preferred center of activity for oral sex, remember that the labia and the clitoral hood are also connected to or part of the clitoris and full of nerve endings, so stimulation there often also feels good. There's way more to the clitoris and sensation with oral sex than just the clitoral glans!

Some people like external licking or sucking of the vulva. You can circle the clitoris and vaginal opening with your tongue, lap at it top to bottom or side to side, flick at it with your tongue, suck on it and the labia, even give your partner's vulva loads of soft kisses. Some people enjoy having their vaginal opening, or even more deeply into the vagina, explored with the tongue. Even teeth, with *gentle* nibbling or grazing, can feel good. You may wish to hold your partner's outer labia open (and they can also do it with their own hands), to be able to see where you're going or provide more intense sensation to the whole area. Sensitivity of the vulva and vagina varies, so you need to adapt for your own partner.

Some people also enjoy vaginal or anal stimulation during oral sex, either with fingers or a sex toy, and some also enjoy oral stimulation to the perineum or anus (see rimming, below). If you're using a latex barrier for oral sex and are going to incorporate anal play, just be sure to use a new dam for that area rather than sliding the same one back and forth.

STI risk: Moderate risk.

Pregnancy risk: No risk.

[ORAL SEX: FELLATIO]

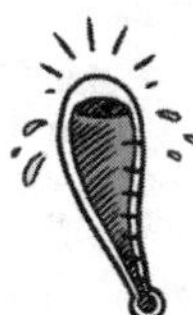

AKA: Blow job, blowing, giving head, sucking off, hummer, tea-bagging (for oral sex on testicles).

What is it, and how do I do it? When the penis is stimulated with the mouth, tongue, lips, and, often, hands at the same time. There isn't usually any actual blowing involved; in the 1950s and 1960s, *blow* was slang for ejaculate, which is probably the source of *blow job* as slang for fellatio.

Generally, fellatio involves licking, lapping, and sucking the head of the penis,

DON'T CHOKE

If you're the receiver of fellatio, a quick etiquette tip: imagine, if you will, someone roughly shoving an unpeeled banana fully into your mouth and throat. Not a pretty picture, is it? Holding a partner's head gently or guiding their mouth with your hands during fellatio is completely fine if they're down with it (not everyone is). Pressing your pelvis very intensely or quickly into a mouth isn't anything but a good way to choke somebody, so just be sure to be attentive, if holding a partner's head, to what your hands are doing and to what their limits are. Check in with a partner often to be sure it's all good.

the ridge beneath it, and the shaft. It can also include oral contact with the testicles, perineum, and/or anus.

There's all sorts of crude commentary on what *not* to do when giving head, but we can sum it up, far more respectfully, by merely saying this: a penis is part of a person, not an object, and a sensitive part at that.

Guard your teeth behind your lips: teeth on delicate and tender genital tissue can hurt, especially if you're not being supercareful and mindful about it. Don't suck on a penis too roughly; start slowly and softly, and then change it up based on your partner's feedback. Even when you use a little more intensity, remember that the skin is delicate there. If you're giving fellatio, know this: you do *not* have to try to fit the whole penis into your mouth or throat. You can use your hands as an extension of your mouth, instead, to stimulate the parts of the penis not covered by the mouth, and that's a mighty common way people go about this.

Although the penis may look simpler than the vulva, as you know from Chapter 2, it really isn't; just like the vulva, it is also a sum of several different parts that people can, and do, experience differently. Don't be in a hurry: take time to get familiar with your partner's unique genitals, starting slowly and gently, and changing things up as you learn together what feels best for the both of you.

There's a pervasive myth out there that every single person with a penis not only loves blow jobs but also loves them more than any other sexual activity or anything else on Earth. The truth is that many, if not most, people of *all* genders enjoy oral sex. And there are also plenty of people, of all genders, who just don't like it or who prefer other things at other times.

STI risk: High risk.

Pregnancy risk: No risk.

[ORAL SEX: ANALINGUS]

AKA: Rimming, rim job, tossing the salad, hitting it.

What is it, and how do I do it? One partner orally stimulates a partner's anus or rectum with their lips or tongue. Rimming is one of those activities often assumed to be practiced only by gay men, but people of all genders and orientations may enjoy rimming as well as stimulation to the perineum. The idea that only gay men—and all gay men—like and want any kind of anal sex is based more in stereotype than in reality.

It's strongly advised to use a latex barrier during analingus, because traces of fecal matter that everybody's butt has at any time often carry bacteria that can cause infections, especially if you're also using your mouth on other portions of your partner's genitals. Although it's unusual to have direct contact with substantial amounts of fecal matter during anal play, bacteria and infections are often present because feces have passed through the rectum and anus, so pathogens have, too.

Culturally or personally, some people may find the idea of anal play repulsive because they have such negative associations with fecal matter (poop) or that part of the body and because of some strong cultural stigmas. For some who only associate anal stimulation with gay

ORAL SEX FREAKOUTS

A lot of people are concerned about tastes and smells during oral sex, especially with new partners or when they haven't had much—or any—exposure to genitals besides their own. If you're with someone you haven't been with exclusively (and they you) for at least six months, practicing safer sex throughout, you should use a barrier method to avoid STI transmission, so taste is really a non-issue. When that kind of time has passed, you'll likely feel more comfortable with your partner and less worried about that.

Healthy body fluids tend to taste like . . . well, body fluids. Like sweat, they're a little salty, sometimes a bit bitter or sweet. Same goes for smells: nobody's vulva or penis smells like roses because, although your body may well be a wonderland, it's not a perfume counter or a sanitized hospital room. Genitals often smell a little musky and more intense than our other body parts. Ultimately, no one in sound sexual health is going to taste or smell "bad." If you know or suspect you do, check in with your sexual healthcare provider: a seriously foul, fishy, or overly strong taste or scent often signals an infection. Treating the infection will take care of the funky smell or taste it brought with it.

If you're curious, it is safe and okay to taste and smell your own genital fluids. If you feel funny about them, that's a good reason to hold off on partnered sex that involves your genitals; until you can enjoy and feel comfortable with all the aspects of your own body, it's awfully hard to do so with someone else.

Last, if you feel fearful, intimidated, or in some way freaked out by getting up close and personal with your partner's genitals—or by having someone get up close and personal with yours—by seeing, tasting, or smelling more of them during oral sex than you might with other activities, or if you feel that some form of oral sex is required of you, have a think. Let's come out with it: there's no need to tiptoe around issues many of us know can be common problems. Some prevalent attitudes about oral sex are pretty unhealthy, especially between cisgender men and women. Some men who sleep with women don't want to engage in cunnilingus (and often, that's more about feeling intimidated than anything else). Some are influenced by cultural attitudes that say that giving a woman oral sex is somehow subordinate, dirty (despite the fact that the vulva is no more or less clean than the penis), or unmasculine, while others just aren't into oral sex; it's just a preference. Some women who sleep with men feel that their partners don't really make fellatio optional. Women may also sometimes give blow jobs as a way to say no to something else—for instance, to get a partner to cease pressures to have intercourse—or they may come up against cultural attitudes about serving "male needs," being dominated, or women being responsible for getting male partners off.

If you've gotten this far into this book, none of these people should be you. You understand the anatomy, you understand crappy cultural and gender mandates and roles, you understand that part of sexual readiness is feeling ready to get very intimate with all of your partner's body. You already know that it's not such a swift idea to do one activity with a partner as a means to try to "earn" the same for yourself. You should always be doing only things you want to do, but it's also smart to evaluate why you do or don't want to do them and make sure your reasons for either are sound, healthy, and in alignment with the kind of sexual life and ethos you're really after. ■■

men, any homophobia may make anal play unappealing. As with anything else, it's perfectly okay *not* to want to engage in anal play. But it might be a good idea, even if you pass on it, to reevaluate how you think, even just about your own anus. No parts of the body are dirty or bad, and learning to be cool with *all* of our parts is pretty essential to accepting our bodies and feeling at home in them.

STI risk: High risk.

Pregnancy risk: No risk.

[VAGINAL INTERCOURSE]

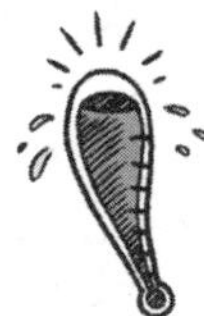

AKA: Sexual intercourse, heterosexual intercourse, having sex, screwing, fucking, making love, shagging, hitting it, nookie, getting laid, the horizontal mambo.

What is it, and how do I do it? Vaginal intercourse—and specifically, penis-in-vagina intercourse—is often the assumed "default" sex, as in, that's what many people mean, and assume others mean, when they say they're "having sex." Vaginal intercourse is when the vagina interlocks with something that can go inside of it, like a partner's penis or a sex toy. Partners then generally move about while interlocked in whatever ways feel best to everyone involved. When vaginal intercourse is something people are doing with a sex toy rather than the penis, there aren't any pregnancy risks, but a shared toy that hasn't been or cannot be properly cleaned and that is not covered by a condom poses moderate to high STI risks, and a hand not washed or gloved also poses those risks.

As with any form of vaginal entry, it's key to take things step by step. An erection of the penis is required for penis-in-vagina intercourse; relaxation, sexual arousal, and lubrication—which often means extra from a bottle—beforehand and during are usually needed for intercourse to feel good to the person whose vagina is being entered.

Take your time working up to intercourse, with other sexual activities beforehand, maybe even to the extent of both partners reaching orgasm or feeling fully satisfied with those other activities *first*. It's just so easy for genital entry to feel crappy instead of awesome, particularly for the receptive partner. The time to move into intercourse is pretty much the time when both people—not just one—feel like they are absolutely aching to do that and their bodies are giving them a green light in ways they recognize. If a person with a vagina is aroused and intercourse is likely to feel good, a few fingers inside the vagina and a penis or dildo entering the vaginal opening feels good and aren't a struggle or strain. There is a very pervasive idea out there that intercourse is supposed to be painful or uncomfortable for a receptive partner, especially the first time or two. Even though a lot of people think that, it's not supposed to be painful, and when a person is relaxed, sexually excited, well lubricated, really *wanting* intercourse, and doing anything extra they need to feel comfortable or good—like giving a partner some directions or making adaptations for disabilities—it usually doesn't hurt, including the first time. But so many of those things aren't in play with a lot of people's first times with intercourse that it does feel painful to a lot of people. It just doesn't have to.

If a partner feels too "tight" (to themselves or a partner) or if that initial entry is painful, unless they have a health issue at the root of the pain, like an active infection or a genital pain condition, chances are very good they're just not yet fully aroused.

How deeply to have intercourse is up to both partners, but the receptive partner is the one most likely to experience discomfort if something is inside their body too deeply or is moved too deeply too fast, so be mindful and stay in communication throughout. (And if discomfort from depth is an issue for a receptive partner, choosing a position where they have more control over that, like on top, can be helpful.) People may find the most sensitive stimulation they feel from intercourse is from shallower depth, because more fine-touch sensory nerve endings are present at or near the front of the vagina and at or near the top of the penis.

Because different people are different shapes, including their genitals (which also don't stay the same shape all the time: they're so tricky!), a position that was great with one partner may not work at all for or with another. A gazillion books out there contain huge lists of sexual positions, but most can be summed up simply: bodies can fit together a whole lot of different ways, and which ways are best generally depends on what feels best for the specific bodies involved. To find out what's good for you and yours, you've just got to experiment a lot, which should be a fun part. If experimenting feels like a drag, sex of any kind with a partner probably isn't going to be so hot because experimenting

Vaginismus

Vaginismus is a persistent condition in which vaginal contact, entry, or intercourse causes the muscles of and around the vagina to essentially clamp up or close, which can make intercourse or manual sex with vaginal entry very painful. It's relatively uncommon, affecting less than 5 percent of people, and may be caused by previous sexual trauma or abuse, by repeated incidents of painful or uncomfortable sexual intercourse, or by intense fear or nervousness about intercourse or other vaginal entry. Because people with vaginismus expect pain, repeated attempts or pressure to engage in intercourse can create anxiety, which only makes things worse. If you are having intercourse only when full arousal and relaxation are present, with plenty of lubrication, but vaginal entry, manual vaginal sex, or intercourse is still painful, check in with a healthcare provider. Various available therapies are effective for the majority of vaginismus patients. Be sure, in the meantime, though, to just engage in other, external activities, because continuing to try over and over again when it hurts can make vaginismus more persistent and intense.

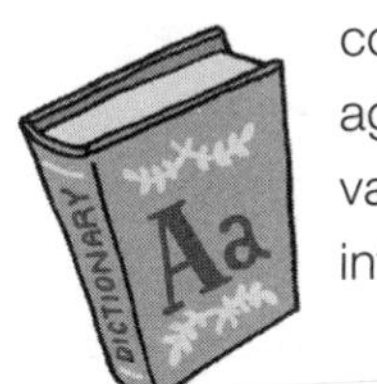

Remember that if a receptive partner is not fully aroused, is scared or nervous, doesn't really want to be having intercourse, or isn't properly lubricated, intercourse is likely to be uncomfortable or painful. That isn't vaginismus or any other medical condition; that's just basic sexual physiology.

and exploring are what make and keep sex anything but an autopilot bore in the first place. In fact, for sexual relationships that last for years or decades, one of the most common sexual sticking points is when exploring and experimenting stops, and people are only doing, often quite dispassionately, what they know "works."

Some schools of sexual thought concern different ways to engage in intercourse to meet certain ends. Tantric practice, for instance, focuses on slowing down movements during intercourse and delaying or withholding orgasm or ejaculation. But overall, most people generally find that what they like has some constants (depth or angle, certain favorite positions) and some variances (how fast or slow, or additional sexual activities) from day to day and partner to partner.

STI risk: Very high risk.

Pregnancy risk: Very high risk.

Hip to the Hype: Common Intercourse Problems and Expectations

A lot of people are raised with the idea that not only are all sexual activities only a lead-up to penis-in-vagina intercourse but also that kind of sex is *the* sexual big deal, *the* one thing we'll all like best (or the ginormous thing we'll be missing out on if we don't ever have partners with whom we can even do that), feel most intensely, and have the most emotional connection during. Many heterosexual people, when they talk about "sex," are only talking about intercourse, and they might not have even had any other kind of sex themselves to know if it does (and it usually doesn't) feel like some totally different animal than any other way of having sex. The media often depict intercourse as falsely as they depict most anything else. We're told, all over the place, that intercourse is the most special, the most intimate sexual thing we can do with another person, which is why a lot of young people are also told that it is *the* thing to save for only The Most Special Person In All Of Human History. That's some pretty intense advance billing and mighty hype.

So, it's not too surprising that when many people do have intercourse, and it's like it is in plain old real life with plain old real people, they're scratching their heads wondering what they did wrong or trying to figure out what all the fuss was about. For some people, it really is everything they expect the first time round, physically, interpersonally, emotionally, or all of those ways. But for many, it isn't, and for most, there are going to be at least a few times—if not a lot of them—when heterosexual intercourse just isn't all it's cracked up to be.

For the majority of people with vaginas—as well as some people with a penis, instead—intercourse, all by itself, is not entirely satisfying, nor is orgasm likely to occur from just intercourse. The primary reason for this is simple: the design of the vagina is such that most of the vaginal canal is not rich with sensory nerve endings, unlike other parts of the vulva, including the external clitoris.

That doesn't mean intercourse can't be or isn't otherwise enjoyable for people who aren't digging it or responding to it when it's the only activity going on or that all enjoyment from it is only emotional or intellectual. It's just to say that pairing intercourse with *other* sexual activities—before, after, and/or during intercourse—is what's optimal for most people, especially if that person has a vagina.

People with penises, as well, may not always find that vaginal intercourse is the very best sexual activity for them or even something they like. Some find that not being able to feel where they end and a partner begins, which is common during intercourse, is too vague for their enjoyment or that more friction is desired for more sexual sensation on their part. People, whatever their genitals or gender, often need or like a varied combination of sexual activities to enjoy themselves and feel satisfied, not just intercourse alone.

That isn't to say that all cheers for intercourse are hype and bluster. Lots of people enjoy intercourse. Many people express it feels more intimate for them than other sexual activities, perhaps because the experience of interlocked genitals and the positions assumed for intercourse can give the feeling of an incredibly full and complete whole-body connect.

Design Flaws

One of the major issues is that intercourse—or manual vaginal stimulation—all by itself usually doesn't excite some of our most sensitive parts. Most of the vaginal canal isn't all that rich with nerve endings. That's a serious bonus for pregnant people in labor: it's already uncomfortable enough! But it's not so great for people who expect and want intercourse to satisfy their every sexual need or who want to be sent physically out of this world.

The other thing is that penis-in-vagina intercourse requires an erect penis that stays that way. Penises don't always get or stay erect, though, even when someone is feeling turned on. So, if a couple attempting intercourse hits a snag and erection doesn't occur or stay present, that may be viewed as failure, which can put a lot of pressure on people, making enjoyment of this kind of sex more difficult for everyone than it needs to be.

Statistically speaking, it also takes people who have vulvas rather than penises at least a couple minutes longer to reach orgasm, from any activity, than it does for people with penises, and sometimes more than that. More times than not, one person will "cross the finish line" first. Thus, a single act of intercourse, all by itself, doesn't commonly equal orgasm or full satisfaction for both partners, even for those who can reach orgasm from intercourse alone. One of the most common complaints about intercourse from receptive partners is that their partner "finishes" before they're done, and that complaint sometimes comes with character indictments, like the person who reached orgasm first is being selfish. Now, if someone is reaching orgasm from intercourse and is all "Seeya, good luck getting off, buddy!" *then* it makes sense to talk about selfishness.

For the record, a way couples who have intercourse—or any other kind of sex—and who both reach orgasm or don't can continue sex until both feel satisfied is by not putting all the eggs in one sexual activity basket and by not trying to have orgasm at the exact same time (that's pretty rare). How people achieve mutual sexual satisfaction is by doing a range of sexual activities and by shifting to a different one when a partner is, in any way, finished with the previous one, until everybody either reaches orgasm when they want to or feels generally satisfied and done. And when a partner is just plain done or is spent—or isn't—masturbation is what people will typically do to get themselves there.

When Intercourse Just Won't "Work"

It's not abnormal to discover that the first couple of times you attempt intercourse, it just won't "work." With everybody nervous and keyed up for an activity that's unfamiliar, it's so easy to space out the simple stuff or to get stressed so that the easy fixes aren't obvious. This can happen with any number of other genital sexual activities, too. Here's what to do:

▶ **Where to go:** Having trouble finding the vaginal opening? Ask your partner to guide you with their fingers, or turn the lights on and have a look. If no one knows, has, or can get any sense of where to go, it doesn't make a lot of sense to try to have intercourse. Instead, better to go all the way back to the starting line with education about your bodies and with exploring them, alone and together, much more gradually.

▶ **Getting inside:** If vaginal entry is problematic, chances are good it's one of these things: lack of adequate lubrication, relaxation, or arousal (for one or both partners); an angle that just isn't working out; or someone not wanting to have intercourse. If the vaginal opening feels uncomfortably tight for one or both people, it's most often a strong signal of fear, nervousness, or someone not being very aroused. Fear or stress makes us tense and tighten our muscles. Feeling relaxed and unafraid relaxes our muscles, including those of and around the vulva and vagina. Arousal also causes the vaginal opening and canal to loosen, become more flexible, and self-lubricate so that intercourse is possible, comfortable, and pleasurable. So, be sure you've taken the time—step back from intercourse and take more if need be—to engage in other enjoyable activities first, and create an environment where both of you can be relaxed, not overly nervous or anxious. Use and add

IS SEX BETTER WHEN PARTNERS REACH ORGASM AT THE SAME TIME?

Not necessarily, and sex therapists advise couples *against* aiming for simultaneous orgasm. Trying to have sex like synchronized swimming isn't such a great idea because it makes it harder for both people to simply enjoy themselves, thereby making any orgasm more difficult, let alone orgasming at the same time. When it happens on its own, it's often a happy accident, but it just doesn't happen all that often. It's also more likely to happen without trying than to be forced. More times than not, when people try to force it, one or both partners end up faking an orgasm, which sets a bad sexual pattern and isn't any fun for anyone. Really, going into any kind of sex with a goal that's anything but "I aim for all of us to enjoy ourselves" is problematic.

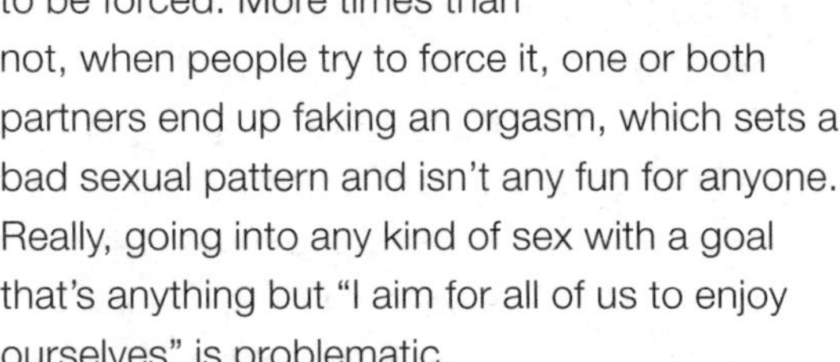

as much additional lubrication as needed; more people than not need more than their body makes all by itself, and most receptive partners also find it makes things feel better for them, even when they already feel mighty nice.

If both of those things are under control, you may need to adjust your angle. Experiment.

▶ **When to take a break:** If intercourse is uncomfortable or painful (or just a big yawner) for either party, at any point, just stop. It's never a good idea for anyone to keep going with anything when they're in pain. Some people try a different position, add more lubricant, slow down, or add other sexual activity, like clitoral stimulation with manual sex, masturbation, or a vibrator. If a partner is having a hard time maintaining erection, give it a rest. Engage in other sexual activities that don't require an erection and that are enjoyable for both of you, or just talk, make out, or cuddle for a while. If you've been going at intercourse for a while and one or both partners isn't reaching orgasm or is starting to feel less aroused, stop for now. You can engage in other sexual activities or just halt sex altogether until another day; sometimes we just hit peak capacity for sex and feel finished, even if orgasm hasn't taken place, and that's perfectly okay.

[ANAL SEX/INTERCOURSE]

AKA: Buttfucking, asslove, backdoor action.

What is it, and how do I do it? Anal sex is entering the anus and rectum for sexual satisfaction of both partners.

Butt B.S.

- Men who enjoy anal sex—whatever their orientation or their body parts—may enjoy being the person doing the entering, the person whose body is being entered, or both. The idea that it's only masculine to put yourself into someone else's body parts, but not to allow sexual partners into any of yours, is just gender stereotyping and other kinds of silliness.
- If you're using toys or dildos for anal sex, be sure the object has a flared base that is a good deal larger than the anus. Although things can't get "lost" inside the vagina, they *can* inside the rectum. As with use of sex toys for anything else, be sure you are either covering toys with a condom or only using toys that can be sanitized; otherwise, bacteria from the rectum can make a toy a vector for infections.
- Anal sex is not "safe sex"; it's not a less risky alternative to vaginal intercourse, nor, like vaginal intercourse, an activity that's wise to engage in unprotected, especially with new, untested, or nonexclusive partners. Both kinds of intercourse have high levels of physical risks, including nearly identical levels of STI risks.

Some young people engage in anal sex, though it's less common than many might think. Data drawn from the National Survey of Family Growth show that for teens fifteen to nineteen years of age, 50 percent had ever engaged in vaginal intercourse; 55 percent had ever engaged in oral sex; and only 11 percent had ever engaged in anal sex. Some young people choose anal sex because they believe it is less risky than vaginal intercourse. This isn't true. From an STI standpoint, it's as or more risky, and because ejaculate + gravity can mean contact of semen with the vagina, it's not always free of pregnancy risks either.

Because of the anatomy of the anus and rectum—they don't self-lubricate, they're surrounded by stronger muscles, and a lot of people don't have any practice relaxing that area of the body—anal intercourse involves *more* patience, preparation, and precaution than vaginal intercourse, not less. So, if you or anyone else doesn't want to go that extra mile or is only doing this because they don't feel ready for vaginal intercourse, I'd suggest a rethink.

Anal sex, like any other kind of sex, shouldn't hurt. But if it isn't done carefully, or happens too quickly, it can be painful for the receptive partner. Doing it in a way likely to feel good for everyone, and hurt no one, involves a few things. First, *both* partners need to actually be

LET'S TALK TECH SEX

What if there was a camera on in your bedroom that recorded any sexual activity you had, and you or your partner could push a button that sent it out to certain people or even just pretty randomly, to anyone, anywhere, anytime? That you—or anyone else who gets it—could edit or change in almost any way you, or they, wanted, today, tomorrow, or ten years from now? That's kind of what sexting—sexual digital texts, images, or videos people who are or want to be sexual with each other make and share—is like.

I don't say that to freak you out, I promise. If you want to be fear-factored about sexting, all you need to do is put it into a search engine or mention it to a group of older adults, and you'll find no shortage of that. What I want to do is give you something that's harder to find: some quick-and-dirty (as it were) realistic information about it so that, like anything else you'll find in this book, you can make informed choices about it that are best for you.

Pros

- Can provide creative ways to explore and express your sexuality, your sexual desires and feelings, and how you present your sexuality or your sexual self in words or images
- Can give long-distance partners, partners who don't have much privacy to be sexual together in person, or partners for whom being sexual in person has high stakes (like people who aren't out yet and for whom it's not safe for them to be out yet) ways to be sexual together
- Can be something that creates sexual anticipation, excitement, and intimacy
- Can increase sexual confidence
- Poses no risk of pregnancy or STIs
- Can provide practice with sexual communication and help develop skills of sexual communication
- Can feel like an emotionally safe way to try out certain sexual things without some of the same emotional or physical risks those things can pose in person
- Is a way of making your own erotica or pornography

interested in it and relaxed about it. Second, anal intercourse should be **very** slow and gradual.

The rectum doesn't produce its own lubrication. The anus is also a tighter, smaller orifice. So, **plenty** of lubricant is *essential* with any anal sex, not optional. Because of the risks of infection *and* small tears or fissures resulting from rough hands during manual anal play, gloves or finger cots are also essentials.

If one or two gloved, lubed fingers feel good to the receptive partner, and they want to move up to a fuller sensation, then you can do that—again, slowly and gradually, and with a condom on the penis or other object. The person doing the anal entry shouldn't be pushing or forcing their way in: if they/you go slow, the anus will slowly "accept" and pull in more of what's introduced to it, and that's something you can feel with whatever body

Cons

- Sharing something digital with one person opens the door to it being shared with others, be those friends or other partners (present and future) of any person you've shared with—two or twenty thousand—you don't know.
- Can often easily be found by parents or others just by clicking around a bit on a cell phone or computer.
- Can be used maliciously by anyone you shared it with if and when a relationship changes or feelings change, like by distributing it within your peer group, to employers or parents, or more widely online.
- Tends to be potentially more dangerous the more vulnerable a person you are; for someone who is a member of a group for which simply being sexual at all or being sexual in media has higher social stakes—like women and people who are queer, transgender, of color, or with certain disabilities—digital sexual media being found or shared widely can be devastating.
- Can be illegal; depending on the content and your age, it may not be lawful for you to make or distribute sexual media. Some of the legal consequences are as serious and awful as serious and awful get. Particularly for legal minors, asking for, creating, or distributing digital sexual images or videos is currently considered child pornography by the law in most areas, so it is a felony that can result in lifelong sex offender legal status and other serious legal and social ramifications.
- Is a way of making your own erotica or pornography (this is in both columns because it can be something one person thinks is awesome but another feels totally creeped out by).
- Can sometimes be an impediment to good sexual communication if anyone involved feels like what they're supposed to say or do or their presentation of sexuality is scripted rather than made-to-order content and exchanges that are expressions of their unique sexuality, desires, and sexual relationships and interactions. In other words, if someone feels that in a medium like this everyone is only allowed to act like a porn star, that won't help with communication.
- Similarly, if anyone involved feels like digital sexual media is automatically an expression or promise of someone wanting or being willing to do anything in person, it can create feelings and dynamics of sexual pressure.

part you're putting inside the anus. After that, how deep, fast, or slow one should go is up to the person on the receiving end, so communication is as important here as ever. Like other sexual activities, anal play or intercourse can be combined with oral sex, manual sex, or even vaginal intercourse by using fingers or sex toys such as butt plugs.

STI risk: Very high risk.

Pregnancy risk: Low risk.

SEXTING, CYBERSEX, OR PHONE SEX

What is it, and how do I do it? Expressing and exploring sexuality with someone else through words or images via telephone, online, or mobile technologies. This way of being sexual has produced some of the most hubba-hubba love (or lust) letters throughout history. Although these ways of being sexual, through words, images, or both, are often presented as being entirely new-millennium, they're so not. People have explored sex and sexuality together through words and images, in person and through media, for probably most of our human history.

Some people engage in this kind of sexual behavior as a warm-up, minutes, hours, days, or even weeks before an in-person sexual encounter. For others, it's an end unto itself or something to do with someone while masturbating. For partners in long-distance relationships, it can be one way of enjoying sexual intimacy between visits.

What language or kind of media or medium—e-mails? Phone calls? Video chat? Sound files? Texts? Social media?—is used is up to the both of you. In terms of what media you use, that'll depend on what you each have access to, your limits, or just-nopes when it comes to your personal safety or privacy and what feels like the right tool or context. In terms of language, some people are turned on by explicit or directive lingo, while others find they're more excited by a subtle approach. The same goes with anything visual; this has the most to do with people's comfort levels as well as what is or feels safe and sound for them. What each person finds more or less arousing or feels in the mood for is going to vary.

One of the tricky parts of some of these ways of being sexual is that most of us hear a lot of scripts—in our culture, in media, from friends—and see a lot of imagery that kind of tells us what to do when we're expressing ourselves sexually through media. Just like it can be easy to initiate or do only sexual activities we've learned are what we're supposed to do, we tend to use media sexually to playact or follow what we've seen or read before, which is usually pretty narrow. Some people even feel like how they express themselves through media is in competition with other sexual media, from previous partners or in commercial pornography and other forms that show a narrow standard of bodies and sexuality.

That places an awful lot of pressure on and influences something that should really be about expressing and exploring yourself and as something for yourself—something that is not likely to be very exciting or interesting to everyone involved unless what people bring to it is imagination, creativity, and their own sexuality and expressions of it.

So, if any of these ways of being sexual are safe for you (including not setting you or anyone else up to potentially commit serious crimes), something you and yours want to explore, and you want it to actually feel fun and unique, not like one or both of you has to put on a show and play a part, think about it as a creative pursuit. Use your imagination; *share* your imaginations. Be you, not someone else.

Like any other way of being sexual with someone, just bring the same respect and care you do or would with in-person sex, and see where that takes you.

STI Risk: No risk.

Pregnancy risk: No risk.

[SENSATION PLAY]

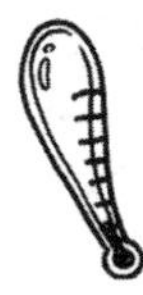

What is it, and how do I do it? Experimenting with different sensations, throughout the body, not just genitally (in fact, it need not be genital at all).

Some people do this by applying hot and/or cold items to the body, by stroking the body with different items, such as feathers or silky or rough fabrics, and by adding food or liquid items to sexual play. Others might use clothespins for a pinching sensation, snakebite kits for "cupping" certain areas of the body for a feeling of suction, safe forms of electrical play with static electricity machines configured for sexual use, or hands, whips, or paddles to strike the skin.

Some use sensation play as part of SM or BDSM activity (see page 245). But those roles or structures aren't at all required for sensation play; many people engage in sensation play without incorporating them at all.

So long as skin isn't broken in any way or direct oral or genital contact isn't being made sensation play is 100 percent safer sex.

STI risk: No risk.

Pregnancy risk: No risk.

["KINKY" SEX]

Just about everybody's heard of it, but no one really knows what it means. That's because *kinky* (like *deviant* or *perverse* or *obscene*) is a pretty arbitrary term; everyone defines it a bit differently. One person's kink is another person's not-kinky-at-all. But what most people mean when they refer to "kinky" sex is either an uncommon practice or one typically thought of as unconventional. Typically, bondage and restraint, fluid or blood play, the use of sex toys, "edge" play, powerplay or role-play, and some sensation play are often filed under "kinky." Whether you feel that any or all of these are "kinky" or not is completely your call.

Role-Play

What is it, and how do I do it? Just like "make-believe" or "playing doctor" as a kid, some people do the same in a sexual context with partners. That may mean a couple pretends that they're in a different place, that someone is watching, or that they're different genders—what have you. Some bring costumes and props into the scene; for others the fantasy is solely in the imagination. Role-play can be a way for couples to play out sexual fantasies together. Sexual cosplay is a kind of role-play, as is most sex that incorporates domination or submission (which sometimes is about an abusive relationship where that's for real, not about consensual sexual role-play).

Some people may incorporate hierarchal roles into their fantasy scenarios; some may be about "powerplay," in which partners explore different power relationships between them or sexual fantasies in which power or hierarchical elements are in place, such as student/teacher or employee/boss. Some people explore scenarios that would either be harmful, dangerous, or taboo in actuality, such as incest, rape, or sex with strangers. Others may use role-play to explore existing gender roles or stereotypes or to enjoy sillier fare, like playing doctor, cops 'n' robbers, badass super(s)hero and captured bad guy, Bert and Ernie—whatever floats your boat.

Role-play that plays with risk, consent, taboo, hierarchy, and power can be very charged and loaded, and more easily coercive. After all, many of those things are problematic in our culture and/or based on violence or abuse, and it's really easy to have unacknowledged, internalized ideas about sexual roles that can limit our awareness of real problems.

Be mindful. Talk about limits and boundaries in advance, and be open to adaptations over time. For instance, you or your partner may find that, although certain activities within a given role-play session are just fine, certain language may be unpleasant, scary, or unwanted. As well, one person's idea of what a given role entails or involves can be pretty different from another's. So, not only is it important to discuss expectations, limits, and boundaries but also it's a good idea to put fail-safes in place that allow either partner to make clear immediately when and if something isn't okay and the action needs to stop. It's also worth talking about where the role-play stays. For instance, if one partner agrees to being submissive during a given scene, make sure both parties understand that there's no obligation or agreement for that partner to always be that way or bring those roles into other aspects of the relationship.

Sometimes, people find that role-play isn't so good for them, especially if the roles they're playing aren't completely wanted or consensual or they're sexualizing or reinforcing negative or destructive patterns. For example, a rape survivor wanting to reenact a rape again and again may be trying to process issues via sex that would be more productively and healthily processed in nonsexual situations.

Last, it's not unusual for a lot of role-play to be hierarchal or based on roles of dominance and submission. One reason that is so common is that this power structure has been the most pervasive through much of our documented history and in our society and culture; those are the roles nearly all of us learn, internalize, and even find to be the only way we've learned to conceptualize power and interpersonal dynamics. But you can also explore sexual role-play that's outside those structures; nobody has to be tied to any given roles if they don't want to be. If your sexual role isn't 100 percent optional, it's safe to say it

BDSM

D/S is a term usually used to describe sexual dominance and submission play, in which one partner "tops" and another "bottoms" and/or one partner is dominating and another submitting. The top or bottom may be of any gender, and the action may involve extending pleasure past a point of physical or emotional comfort; "punishing" a partner via humiliation, sexual play, or withholding of sexual activities; and utilizing bondage, sensation play, or verbal enactments. *SM* or *S/M* is an abbreviation for sadism and masochism, or sadomasochism, which means that one partner is giving pain (*sado–*), and the other is receiving it (*–masochism*). The *B* in BDSM usually refers to bondage.

BDSM educators recommend what's often known as the *SSC rule:* safe, sane, and consensual. In other words, whatever is being done is agreed upon by both partners and is performed in ways that are both physically *and* emotionally safe and sane—the same sort of guidelines advised for any kind of sex. Safe and sane include partners truly being able to consent (including legally) and fully understanding what they're agreeing to, both in the short term and the long term (that is, how these sexual choices may affect the individuals, their relationship, and the other areas of their lives). Any sort of sex or role that is forced, coerced, or malicious through the use of power roles or sex is *not* safe, sane, or consensual.

D/S play may involve sex acts most people are familiar with, such as oral sex and intercourse. D/S may also incorporate sensation play, bondage, or other "kinky" sexual activities. Many people engaging in D/S play incorporate *safewords* into their play: phrases or gestures understood by both to express thresholds, limits, and boundaries. Saying a safeword stops the role-play or sexual activity at any time, immediately and without question. Like polyamory, D/S or BDSM play often requires more discussion and negotiation than other sexual activities might. D/S roles shouldn't be dictated by sex or gender: people of any gender can be tops, bottoms, or "switches," people who enjoy both roles. What role someone should choose is the role that they want.

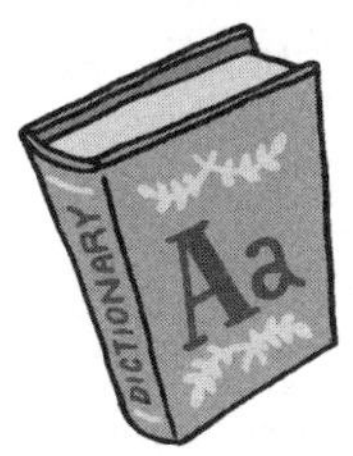

Stay self-aware if you're considering or involved with D/S play. Some people do use D/S as a way of making an abusive relationship seem acceptable or sexy or to employ it as a means to extend self-injury or controlling behavior, even unconsciously. If your partner is in any way physically abusive in the whole of your relationship or you're not having deep discussions negotiating sexual roles; if your partner verbally abuses or humiliates you outside a "scene" or as a general practice; if you feel that there's a required, implied, or given—rather than agreed upon and optional—power dynamic or imbalance, then it's entirely possible that D/S or S/M play is merely an extension of abuse. With relationship abuse as prevalent as it is, it's not sensible to entertain the delusion that somehow BDSM relationships or communities are immune.

isn't healthy (and that goes for our sexual roles even when we aren't role-playing).

STI risk: Risk levels depend on what sexual activities are engaged in during role-play.

Pregnancy risk: Risk levels depend on what sexual activities are engaged in during role-play.

Bondage/Restraint

What is it, and how do I do it? Bondage or restraint is the practice of having one partner (or less often, both partners) restrained in some way, usually with ropes, cords, other types of fabric or cuffs, and other restraints, during sexual activity for the purpose of increasing pleasure. Some people self-restrain during masturbation. Others use rope or cord to create intricate and creative patterns of knot-tying on the body.

It's really important to understand that tying up or restraining a partner against their will is an absolute Big No. **That is assault and kidnapping, and it is both criminal and abusive.** As with any other sexual activity, for this sort of play to be at all emotionally safe, it's vital that *everyone* feels *good* about it and consents to it, that everyone is clear on their limits, and that the intent isn't malicious or punitive but about pleasure and intimacy.

Like sensation play, sometimes bondage and restraint are incorporated into BDSM or role-play, but just as often, they aren't. Bondage can be used to allow a partner to be selfish in terms of being given all the pleasure, being unable to reciprocate during a given sexual activity, because they can't use their hands or mouths. Some people enjoy being bound or restrained in certain ways that keep them from engaging in behaviors that may be habitual for them, as a way to seek out other avenues of pleasure; for instance, a person who typically masturbates during intercourse may enjoy having their hands bound and then having to seek out other forms of extra stimulation.

Discussing bondage in advance of the activity is important, as is establishing some code or means of communication so that if the bound partner begins to feel uncomfortable or unsafe, it's easy for them to clearly express that and halt the action.

If you're going to be tying or restraining a partner, remember that circulation is a good thing, and cutting it off isn't. To assess healthy circulation, especially in limbs, doctors and nurses use the code CSM: **color, sensation, and movement.** *Color* should be normal, a person should be able to feel the same *sensations* on that limb as anywhere else, and they should be able to *move* extremities easily. Make sure whatever restraints you're using are comfortable for your partner and that they still have at least some mobility. If they are tied to something, make sure that it's stable and safe and that they are not left alone. Although some people like the feeling of some restraint on their neck during sexual activities, restricting the airway, for a partner or yourself, is incredibly dangerous.

Not everybody wants to engage in activities like bondage. For plenty, it may ring of servitude, slavery, or imprisonment, conditions that many people don't find erotic or pleasant at all. For others, consent and care being present erase those negative associations. As with anything else, if you're interested in an activity and your partner just really isn't, don't push.

STI risk: No risk (as long as skin is not broken and items used or shared are clean).

Pregnancy risk: No risk.

Body Fluid or Blood Play

What is it, and how do I do it? Some people enjoy any number of body fluids sexually: ejaculate, vaginal fluids, menses, urine, or blood. They may simply enjoy tasting, feeling, or smelling them during sexual activities, or they may engage in activities specific to enjoying those fluids, such as "golden showers" (being urinated on) or having a partner ejaculate on them. Some enjoy this because it feels taboo, or naughty, to have intimate contact with body fluids. For others, fluid play may be enjoyable because a certain intimacy or sacredness is experienced in fluid bonding.

But from an infection and disease perspective, fluid play can be dangerous, especially when body fluids have contact with incredibly sensitive sites like the eyes. Whereas urine itself is sterile, it does pass through the urethra, where an infection may be present. Ejaculate can carry several different infections. Contact with blood, or cutting or piercing partners in any way, opens the door to some of the deadlier diseases and infections out there, like hepatitis B and HIV.

So, for the most part, this sort of play is quite risky, especially for younger couples, the majority of whom have not had sound or regular sexual health care. Most younger people have not had safer sex with a monogamous partner long enough to be safely "fluid-bonded."

STI risk: Very high risk.

Pregnancy risk: No risk, unless semen comes into contact with a vulva.

Sex Toys

What is it, and how do I do it? Sex toys come in many varieties. From vibrators—electric and battery-operated, big and small, swanky and silly—to silicone dildos, anal plugs to masturbation sleeves, cock rings to clitoral suction devices, toys and tools run the gamut. People use them for masturbation as well as for partnered sex, by themselves or in conjunction with other activities.

Generally, sex toys aren't available for purchase by minors and are sold in sex toy shops, through catalogs, and on Internet sites. Some people also make their own sex toys or use household objects as sexual toys or aids: electric toothbrushes, plastic bottles, socks, pillows, and all sorts of other objects.

So long as simple directions are followed for items sold as sex toys, they're usually safe for use. For instance, using something electrical in a bathtub isn't safe or smart, and using an item not designed for anal use—and without a flared base—in the anus is a bad idea. Anything with sharp edges should generally not be used on or in the genitals. You must be able to cover with a latex barrier anything that is being used as a sex toy, especially if it is shared, or be able to boil it; otherwise, you could brew and pass around infections and bacteria. Shared (and uncovered) toys are often a very common route for infections to be spread between female partners, something lesbian women often aren't

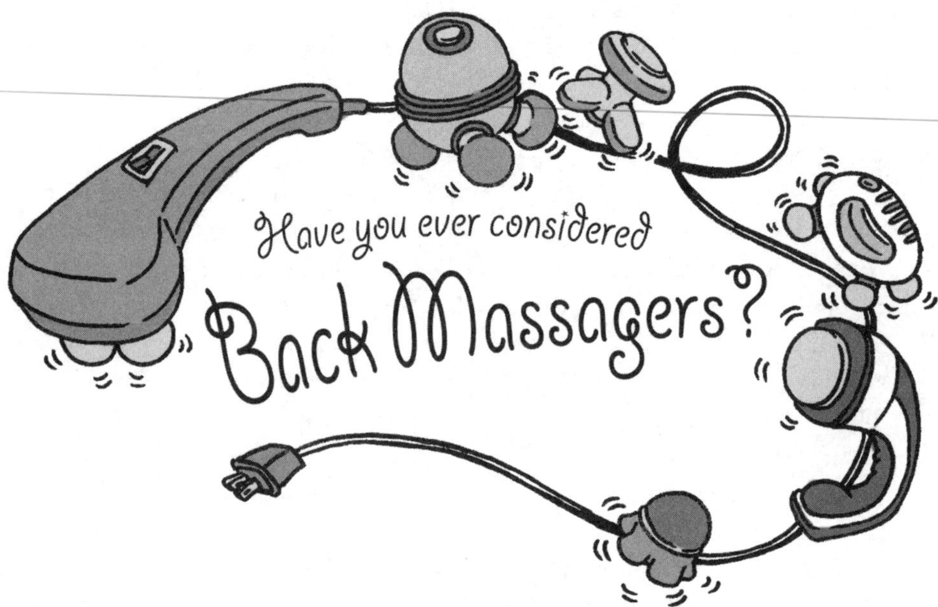
Have you ever considered
Back Massagers?

even aware of. Using household items—such as electric toothbrushes, the zucchini for dinner, or shampoo bottles—as sex toys, when they *are* shared by household members, who are unaware of what they're being used for by you, is decidedly on the Not Okay list.

There are so many different kinds of toys, and so many different ways to use them, a whole separate book would be required to cover all the bases. But people of all genders can and do enjoy a multitude of toys, and many people, and often especially women, who have trouble first reaching orgasm find that a vibrator can help get them there. People may like vibrators or suction toys used on their clitoris or labia, on the penis or testes, on the perineum or anus, or the nipples, or almost any other body part. Dildos, plugs, and insertable vibes can be used inside body parts or body parts can be put into them. People can use dildos paired with harnesses worn on the hips for intercourse.

People often ask whether vibrators can permanently desensitize areas they're used on: the answer is no. Very fast or intense friction or sensation can *temporarily* cause less sensation to be experienced in the genitals, because heavy friction tends to numb things slightly. A person can experience that with a vibrator but also with oral sex or by riding a motorcycle. Clap your hands together very intensely for a while, for instance, and you can get an idea of how loss of sensation can happen and how quickly sensitivity usually returns. Right after the clapping, the tingling in your palms will be intense, and touching your palm with fingers may not feel like much, but shortly the tingling subsides and your touch will feel more sensitive again. No big. Too, any one form of stimulation can, after a while, feel old or become a mere habit. But vibrators and other sex toys don't damage people's bodies or genitals in any way simply by being used, even when used frequently.

Some partners feel insecure about a suggestion to use sex toys together, feeling like if a toy is "needed," they or their genitals or other body parts are inadequate in some way. Generally, some people mistakenly think that they are supposed to be their partner's absolute sexual everything and that their body is the only playground. Explaining the difference between "need" and "want," in these situations, is often helpful, as is making clear that wanting to add toys to play is really no different from wanting to try any new sexual activity.

Also, toys that all partners can enjoy, in whatever ways, are often helpful for dealing with feelings of insecurity about sex toys: when everyone involved uses them, instead of just one person, that can help a partner who wants to use a toy but feels self-conscious about being the only one. Some partners may feel that sex toys are "unnatural," but nowadays, so much of our environment, from our sex lives to the foods we eat to what we put on our hair, is man-made or synthetic that, although the desire to stay close to nature is understandable, sex toys aren't holding the world back from that. Too, people with some kinds of disability often *need* sex toys or devices to engage in the sexual activities they want to. There are a lot of tricky attitudes out there about sex toys or aids.

Of course, if someone just doesn't want to use sex toys, alone or with a partner, all that's to be done is to accept and honor that. Even though a resistance to sex toys doesn't always come from a place of confidence, that doesn't change the fact that we always simply accept any sexual no someone gives us.

If you're a minor without access to manufactured sex toys, life *will* go on without them for the time being. You can also do a little DIY if you like: a lot of people use "back massagers" (and two of the most popular vibrators ever sold, the Hitachi Magic Wand and the Wahl Coil are such "massagers"), the backs of electric toothbrushes, or other self-fashioned toys. So long as it belongs to you (or you can throw it away), no part of it can injure you, and you can make it sanitary, it's probably safe, fine, and someone else has probably also made it work for themselves before.

STI risk: No risk to moderate risk.

Pregnancy risk: No risk.

Phthalates

Some sex toys may contain toxic substances, such as phthalates—a family of chemicals that has been linked in some studies to reproductive problems for men and women and potential cancer risks. Some toys say that they are phthalate-free on their packaging, and sex toy sellers can usually direct customers to phthalate-free goods, but many manufacturers do not list these ingredients. Because many sex toys are sold "for novelty-use only," manufacturers can dodge health regulations. Toys that are made of "cyberskin" or "jelly toys" are most likely to contain these substances; silicone, hard plastic or acrylic, glass, and metal sex toys usually do not.

YES, NO, MAYBE SO: A WHAT-YOU-WANT-AND-HOW-YOU-WANT-IT SEX CHECKLIST

Because what sex can be—and how we can go about all that it is—is so vast, it can be hard to get a good sense of what we want and how we want things if we're trying to keep it all sorted in our heads. A checklist like this can help you consider all of this more tangibly and can be something you just do by and for yourself or do together and share with partners. Your answers to this list will probably change and shift over time or from partner to partner. For now, consider it a sexual snapshot of this point in time and an ever-evolving work in progress, just like you and your sexuality are.

Code Guide

Y	=	Yes
N	=	No
M	=	Maybe
IDK	=	I don't know
F	=	Fantasy
N/A	=	Not applicable

Body Boundaries

____ A partner touching me without asking first

____ Touching a partner without asking first

____ A partner touching me affectionately in public

____ Touching a partner affectionately in public

____ A partner touching me sexually in public

____ Touching a partner sexually in public

____ Having my shirt/top off with a partner

____ Having a partner's shirt/top off

____ Having my pants/bottoms off with a partner

____ Having a partner's pants/bottoms off

____ Being naked with a partner

____ A partner being naked with me

____ Direct eye contact

____ Being looked at directly, overall, when I am naked

____ Talking about a partner's body

____ Some or all kinds of sex during a menstrual period

____ Seeing or being exposed to other kinds of body fluids (like semen, sweat, or urine)

____ Other:

____

____

Some parts of my body are just off-limits. Those are:

____

____

I am not comfortable looking at, touching, or feeling some parts of another person's body. Those are:

____

____

I am triggered by (have a post-traumatic response to) some thing(s) about body boundaries. Those are/that is:

____

____

Words and Terms

I prefer the following gender/sexual identity or role words for myself:

____

____

I prefer the following words for my chest, breasts, genitals, and other body parts:

____

____

Some words that I am not okay with to refer to me, my identity, my body or that I am uncomfortable using or hearing about with or during any kind of sex are:

____

____

I am triggered by certain words or language. Those are/that is:

____

____

Relationship Models and Choices

____ A partner talking to close friends about our sex life

____ Talking to close friends about my sex life

____ A partner talking to acquaintances, family, or coworkers about our sex life

____ Talking to acquaintances, family, or coworkers about my sex life

____ An exclusive sexual relationship

____ Some kind of casual or occasional open/nonexclusive sexual relationship

____ Some kind of serious or ongoing open/nonexclusive sexual relationship

____ Sex of some kind(s) with one partner at a time, only

____ Sex of some kind(s) with two partners at a time

____ Sex of some kind(s) with three or more partners at a time

____ A partner directing/deciding for me in some way with sex

____ Directing or deciding for a partner in some way with sex

____ Other:

____

____

Safer Sex and Overall Safety Items and Behaviors

____ Sharing my sexual history with a partner

____ A partner sharing their sexual history with me

____ Doing anything sexual that does or might pose high risks of certain or all sexually transmitted infections (STIs)

____ Doing anything sexual that does or might pose moderate risks of certain or all STIs

____ Doing anything sexual that does or might pose low risks of certain or all STIs

____ Using a condom with a partner

____ Putting on a condom myself

____ Putting a condom on someone else

____ Someone else putting a condom on me

____ Using a dental dam with a partner

____ Putting on a dental dam for myself

____ Putting a dental dam on someone else

____ Someone else putting a dental dam on me

____ Using a latex glove with a partner

____ Using lubricant with a partner

____ Applying lubricant to myself

____ Applying lubricant to a partner

____ Someone else putting lubricant on me

____ Getting tested for STIs before sex with a partner

____ Getting regularly tested for STIs by myself

____ Getting tested for STIs with a partner

____ A partner getting regularly tested for STIs

____ Sharing STI test results with a partner

____ Doing things that might cause me momentary or minor discomfort or pain

____ Doing things that might cause a partner momentary or minor discomfort or pain

____ Being unable to communicate clearly during sex

____ Having a partner be unable to communicate clearly

____ Other:

____

____

I am triggered by some thing(s) around sexual safety or need additional safety precautions because of triggers. Those are/that is:

____

____

Sexual Responses

____ Experiencing or expressing unexpected or challenging emotions before, during, or after sex

____ A partner experiencing or expressing or challenging emotions before, during, or after sex

____ Feeling and being aroused (sexually excited) alone

____ Feeling and being aroused with or in front of a partner

____ Having genital sexual response, like erection or lubrication, alone

____ Having genital sexual response, like erection or lubrication, seen or felt by a partner

____ Not having or "losing" erection or lubrication alone

____ Not having or "losing" erection or lubrication with or in front of a partner

____ Being unable to reach orgasm alone

____ Being unable to reach orgasm with a partner

____ Having orgasm alone

____ Having orgasm with or in front of a partner

____ Ejaculating alone

____ Ejaculating with or in front of a partner

____ Having a partner ejaculate with me/while I'm present

____ Having an orgasm before or after I feel like I "should" with a partner

____ Having a partner have an orgasm before or after you feel like they "should"

____ Making noise during sex or orgasm alone

____ Making noise during sex or orgasm with a partner

____ Having sex interrupted by something or someone external or your own body or feelings

____ Other:

____

____

I am triggered by certain sexual responses of my own or those of a partner. Those are:

____

____

Physical and/or Sexual Activities

____ Masturbation

____ Holding hands

____ Hugging

____ Kissing

____ Being kissed or touched on the neck

____ Kissing or touching a partner's neck

____ Giving hickeys

____ Getting hickeys

____ Tickling, doing the tickling

____ Tickling, being tickled

____ General massage, giving

____ General massage, receiving

____ Having my chest, breasts, and/or nipples touched or rubbed

____ Touching or rubbing a partner's chest, breasts, and/or nipples

____ Frottage (dry humping/clothed body-to-body rubbing)

____ Tribadism (scissoring, rubbing naked genitals together with a partner)

____ A partner putting their mouth or tongue on my breasts or chest

____ Putting my mouth or tongue on a partner's breasts or chest

____ Masturbating in front of/with a partner

____ A partner masturbating in front of/with me

____ Manual sex, receiving

____ Manual sex, giving

____ Ejaculating (coming) on or in a partner's body

____ A partner ejaculating (coming) on or in my body

____ Using sex toys (like vibrators, dildos, or masturbation sleeves) alone

____ Using sex toys (like vibrators, dildos, or masturbation sleeves) with a partner

____ Oral sex (to vulva), receptive partner

____ Oral sex (to vulva), doing to someone else

____ Oral sex (to penis or strap-on), receptive partner

____ Oral sex (to penis or strap-on), doing to someone else

____ Oral sex (to testes), receptive partner

____ Oral sex (to testes), doing to someone else

____ Oral sex (to anus), receptive partner

____ Oral sex (to anus), doing to someone else

____ Vaginal intercourse, receptive partner

____ Vaginal intercourse, insertive partner

____ Anal intercourse, receptive partner

____ Anal intercourse, insertive partner

____ Using food items as a part of sex

____ Wearing something that covers my eyes

____ A partner wearing something that covers their eyes

____ Having my movement restricted

____ Restricting the movement of a partner

____ Being bitten, scratched, slapped, or spanked by a partner in the context of sexual pleasure

____ Scratching, biting, slapping, or spanking a partner in the context of sexual pleasure

____ Pinching or having any kind of clamp used on my body during sex

____ Pinching a partner or using any kind of clamp on them during sex

____ Other:

____

____

I am triggered by certain sexual activities. Those are:

____

____

____

I want or need to use safer sex barriers or methods of contraception with the following activities:

____

____

____

Nonphysical Sexual Activities

____ Communicating my sexual fantasies to/with a partner

____ Receiving information about a partner's sexual fantasies

____ Role-play

____ Sexting, cybersex, or phone sex

____ Reading pornography alone

____ Reading pornography with a partner

____ Viewing pornography alone

____ Viewing pornography with a partner

____ A partner reading or viewing pornography

____ Giving pornography/erotica to a partner

____ Getting pornography/erotica from a partner

____ Other:

____

____

I am triggered by certain nonphysical sexual activities. Those are:

____

____

____

THE OL' GIVE-AND-TAKE: SEXUAL SYMMETRY, RECIPROCITY, AND EQUALITY

Inequities, imbalances, and mismatches in love and in sex can manifest in many ways. Maybe you performed oral sex on a partner and so feel they "owe" you the same, even if they aren't as interested in it as you are—or maybe you only performed that oral sex to try to earn some for yourself. Or you find you feel guilty about a partner rubbing their genitals with your hands when you don't want to or don't feel ready to yet, and you think you're being unfair in some way. Perhaps you always initiate sex in your partnership and would really like the shoe to be on the other foot for a change. One partner might feel that the other always gets what he or she likes but that they never get what's good for them. And, sometimes, one partner may have a satisfactory experience, while the other just doesn't, and that might feel unfair.

Reciprocity, Reloaded

I'm going to suggest you look at reciprocity in sex—the idea that one person gives something, so the other should get something of equal value back—in a different way than you might be used to.

With activities like sexual intercourse, dry sex, and kissing, where the same or similar parts are getting used and stimulated at the same time, we assume reciprocity: that both parties are giving and getting the same thing. That in and of itself is often a false assumption, because no activity guarantees that both partners are having the same experience or that their enjoyment in that activity is identical.

With activities like oral and manual sex, people usually assume that one partner is giving and the other getting and that the giver and the getter can't be both giving and receiving unless they're "performing" the same activity on each other simultaneously. Assuming that assumes a lot. For starters, the assumption that only one partner is sexually engaged or pleased is based on the flawed idea that our genitals are our only pleasure center and that when one person's genitals aren't involved in a sexual activity and someone else's are only the person whose genitals are getting some action is "getting" sex.

If during any partnered sex activity either partner feels they aren't getting *anything* out of a given sexual activity or getting pretty equal satisfaction, then you'll want to figure out how to change or make room for that.

Partnered sex involves more than just you, and there can be many things going on for each person—both giving *and* receiving pleasure. If we're with someone who is a good partner for us, we're not just getting off on being pleased, we're getting off on our partner experiencing pleasure. If both the giving and the receiving aren't pretty fantastic, no matter what role you're in during a given activity, that's something to evaluate. Check to make sure you're sleeping with someone you really like, for instance, and who you know likes you—inside *and* outside the bedroom. Be mindful of hidden trouble spots in the relationship, like feeling taken advantage of, that your needs are ignored, or that you always have to be the leader. Double-check with yourself to be sure that partnered sex rather than masturbation is really what you want at the moment and that you're not engaging in any sexual activity out of obligation rather than desire.

It's also worth making sure that neither of you is just being a selfish creep. It happens, even to the best of us, sometimes—even otherwise good, sharing partners can get so caught up in having sex that's all about them that they space out their partner's wants, needs, or limits.

[SEX AND OBLIGATION]

Nobody "owes" anyone sex. We don't lend and borrow sex the way we lend and borrow our favorite sweaters or a cell phone, nor do we "owe" someone a blow job for going out with us like we owe someone who fixed the toilet payment for their services. Yet, some people engage in sex or certain sexual activities out of feelings of obligation. Obligatory sex usually feels crappy and boring, at best, and horrible—emotionally and physically—at worst, especially over time if it becomes habit. When your partner is doing their homework in their head during sex rather than being fully present with you or is just saying yes to avoid an argument, it can feel pretty weird and create some unhealthy patterns.

Maybe your partner performed oral sex for you, so you feel that you're obliged to perform a similar or understood-to-be-equal activity, whether you like it or not. You may feel that your boyfriend or girlfriend is someone you don't deserve or is somehow above you, and sex seems like a good way to even the scales. Friends may push you to become sexually active for their own agendas. Perhaps your partner has had a level of previous sexual experience you feel you've got to live up to. Maybe you've been together for some time, and it seems sex should happen, by some arbitrary and invisible timeline, or it's been a few weeks since you had sex, and even though you're not in the mood, you feel you owe it to your partner to have sex with them.

If your partner engaged in oral sex with you and your genitals, and they're expecting something in return that you aren't interested in, let them know you aren't interested in whatever that is, and fill them in on the things you *are* interested in instead. If you feel that your boyfriend or girlfriend is too good for you and you've got to compensate by engaging in sexual activity they want, then deal with the self-esteem issues or relationship imbalances that are causing you to feel that way. If you've been together a

ONE YES (OR NOT) AT A TIME

Once you or your partner engage in any given sexual activity, you're not then forever obligated to keep doing it. If you find there's something you just don't like or have no interest in; if at any given time something you usually like just doesn't have appeal; if at any point you feel you want or need to take a break from sexual activity or partnership altogether, it is *always* okay. If we make someone breakfast once, we aren't obligated to do it it every day or always on Sunday or to always make pancakes, and the same goes for any sort of sex.

while, and some arbitrary timeline seems to require that sex should happen, start talking to your partner about feeling that way, and discuss, between you, what your own individual timelines are and what you feel ready for and want. If it's been a few weeks since you had sex, and you're still not in the mood, start talking: look into why that might be, like relationship or sexual problems, stress, depression, low libido, or just not feeling up to sex. You owe your partner communication and honesty, not sexual favors, and they owe you patience and understanding.

If you find yourself in a situation where anyone feels owed or obligated, regardless of *any* actual shared desire, you two need to do more talking before having anymore sex.

[FAKING IT]

Plenty of people (and not just women!) fake orgasm, for a variety of reasons: They may feel that if they don't "come," they are ruining something for their partner; they may be worried that they'll look sexually immature or inexperienced if they don't have an orgasm or that they'll hurt a partner's feelings. Whatever the reason, although you'd be hard-pressed to find a person who has never once in their life faked it, it's a bad habit to get into. Faking orgasm is not only a sort of dishonesty that can break down the trust and intimacy in your relationship, it gives a partner false cues about what is turning you on. You fake it a few times, you may find you've created big barriers to building the sexual communication you need to make a real orgasm happen with a partner. Eventually, to get back on track, you may have to 'fess up that you've faked it, setting both of you up for hurt feelings and a loss of trust, both in and out of bed.

If you've never faked it, do yourself and your sex life a favor and don't start. If you feel that you have to fake it or are stuck in a pattern of doing so, talk to your partner. It's sure not the easiest conversation to have, but it can be done sensitively. Make it clear that your faking isn't about your partner being "bad in bed" but about your failure to explain or explore what does work for you, or maybe it's about trying to live up to unrealistic expectations one of you has. Make clear that you don't *want* to fake it; you want to work on communicating and exploring what you both *do* enjoy, with or without orgasm. Be sure to express that it's okay if either you or your partner doesn't have an orgasm; your self-esteem doesn't (or sure shouldn't) depend upon their orgasm.

People just don't always reach orgasm, even with very satisfying sex. They may be tired, stressed out, emotionally overwhelmed, or physically exhausted. If you're expecting yourself or your partners to achieve orgasm with every sexual experience, you're being unrealistic in your expectations.

[HAVING TROUBLE REACHING ORGASM OR FEELING AROUSED WITH A PARTNER?]

Take a look at these common culprits (even just one may be your roadblock):

▶ Are you moving too fast—not just in terms of getting sexual with someone but in the way you are sexual? Are you giving yourself time to savor *every* nuance, or are you in a big hurry because one or both of you are nervous, in an unsafe place, or afraid of being caught?

▶ Can you have a good sense of humor during sex, or are you afraid to laugh with your partner? Does the context of your sex life or the way you're going about it feel more like a funeral than something more fun and light?

▶ Are there aspects of your sexuality or sexual choices that feel forbidden or taboo? If so, are they enhancing your experience or keeping you from satisfaction? Do you feel ashamed or guilty before, during, or after sex?

▶ Are you comfortable with the power roles between you and your partner? Do you feel that you're pretty equal, for instance, in initiating sex, setting limits and boundaries, and reciprocating sexually? Do you feel that either of you is passive or not fully included in any aspect of your sex life?

▶ Do you feel safe, physically and emotionally? Can you say no and have it be respected, without argument? Do you have protection from pregnancy and STIs?

▶ Are you comfortable communicating with your partner, and do you feel they're communicating with you, in terms of what you both want and need, like and don't like? Can you discuss what could be better, what you'd like done differently, what you need included in your sex but aren't getting?

▶ Do you feel under any pressure to reach orgasm, to be or feel "sexy," or to please your partner?

▶ Do you have any current conflicts, doubts, or worries about your relationship?

▶ Are you comfortable with your sexual fantasies, wants, and needs? How about your partner's?

▶ Are you really recognizing and communicating that you are or are not aroused? Do you feel 100 percent comfortable saying no when you're not aroused, or do you feel obligated to go ahead anyway?

▶ Are you dealing with depression, anxiety, recent illness, surgery, a major health complication? Are you sleep-deprived, or have you not been resting well recently? How about recent stress or trauma, like college acceptance issues; tests or grades; arts or sports competitions; a death, illness, or separation in the family; sexual or other assault?

▶ Do you feel that your partner has to supply all of your sexual satisfaction, or are you down with providing it on your own via masturbation, both when you don't have a partner and when you do? Are you comfortable with having or trying masturbation as part of your partnered activities?

▶ Do you feel comfortable reaching orgasm or being aroused, or do you feel self-conscious about aspects of arousal or normal body functions (like erection or ejaculation, clitoral enlargement, vaginal lubrication, menstruation, farting, body scents, or the effects of orgasm)? If you have a disability, do you feel comfortable making needed modifications or adjustments with your partner?

▶ Does sexual response make you feel uncomfortably out of control; do you trust yourself when aroused or sexually engaged? Do you feel overexposed physically with a partner, nervous about nudity? Do you experience body-image problems with a partner?

▶ Are you getting hung up on things that appear to be problematic rather than seeing ways in which your obstacles can enhance your erotic experience? Are you overthinking sex and finding yourself unable to relax enough to turn off your analytical brain for a bit so you can actually enjoy yourself?

Who's in Charge?

The structure of our society often gives us the impression that relations between people have to be hierarchical: leader/follower, top/bottom, boss/employee. But they don't. In a healthy sexual relationship, *everyone* should be active partners, in initiation, in decision making, and in performing actual sexual activities.

Are you worried about asserting yourself, about stepping up and talking about what you really want and need, about taking charge just as much as your partner is? Do you feel that you'd be threatening your relationship by doing so? If you feel threatened or usurped by a partner doing those things, step back and evaluate the situation. Are you and your partner both really ready to be in an intimate relationship with someone else, or not? Are you involved with someone who's really right and appropriate for you, or not? Are you ready to truly make full allowances for someone else's needs and wants and learn to work out yours with theirs, even when it's hard or disappointing, or not? Do you feel confident enough in yourself to both assert your own needs and desires *and* make some compromises sometimes? Do you feel secure and safe enough with your partner to screw up sometimes and to deal with that? All of those things are worth looking at to be sure that you're both able to share the wheel.

[SEXUAL DIFFERENCES VS. SEXUAL INCOMPATIBILITY]

It's very rare to encounter a sexual partner with whom your sexual wants and needs are an effortless, perfect match. More times than not, you will find yourself and your partner making some allowances and minor compromises. That might mean skipping an activity you've liked with other partners, avoiding a position you like that is uncomfortable for your partner, trying something new, or accepting that your favorite fantasy has just got to renew the lease in your head for another year rather than moving out into the real world.

Those things shouldn't be that big a deal. Engaging in a sexual activity with someone who isn't really into it takes the fun out of that activity, and you usually find that fun and satisfaction in activities both partners *do* enjoy.

If a partner is being honest with you about what they like and dislike, what they do and don't want to do, you've just got to accept those things. You can talk it over and work to find middle ground, but pushing, guilt-tripping, or otherwise pressuring a partner into any sexual activity isn't part of healthy, consensual sex.

It ***is*** okay to opt out of or terminate a relationship because of sexual incompatibility. Some people have the idea that doing so is shallow or insensitive, but strong sexual wants and needs aren't different from any other sort of wants and needs, such as wanting to be married or not, wanting a given amount of time alone, wanting monogamy or not. We wouldn't think it was shallow if a person terminated or didn't pursue a relationship with someone who didn't want the level of commitment they did or didn't share their emotional feelings, after all.

It might be hard to fathom that you will encounter people who meet most, if not *all,* of your needs—sexual, emotional, practical—without either of you trying too hard. That can seem especially improbable when you're young, when you've been single for a long time, or when you've had a long run of relationships that didn't even come close to meeting your needs and wants.

But they are out there. And part of finding them is becoming and staying aware of your wants and needs, of reciprocity and equality, of what's genuine and what is forced.

AFTERCARE

Part of what can make partnered sex so intimate and so intense is the openness and vulnerability we experience with each other, no matter what kind of sex we've been part of.

When we've finished with sexual activities, it's pretty common to want a little comfort, to want to reaffirm and extend that intimacy together. Snuggling, kissing, lying around and talking, taking a bath or a walk, going to sleep curled up together, or even good-natured roughhousing and laughing (pillow fight!) are all kinds of aftercare plenty of people appreciate and savor.

It's just as common for some people to want a little personal space or even to feel a little overexposed, a little *too* vulnerable, and to want a *lot* of space. Sometimes, that's the result of not-so-great sexual choices, but it can also be caused simply by differences in personality, chemistry, emotional nature, and style.

Just as people differ in what they want and need during sex, what one partner wants and needs after sex may not be what the other does. We've all heard the complaints about the partner who "just rolls over and falls asleep" as well as about partners who are too "clingy" after sex. But aftercare is just another aspect of sexual compatibility—your partner may naturally fall into the exact sort of aftercare you need . . . or they may not. Communicate your aftercare wants and needs, limits and boundaries, and seek a middle ground when need be, just as with anything else.

"QUEER" SEX AND "STRAIGHT" SEX: WHAT'S THE DIFF?

The sex queer people engage in most often involves the exact same sort of things that it does for straight people: kissing, hugging, snuggling, petting, touching, frottage, mutual masturbation, manual sex, oral sex, and vaginal or anal intercourse and stimulation—the works. Any and all of those activities are just as fulfilling, satisfying, and orgasm-inducing (or not) for queer people and couples as they are for anyone else.

But people can still experience some differences if they've lived in both worlds. The biggest general difference is how the people involved feel about and sometimes treat their partners in terms of gender. It's very easy for people of every orientation to fall into heteronormative roles; it's often harder when your sex life exists outside a heterosexual framework. So, although people of every orientation don't have to assign or perform any given roles around gender or anything else in their sexual lives, people who are straight and who believe those roles are a must sometimes experience a harder time creating a sex life with partners that's different.

For the same reasons, sometimes queer people feel more freedom to be experimental with sex; sometimes not. It's also common for people to feel differently about, or safer with, sex when there's no risk of pregnancy.

But, ultimately, what feels good or doesn't, what one person likes or dislikes in sexual activities, is less about orientation than it is about life experience, individual sensation, and individual attraction and chemistry.

[SEX AND DISABILITY]

Disability is a word that can cover a wide range of things. A person may have a physical, neurologic, psychological, developmental, or learning disability in an obvious way: they might be deaf, blind, or wheelchair-bound; have a missing limb or a speech impediment; or suffer from a condition like narcolepsy or an obsessive-compulsive disorder (OCD). Some disabilities, such as epilepsy, fibromyalgia, eating disorders, depression, attention deficit disorder, and autism, may be fairly invisible or harder to notice.

When it comes to sex and disability, it's pretty simple: most folks with disability are like most people without disabilities. Most disabilities do not remove the desire for sex, sexual partners, and romantic and/or sexual relationships. Partners of a person with a disability may or may not also have a disability themselves. The same sexual risks that apply to those without disabilities usually apply to those with disabilities: people with a disability can contract STIs like anyone else and can often become pregnant like anyone else. Having a disability doesn't take away humanity, nor does it elevate a person to a level "above" being human.

Like most other people, those of us with disability are going to have individual wants and needs, and sometimes some special adaptations need to occur to make sex work for us, whereas some things just don't work. With certain physical disabilities, some sexual positions or activities may be uncomfortable or just not doable. Some medications for mental illness may decrease libido or have other sexual side effects. Some disabilities may require special modifications during sex to make communication possible: for someone with visual impairment, verbal communication is important; for someone with hearing impairment, having the lights off may not always work. If you have a disability, you may find you've got to work a bit harder at communicating with your partner than do those without a disability. That may have its rough spots and get frustrating sometimes, but it's actually a blessing in disguise: the better any set of partners gets at communicating with one another, the better their relationship and their sex life tend to be.

Ask for help managing your sex life when you need it—not just from your partner but also from friends, parents, doctors, or therapists. It's hard enough for many young people to talk to their doctors or counselors about sex, and it may be an even larger challenge for those with a disability—especially if a doctor or counselor thinks that a disability makes someone less of a sexual being. If you have a disability and need to know about issues pertinent to your sexuality (like whether your disability affects your fertility, how to engage in a certain sexual activity with limited mobility, what type of birth control you can use, how to talk to partners about sexual specifics pertaining to a disability), ask questions of your healthcare providers, and insist on getting the answers you need. If you have a healthcare provider who insists on treating you like you must not have a sexuality because you have a disability, find a new one.

If you have a disability, you may also find you have social challenges when it comes to dating, relationships, and sexual partnership. Whether you date or want to date someone with a disability, you may find you have to fight for your right to live, date, and love like anyone else. You may face discrimination or silly questions about your abilities, even when they aren't asked with the intent to be insensitive or malicious. You may find that some people just will not even consider dating a person with a disability, for any number of reasons, both fair and completely stupid.

If you're a person with a disability dating a partner without disability (or you are a person without disability dating a person with a disability), you may both have to deal with tricky and difficult social adjustments. Talk it out among yourselves, your friends, and your families. Ask all the questions you need to, even if they seem stupid. If your partner has a disability, inform yourself about their specific disability. Seek out support groups or help intended specifically for those with disabilities and their partners. Try to be patient, and have a relationship that's full and fun, not tense. No one should feel as if they're walking on eggshells all the time. If a person with a disability tells you something won't break them, hurt them, or make them ill, trust them. If you have a disability and your partner without disability tells you they're cool with adaptations you need or things you can't do, believe them.

THE POPULAR MECHANICS ROUNDUP: THE FIVE MOST IMPORTANT THINGS TO REMEMBER DURING PARTNERED SEX

1. Communicate! Express yourself honestly, openly, and clearly. Let your partner know when something feels good, and let them know—kindly—when something doesn't. Ask them to tell and show you what they enjoy. It's okay to feel shy, but when you're naked in bed with someone being physically intimate, you've pretty much tossed shy right out the window. So, if you don't yet feel comfortable about communicating clearly and openly during sex, then wait to have partnered sex until you *do.* If you feel unable to do so with a given partner, that can be a strong signal that either you're not with the right partner or not at a good point yet to be sexually active with that partner. Sex shouldn't be like a silent movie.

2. Start slow. Something doesn't have to be fast to be intense and charged. Genitals, mouths, hands, and other body parts are sensitive, but too much fast action and friction, especially from the get-go, can actually make things feel *less* intense—or intense in a bad way—rather than more. When you're communicating with your partner during sex, if they want to go faster, all they've got to do is say so. Avoid everything-at-once sex where you go from no sexual experience with someone to trying to do all the things—take your time.

3. Forget about the "right" way. It's fine to feel clueless; in fact, it's better to feel clueless when you really are than to think you know what to do when you really don't. Experimenting is good, asking questions is good, finding out as you go . . . it's all not only good but also the only way to truly find out what you and your partner enjoy most. Sex, alone or with others, should be Choose Your Own Adventure, not the umpteenth sequel to yet another of the same tired, formulaic script.

4. Partnered sex is for mutual enjoyment, pleasure, care, and intimacy. That means that the following are Really Bad Reasons to have sex with someone: to fulfill perceived obligations or expectations, to impress someone or yourself, to try to gain status or a given reputation, to prove your worth or sexual value, to avoid problems in a relationship or to try to keep a partner from leaving, to replace masturbation or self-only pleasure, to "just get it over with," to boost your self-esteem, to comfort someone you feel sorry for, or to get back at somebody else—or any other number of other reasons that are *not* about mutual pleasure, care, and intimacy. That doesn't mean, for instance, that casual sex, sex with multiple partners, or sex with a friend, if that's what you want, has to be a no-go. It just means those scenarios, too, should be about mutual pleasure, care, and intimacy, above all else.

5. Feeling good in terms of sexual activities isn't just about getting off or just about feeling good during those activities. It's also about being intellectually, ethically, and emotionally okay with whatever you're engaging in; about taking care of everyone's hearts, minds, and bodies as best you can. It's pretty easy to avoid regret or other hard feelings about sexual experiences when you're mindful and aware of how the choices you're making and the things you're doing might affect you as well as your partner; when you take care of your sexual health before the fact, and routinely, not just in crisis situations; when you protect yourself from physical and emotional risks smartly; when you're with partners who are attentive and caring, not just before and during sex but afterward as well; when you choose partners who hear and respect "no" at any time and when you can do the same; when you seek out sex for good reasons rather than destructive or self-destructive ones; and when you treat yourself and your sex partners with the respect you all deserve.

10

Safe and Sound: Safer Sex for Your Body, Heart, and Mind

Sexual safety isn't just about avoiding pregnancy, abuse, or the most deadly infections and diseases. It's also about doing what we can to safeguard ourselves and everyone else in body and in mind via basic, preventative sexual and general health care, awareness of physical and emotional risks, and smart sexual habits and practices that make it so we can enjoy any sex we take part in without having to pay a big price for it or add a bunch of extra stress no one needs.

Safer sex, specifically, is a group of simple practices proven to greatly reduce risks of sexually transmitted illness. Some people say "safer sex" when they really mean contraception, or birth control. That's not what safer sex is. For information about contraception, see Chapter 12. I'm going to get into safer sex in this chapter, but I'm also going to talk about a bunch of different ways to get down with sexual safety and reap its benefits.

Whether or not you're having any sort of sex, the best place to get started in protecting your sexual health is with regular, preventative sexual health care and good sexual self-care habits.

[TAKING CARE DOWN THERE: SEXUAL HEALTH CARE]

Sexual health care is like any other sort of health care. If you take care of your sexual health by yourself and in cooperation with healthcare professionals, both preventatively—in advance of any issues—and in response to worries or concerns, it's very likely you'll stay healthy, avoid most infections, and enjoy your sexuality more than you probably would otherwise.

Here's the scoop on what you need from healthcare pros, when, how, and where to get that care; how to keep yourself well *by* yourself; and what steps to take to get started on a life of great sexual health and well-being.

Your Business, Their Business: Healthcare Confidentiality and Privacy

Organizations like the American Academy of Pediatrics have reported that the main reason young people are hesitant to seek out health care is concern about confidentiality: about what they say and what a healthcare provider finds out being private. It's important for doctors who serve young people to develop office policies that ensure confidentiality and instill trust, and those policies—available to patients and staff—should include information about when confidentiality must be waived, guidelines for reimbursement for services, medical record access, appointment scheduling, and information disclosure to public (such as to public health agencies) and/or private parties.

Most areas do **not** require parental notification or permission for STI testing or treatment, birth control services, prenatal care or delivery, or other sexual or reproductive health care. The same is typically true of mental health and substance abuse services. In the case of abortion, laws regarding young adult autonomy and parental notification/permission vary. Your best bet is always to ask your doctor or the office staff about their confidentiality policies before sharing any private information or any exams and about their policies for legal minors when that's your deal; you can even do that on the phone before making an appointment. That way, you can feel more able to share all of your information and history with a provider, which makes it a lot easier for them to do their job and avoid disclosing anything to anyone that you need kept private.

Know that **all** major medical associations advise healthcare professionals to respect and ensure the privacy and confidentiality of patients, including teen and emerging adult patients, and most medical professionals are in strong agreement: they take their patients' confidentiality and

STI and STD

In this book, the term *STI* is used to discuss sexually transmitted infections. Some people use the older term *STD* (sexually transmitted disease). The word *disease,* in medical parlance, usually means illness that is necessarily progressive, that sticks around, gets worse, and has ongoing health impacts. But most sexually transmitted illness isn't like that; most can be treated and don't get worse or have increasing or ongoing impacts so long as they are treated. However, some people, including some healthcare providers, still use *STD,* most often just out of habit. In this chapter, we discuss sexual health care, safer sex, some general infections, and issues pertaining to all the STIs out there. For specific information on each of them—what they are, how widespread they are, what symptoms they involve, how they're tested for and treated—refer to Appendix A.

their legal rights to it very, very seriously. Legal policies in place in most areas—like the Health Insurance Portability and Accountability Act (HIPAA) policy in the United States—provide very strict guidelines for healthcare providers when it comes to patient privacy and confidentiality. Ultimately, the golden rule most medical professionals uphold—echoed in policies like the mature minor doctrine—is that what is best when it comes to young adult health care is what is best for the young adult patient. Most healthcare providers also take advocating for their patients, no matter their patients' age, very seriously. So long as you are clear that your privacy is important and can advocate for yourself and demonstrate a clear understanding and ownership of your health, there is usually no reason to let worries about privacy stand in the way of getting the health care you need. Only if your healthcare provider determines that you do not understand the situation or that your privacy is endangering your health should they discuss notifying parents with you.

If you are using a parent's or guardian's insurance plan, understand that your exam and any other fees may appear on their statements, but perhaps not, or the charges will be listed, but not in a way that makes figuring out what they are easy. If that's a concern for you, you can call your insurance company to find out whether that will or won't happen, ask your healthcare provider's billing office for that information, or possibly just pay for your health care yourself. If the issue is keeping test results private, you can ask to have results sent only to you (such as at a college address) or sent to a friend's house, or see if you can call in to the office for your results rather than having them mailed.

Before Your First Sexual Health Appointment

▶ When you call to make your appointment, express to the receptionist or healthcare provider that it is your first visit, and feel free to let them know if you feel nervous or have any special concerns or needs. Ask any questions you want answered before you commit to an appointment to ensure this is the right place for you. You may also be able to first make a consultation-only visit, if you like, where you can just talk to a provider and first be sure they're someone you even want as your sexual healthcare provider without any kind of exam.

▶ If you feel more comfortable with a healthcare provider of a certain gender, you can ask for one and/or ask for a nurse of that gender to be in the room during the exam. If you are able to choose your healthcare provider, you can ask friends or family for a recommendation of someone they like. If you have any special needs the nurses, doctors, or staff should be aware of, such as any disability access needs or issues stemming from sexual or other trauma, let them know these things in advance of your appointment as well.

▶ If you want a parent or guardian in the room with you, let your healthcare provider know. If you want to keep a parent *from* coming in with you but feel you'll have a hard time asking for it in the office, you can discuss this over the phone in advance and request a note be left for your doctor or nurse to please ask your parent to stay in the waiting room. If you have any specific billing requests—such as whether to bill a parent's insurance plan or you need a payment plan—state them up front.

▶ Prepare a list of all your questions in advance (like whether your genitals look normal, if you can do anything about menstrual cramps, is a lump or bump on your labia or penis okay, why you're experiencing pain during sexual activities, etc.). Sometimes, the healthcare provider's office can feel a little intimidating, and it can be easy to forget things when we're nervous. So having a list in your hands is helpful in being sure to have all your needs addressed.

▶ Do what you can to relax. Tension and anxiety, no matter the situation or your sex, always increase emotional or physical discomfort during exams or other health care.

Who Provides Sexual or Reproductive Health Care?

▶ **A primary care physician/provider (PCP) or general physician (GP):** A PCP or GP is a general doctor or healthcare provider who you probably have already seen in your life for things like immunizations and general checkups. Rather than specializing in a certain system of the body, these kinds of physicians focus on a person's whole health. Most PCPs/GPs can do gynecological or urological exams, Pap smears, STI testing, prenatal care, and labor and delivery of infants. If and when you want someone more specialized (and some people prefer to see someone other than their family doctor for their sexual health care) or this kind of doctor feels you need more specialized care than they can provide, they can also usually give you a referral to a specialist.

▶ **A nurse practitioner (NP or APRN):** Nurse practitioners generally hold a master's degree in nursing in addition to being registered nurses (RNs) and holding other certifications. They have extra training that allows them to diagnose and provide treatment (including writing prescriptions) for many common conditions. NPs may practice generally or specialize in an area like sexual health.

▶ **A physician assistant (PA):** PAs usually have a master's degree and practice medicine on a team under the supervision of physicians and surgeons. They can examine patients, diagnose injuries and illnesses, and provide treatment.

▶ **An obstetrician/gynecologist (OB/GYN):** An obstetrician/gynecologist specializes in managing pregnancy and birth (OB) and health care of the uterus, vagina, vulva, and related structures (GYN).

▶ **A urologist:** A urologist specializes in health care of the penis, testes, prostate, and related structures.

Sexual Health Care for Beginners

There's no one set time for someone to start getting sexual health care. This is a kind of health care people can start either before or after they've been sexual with other people, depending on individual wants and needs. What kind of care you'll get is something you'll work out with a healthcare provider based on your unique sexual history, your body, and your concerns or current issues. You might seek out sexual health care to address concerns about your sexual or reproductive development, to find solutions for menstrual troubles, or to get tested for STIs or obtain contraception.

There's really no need to be scared about your first sexual health visit. It's typical for people to feel awkward about it because the genitals are often something we learn are "special" or "private" parts. But to a healthcare professional, your genitals or breasts are really no different from your elbow, nose, spleen, or any other part of your body. There is no reason to feel this kind of care is shameful, sexual for anyone, or dirty—it isn't. You're just taking care of yourself and your body, and a healthcare professional is there to help you do that.

What to Expect During an Exam

Before you do anything else, you'll usually be given intake forms to fill out. These ask for a bunch of health history and information from you. If there's anything on those forms you don't understand or aren't sure about, you can either ask the person who gave them to you or just leave those parts blank and mention them to your healthcare provider once you're in the exam room.

Because you're seeking out sexual health care, those forms often include some basic questions about your sexual history, including whether you have been and/or currently are sexually active. It's vital that you be honest about this (and volunteer that information if your healthcare provider does *not* ask) so that your doctor can do their job and give you whatever screenings and tests you may need. Being "sexually active" usually means participation in any kind of sex that involves your genitals or those of someone else, so, any manual, oral, vaginal, or anal sex with a partner of any gender.

Once you're called to start your appointment, you'll usually be given a basic physical exam for the healthcare provider to learn basic information about your body, like your blood pressure, pulse, height, and weight. This part of your appointment often is done by clinical support staff. This person may also just check in with you about why you're there and what care you're seeking specifically. They may ask you some questions about all of that, taking notes for your healthcare provider to review before they come in to see you.

This person also often asks you to change into an examination gown (leaving the room to give you privacy while you change), and then heads out, letting your healthcare provider know you're ready when they are. If you're not already sent off to collect urine for any tests, do yourself a favor and go to the bathroom before your exam: having a genital exam when you have to pee is pretty unpleasant.

After you have changed into an examination gown (and sometimes you'll also be given a sheet to drape over yourself before you sit on the table) and once your provider comes into the exam room, the provider may:

▶ Review your reasons for being there, and ask you some more clarifying questions to help them be sure to give you the kind of care you need and are asking for that day.

▶ Give you a breast exam (if you have breasts). The healthcare provider will feel your breasts and chest area in pressing movements to check for any lumps or irregularities. They may also ask if you do regular self-exams and show you how to do so.

▶ If you're there for STI and/or pregnancy testing, they will collect blood, urine, or both for those screenings (see page 285).

If you've got a vulva, part of your exam will probably involve laying on a gynecological table; it's got metal stirrups at the end of it. The provider will pull them out and ask you to move your torso down the table so that your bottom is on the edge of the table and to slide your heels into the stirrups. The healthcare provider will then sit between your legs. Plenty of people find that a gynecologist's table, and the placement of a healthcare provider at the end of it, is intimidating: it does look pretty funky, and this may also even be the first time since you had your diapers changed that someone else is quite *that* up close and personal looking at your genitals, and without mood lighting, no less. The stirrups are there to help make your exam physically comfortable for you (even though they may make you feel emotionally uncomfortable) and to give your healthcare provider a good position in which to perform the exam. However, some gynecologists feel that stirrups and the doctor's position between them make the exam more psychologically uncomfortable for patients, and they may give pelvic exams standing to the side of you while you lie on the table with your knees up and your feet flat on its surface.

If you are someone with a penis rather than a vulva, then you will probably only be sitting on a standard exam table.

CAN YOU HAVE A PELVIC EXAM DURING YOUR PERIOD?

It's often suggested that you do not have annual pelvic exams when you are menstruating because menses tend to make examining vaginal discharges and cervical cells more difficult. However, if your healthcare provider is difficult to get an appointment with, or if you have a serious crisis or emergency, give their office a ring and ask. In some situations, it may be just fine for you to go in with your period.

Your healthcare provider will first do a visual exam of your genitals: looking at the appearance of your vulva, anus, penis, and/or testicles. They don't do that to make you feel uncomfortable: they're looking for any clear signs of trouble, like chafing, redness, swelling, unusual discharge, cysts, lesions, genital warts, or other indications of illness, infection, or discomfort. They will touch your genitals during this exam, like by pressing the vaginal opening to see if the glands around it produce any pus or mucus when touched or by holding your testicles and asking you to turn your head and cough (they do that to check for hernias).

If you have a vagina, you may get a speculum exam and a Pap smear (that's a sample taken of cervical cells to make sure the cervix is healthy) at your first exam. Unless you are coming in with problems that make a speculum exam or Pap needed, those are exams a person needs or currently has recommended either once they've started having sex with partners (or after sexual abuse or assault) or at or after the age of twenty-one, whichever comes first.

A *speculum* (the Latin word for *mirror,* for the language geeks among you) is a sanitary plastic or smooth metal device that is used to hold the vaginal canal open so that your healthcare provider can examine the vaginal walls and cervix. If you're really nervous, or not used to the feeling of the vaginal opening and canal being stretched a bit, this may hurt a little, but your provider will choose a speculum size that is right for you to do their best to ensure it's not painful. If it is very painful, by all means, speak up—maybe the provider's guess about size was off, or you need them to go more slowly or use more lubricant for your comfort. You may feel some pressure in your bladder when the speculum is in; if you do, that's something else to let them know so they can make adjustments for your comfort. Sometimes the speculum might also feel chilly, especially if it's the metal type; you can always speak up about that, too.

To do a Pap smear, or to collect cell samples to test for certain STIs, a long cotton swab or curette is used to collect cells. For a Pap smear, they swab around the opening of your cervix. This shouldn't hurt, but it can feel a little weird, especially if you're not used to feeling something on your cervix.

(If you're curious, you can always ask your provider to get a mirror and show you what your cervix looks like when the speculum is in; it's really pretty cool.)

To do a bimanual exam, a provider will remove the speculum and will insert gloved fingers into the vagina while they put their other hand on your abdomen and torso. They'll press different spots on your abdomen and hips, and ask if anything feels painful or tender. It can be a little strange to have someone you don't really know or feel close to with their hand in your genitals asking you questions, but you can always ask for whatever you need to feel more comfortable, and over time, this will usually start to feel less awkward.

The next thing your provider may do is a rectal exam, which usually involves putting one finger in the anus and another in the vagina. This is so they can see how the uterus is aligned with the other parts of your reproductive organs. In general, this is the part of the exam most people find the most uncomfortable. If the provider knows it is your first exam, you can feel confident they will be gentle and careful, and try to cause you the least discomfort possible. And just like with other parts of the exam, if you're suffering, don't suffer in silence: say something so they can make any adjustments they can. This is supposed to be about caring for yourself, not about torture or punishment.

If you have a penis and testicles rather than a vulva, your provider will also do external examination of your genitals and will feel the penis and testicles with a gloved hand, searching for any unusual lumps or bumps and testing for any pain or discomfort from gentle pressure. They may also perform a rectal exam by putting one gloved finger gently into your rectum, feeling for swelling or tenderness.

Urethral Swabbing

If you have a penis and you're having any STI testing done or have had any sort of urinary problems or concerns, your healthcare provider may want to do a urethral swab test (though STI tests can usually also be done without them). A urethral swab involves a *very* slim, tipped swab inserted a few millimeters into the urethral opening that is turned briefly and then taken right out. Like Pap smears, urethral swabbing shouldn't be crazy painful; it just feels unusual—but the idea of swabbing does freak a lot of people out. Wigging out about it, or any other part of an exam, can create a situation healthcare pros refer to as a *perceived body injury* (or *insult*): if we expect pain, we're much more likely to trick our bodies into feeling it, even when it isn't really there. Your best bet is just to relax. Ask any questions you need to beforehand, or have the healthcare provider show you the swab and explain how it works so that you can feel less stressed about it. Then just breathe, and think about cats riding around on Roombas or something; it'll be over in a flash.

That's it! If you have any questions or concerns that weren't addressed before or during the exam, now is the time to ask them. Remember: part of the service any healthcare provider should provide is *information,* so take advantage of your time there to ask your questions. Results from exams, including any test results, are usually ready in a week or so; if you don't hear anything back in a couple weeks, call in. If all your results come back normal, you won't likely need to have an exam for another year, unless a new issue crops up in the interim.

CHECK, PLEASE!

Many healthcare providers do not give full STI screenings (tests) during exams **without a patient specifically asking for them** (unless they see anything that suggests a possible STI during other parts of the exam), and that's particularly common with teen patients. If you are or have been sexually active, it's very important to get those screenings. Condom and barrier use are only a part of practicing safer sex, and although they do a great job of preventing STIs, they aren't 100 percent effective. And a lot of people don't use barriers consistently, correctly, or for all the activities that pose STI risks. STI screenings are the other essential. Don't just assume your exam includes those screenings; be sure you ask for those screenings, for *all* sexually transmitted infections, not just HIV or a given infection you're concerned about at the time. For more information on STIs and screenings, read on.

Special Concerns

▶ **Virginity:** Unless someone has an STI showing genital symptoms, a healthcare provider (or any other person, for that matter) cannot tell whether someone has been part of vaginal intercourse or other kinds of sexual activity just by the appearance of the vulva or vagina. A gynecologist also cannot "devirginize" anyone via a GYN exam. If virginity is a framework, know that it's not something with an anatomical or medical definition; it's a personal or cultural belief about behavior or life experience. Anyone saying it's something medical or anatomical is either misinformed, lying, or believes things about the genitals and what they can show us about sexual behavior or history that simply aren't true.

▶ **Pubic hair:** Sexual healthcare providers have seen every type of genitals under the sun and about any configuration or amount of pubic hair you can imagine.

▶ **Judgment for being sexually active:** When discussing whether you are or are not sexually active, and with whom, your healthcare provider should not be doling out lectures or heavy-duty value judgments. If yours does, or you feel you can't be honest with your provider about your sexual activity because they're all judgy, find a new provider. For more on this and other types of healthcare discrimination, see page 273.

▶ **Breast or penis size worries or other concerns about how your body looks:** All a healthcare provider is looking for when it comes to your body are signs of health and any signs of illness or other problems. They're not checking you out to figure whether you're hot, and your own ideas of what does or doesn't look normal probably don't square with what really is or isn't common. Having people look closely at your body can certainly make anyone feel vulnerable and uncomfortable, and there's often no getting around at least some emotional discomfort with that. But don't let your own body issues or discomfort keep you from health care you need. Do your best to just let it be weird and get through it. If you find a specific provider is someone you feel extra-uncomfortable with in this regard, see whether you can't swap for someone else.

▶ **Birth control:** If you would like to discuss birth control options, tell your provider or their office in advance of the exam; there's certainly no need to have extended conversations about all your options while you're freezing your buns off in an examination gown. If there are specific methods you're interested in, your provider can be on the lookout for health issues during the exam that may make a given method a bad fit for you. When you're finished with the exam itself, you and your provider can decide on a method that's best for you. If you're seeking birth control that requires a prescription, like oral contraceptives, your provider can tend to that during this time. For specific information on contraceptive options, see Chapter 12.

Transgender and/or Queer Care

If you're a trans guy who still has a cervix, you'll also still need Pap smears. For many obvious reasons, that can be a loaded experience. Queer patients also have some special needs when it comes to sensitivity from and the education of providers. This is a good area in which to screen healthcare providers in advance: if they don't say in any of their office information, before you make an appointment, ask your provider's office if they are sensitive to and educated about the needs of transgender and/or queer patients, and only make an appointment if you feel satisfied with their answers. For more on dealing with any healthcare discrimination or just how to manage it and advocate for yourself when your healthcare options don't seem to leave real room for you and your specific needs, see page 273.

Sexual health care isn't a punishment for being sexual, nor does it need to be something to dread. It's just part of taking care of ourselves, like getting our cavities filled, getting an immunization, or calling a best friend for some love and comfort when you're heartbroken. Your healthcare provider can turn out to be a great source of honest, accurate sexual health information and support for you, for years to come. Keeping our sexual health in tune regularly is just one of the steps that we need to take to help ensure our sexual lives don't make us sick, to take care of us if and when necessary, and to address a system of the body that we need a professional to check on every now and then, just like every other system of the body.

That's really all there is to it! But that needn't be all that happens in your exam. If you have questions about your sexual health, about birth control or reproduction, about genital appearance or sexual function, this is your golden opportunity to ask. You may feel awkward or embarrassed, but pretty much any question you can think to ask is one your healthcare provider has heard and answered before, and that's part of what your healthcare provider is there for.

Sexual Healthcare Discrimination: Roadblocks to Good Health

Because of the strong feelings in much of our culture about teen and young adult sexuality, it is possible you may bump up against some discrimination that makes taking care of your sexual health more difficult instead of easier.

DID YOU KNOW? . . .

Vaccines for some STIs are available, and more are in development. For now, your family doctor likely already takes care of your hepatitis vaccinations, but there is also a vaccine available to help protect you against the most common sexually transmitted strains of human papillomavirus (HPV), a virus that can cause cervical or other cancers. The HPV vaccine is currently administered as a series of three vaccines, so until someone's had all three, they shouldn't figure they have the protection this vaccination can provide. It's ideally given to people before they've been part of any genital-to-genital contact, because then they'll be protected right from the start. However, even if you have been sexually active, you will likely benefit from the vaccine. For more on HPV and hepatitis vaccinations, see Appendix A.

That discrimination may be minor and fairly easy to counter: perhaps your family doctor doesn't want to give you a pelvic exam or prescribe birth control, but you have access to other providers. Your healthcare provider doesn't have to agree with your decisions, but your decisions are your job, not theirs—it's their job to give you information and guidance to be as healthy as possible and to treat or help you prevent any health conditions. It is not their job—nor is it part of their ethical code as professionals—to impose their own values or beliefs on you: it *is* their job to manage their own biases and act like a professional. In situations like these, you can voice an objection or make a complaint, switch to another healthcare provider, or visit a general sexual health clinic

On the Down Low

Honesty with your doctor or clinician includes honesty about the gender or orientation of your partners and specific activities with them. Some people who have partners of the same sex or gender may find it difficult or highly uncomfortable to be fully honest. Just remember that a healthcare provider isn't a priest or a parent: it's not their job to sit in or dole out any sort of judgment about your sexual behavior or your sexual identity when it is not directly related to health issues or concerns, and it is their responsibility to respect your privacy and to treat you with respect, including for who you are and who you love (or just lust). Their job is to assess and safeguard your health, and to help them do that, you need to be forthright. If you don't feel safe doing that with any given provider because of your orientation or sexual history around gender (or anything else), ask for someone different or seek out a different provider.

instead, where sexual health services are provided without judgment by design.

It's important to learn to be your own advocate. Find out what your rights are, based on your age and what you're seeking (STI screenings, GYN exams, birth control or emergency contraception, abortion, confidential testing, sliding fees): your rights will differ some from country to country and state to state. For instance, confidentiality requirements and obligations in terms of services, records, and results vary in certain situations and areas based on local laws, your age, and general practice or clinic guidelines and approaches.

Queer or gender-nonconforming patients often face additional challenges. Discrimination can manifest in many ways. A given healthcare provider or clinic may go overboard in panicking about sexual health risks for gay men while completely dismissing or ignoring lesbian STI risks and concerns. Patients who are not out yet may have special concerns about confidentiality. Bisexual patients may experience assumptions that their orientation means they're having sex with the entire city or are sexually irresponsible. Transgender patients may find it difficult to have their boundaries or their identity honored, even with something as seemingly small or easy as asking for healthcare providers to just use their right pronouns or to recognize that their thorny feelings about puberty may be particularly complicated and challenging.

All that said, finding health care that is accepting, informed, and appropriate for queer or gender-nonconforming patients is absolutely possible. Look in the phonebook or online for clinics that expressly serve your population or populations, or call community centers, therapists, or groups that clearly advertise themselves as LGBT-friendly and ask for help finding safe, welcoming health care. Some Internet sites, groups, and resources can also be of help (see the Resources section for some organizations). You can use a couple great online databases to find queer or transfriendly healthcare providers.

If you do encounter discrimination, the best approach is to find a better healthcare provider, practice, or clinic first, and then deal with any reporting you want to do about the discrimination later. Your health and safety come first. What's most important is the quality of your health care and your ability to be honest and open with a healthcare provider so that you can be sure to get what you need.

KNOW YOUR RIGHTS!

You have a right to seek and receive quality sexual health care, no matter your age, location, gender, orientation, or income bracket.

You have a right, when you choose sexual health care, to choose that which is in your best physical and emotional interest from a healthcare provider who will be your sexual health ally. Shop around with clinics and healthcare providers when you can. Before making an appointment, call a few different offices. Voice concerns—whether about having access to the services you need or simply finding a doctor or clinician who'll treat you with respect. Bear in mind that *respect* may not always mean unconditional or quiet acceptance of everything you do. A good doctor or nurse, for instance, isn't likely to stay mum if you're engaging in high-risk activities without any protection or are playing Russian roulette with pregnancy when you make clear you don't want to become pregnant. But you should always be treated with courtesy and objectivity, no matter what.

A good way to find a good provider clinic is to ask peers or trusted adults for a referral. In a particular group practice, one of the best ways of finding a good doctor is to talk to the nurses who work there, and let them know what exactly you're looking for. Nurses are often incredible patient advocates.

Bringing a friend or someone else with you to health care, someone you know has your back, can be a great help. It's easy to feel intimidated in healthcare settings even without possible—or actual—discrimination or invisibility issues. When we add those to the mix, it can feel really daunting and be harder to advocate for ourselves. Having someone else with you who can step in if and when you need them to can be everything. Supportive friends or family can also help you seek out health care in the first place; sometimes even that part of the process can be tiresome and distressing to go at alone.

If health history or other forms don't include you, you can go ahead and modify them as necessary to make them fit better; they're not like SATs where you can only work with the options you're given. If you need to add a relationship construct, gender, or pronoun that isn't listed, write in a different word or name than they have on your paperwork. If anyone who provides health care or who works in the records section of your healthcare office doesn't understand and needs you to clarify, they can always ask you. Health forms are also a great place to make a clear note about what you want your body parts to be called, which pronouns you prefer, and what name you prefer be used for you (when it's different from your legal name).

Sometimes, harassment and other abuse, sexual and otherwise, can occur in the healthcare system. In those instances, do *not* go back to that healthcare provider or clinic. Speak with your parents or another trusted older adult and/or contact the medical board, police (if that feels necessary, and always in cases of any sexual or physical abuse), a private lawyer, or a legal aid service. For more on how to handle abuse or assault—from anyone—see Chapter 11.

[DIY SEXUAL HEALTH CARE]

A big part of keeping yourself sexually healthy is maintaining your sexual and reproductive wellness in the first place. Pay attention to your sexual health as a habit so that you can get the jump on any problems. Although having sexual and general health checkups every year, as well as using safer sex practices, is important preventative care, so are these basic ways of caring for yourself every day, for your whole body, not just your genitals:

▶ **Would you really want to be what you eat?** Poor eating habits and nutrition can take a toll on your sexual health. Sodas, refined sugars, fried foods or junk foods, alcohol, chocolate, caffeine, nicotine, and foods that have been treated with chemical pesticides can all contribute to yeast infections or jock itch; bacterial urinary tract infections (UTIs), or bladder infections; menstrual problems (such as severe cramps and PMS); and issues with sexual desire and sexual response. They also can interfere with your overall sexual health and enjoyment and your overall physical and mental health. A poor diet often compounds mental health issues like depression and anxiety—which already can take a toll on a sex life—and can contribute to poor functioning of neurotransmitters that send sexual messages to the body that create sexual responses like arousal and orgasm. A poor diet also keeps your immune system from working at its best, which can put you at an increased risk of STIs. The same goes double for smoking and drug and alcohol abuse.

▶ **Rest and motion:** Rest and physical activity are both big parts of staying healthy. Good circulatory, cardiovascular, respiratory, and endocrine health and reduction of stress support a satisfying sexual life. When any of those things aren't doing so well, our bodies will often struggle with sexual desire and response.

▶ **Cleanup—daily genital hygiene:** When washing your genitals, you only want to use a gentle, unfragranced soap. Even using just warm water is totally fine. Fragranced or deodorant soaps, or vaginal "cleansers" and douches should be avoided. Sometimes a healthcare provider with prescribe a douche (a fluid mixture used to rinse out the vagina) for a given condition, but that's the only time douching should be done. The vagina is self-cleaning (*how cool is that!?*), and douching is associated with infections and other health problems, not with sound health and hygiene. People, whatever kind of genitals they have, only need to concern themselves with cleaning the external genitals, not inside genital orifices like the vagina, anus, or urethra.

For people who have a foreskin, to clean, you just gently pull back the foreskin (only as much as feels comfortable; this shouldn't ever hurt) and clean lightly beneath or around it with warm water to get rid of the normal dead skin cells and secretions from the sebaceous glands (otherwise known as *smegma,* which also may be found inside or around parts of the vulva), which help keep the foreskin lubricated for comfort and often accumulate beneath the head of the penis and foreskin.

DID YOU KNOW? . . .

Adolescents need a *lot* of rest—usually way more than most are getting. That common feeling during adolescence when the amount of sleep you're getting doesn't feel like as much as you want is probably just your body being very smart and trying to let you know that, indeed, you need more sleep or rest. A lot of parents or guardians don't know this, or they have picked up on tropes that claim sleepy young people are being apathetic or lazy and believe them. If you're not being supported at home in getting the amount of sleep you really require, you may need to do some educating and then some standing up for yourself. Sleep deprivation can really mess up our physical and mental health.

If at any point your genitals just feel, look, or smell superfunky, and this kind of basic hygiene doesn't change that up fast—like a foul smell (genitals smell like genitals, not air freshener, but although that's often a musky smell, it's not something that should turn anyone's stomach), profuse or discolored discharge, itching, or the like—talk to a healthcare provider and make sure you aren't dealing with an infection or other issue you need health care for.

What's good for your general health is what's good for your sexual health. Healthy, fresh foods that are both enjoyable *and* good for you, a moderately active lifestyle, plenty of sleep and rest, and basic daily hygiene and other habits that support your overall health and well-being are great big deals if you want to be healthy and feel healthy sexually.

Check Yourself Out!

Check Out Those Testicles

Testicular cancer is the most common cancer for those with penises age twenty to twenty-five, so for those with testes (whatever your gender) a testicular self-exam each month is a must. It's best to perform self-exams after a bath or shower, when the heat has relaxed the scrotum. Standing in front of a mirror, first look for any unusual swelling. Then, using both hands, check out each testicle, one at a time. With your index and middle fingers under a testicle and the thumbs on top, roll the testicle gently between your thumbs and fingers, comfortably. Feel around for any unfamiliar lumps; it's normal for the testicles to already feel a little lumpy, and the epididymis, which is behind the testicle, normally feels a little lumpy. Lumps that can be cancerous are usually on the sides or front of the testicles, not the back. Remember, too, that a difference in size between testicles is normal.

If you discover any small, pea-like lumps that are unfamiliar to you, seem unusual, or are painful to the touch, then talk to your healthcare provider. Same goes for any general discomfort, soreness, swelling, or feeling of heaviness of the scrotum or testes that lasts for more than a couple of days.

Check Out Those Breasts

Every month, people with breasts should do a breast self-exam to check for any possible signs of breast cancer. These are best done lying down and then standing, with the arm raised on the side of the breast you're checking, or in the shower.

With your three middle fingers of the hand from the opposite side (if you're checking your left breast, raise your left arm, and use your right hand to check that breast), you want to feel for lumps in the breast. Use enough pressure that you can feel the different textures of the breast tissue, starting with light pressure, just to move the skin, then a bit more to feel more of the tissue, and finally the most pressure, to be able to feel your ribs beneath the breast.

Feel around the whole breast in circles, from the outside in, or by going up and down from one side to the other. It's best to pick one way to do your exams and stick with it, because then you'll become familiar with how the breast feels in that pattern, which makes it easier for you to recognize anything abnormal. You need to do this for both breasts. If you did the exam lying down, you want to stand or sit up when you've done the exam and go through it once more; some parts of the breast feel different when standing.

Do a visual exam as well, keeping an eye out for any changes in your nipples, skin dimpling, puckering, unusual redness, or swelling.

Should you find an unusual lump, see your healthcare provider. Most breast lumps are not cancerous, so if you do find something, don't panic, just get it checked out.

Breast cancer doesn't just happen to women or people with a vulva, by the way. Although it's much more rare, it is an illness that people can develop who don't have the kind of breast tissue most people with a vulva and breasts have. So, it's a good idea for everyone to get in the habit of doing breast—or chest—self-exams.

Check Out Those Genitals

Genital ingrown hairs and pimples are pretty easy to identify, because they'll look pretty much the same way they do when they show up on other parts of your body. They either have a small white head, or they are just tiny bumps, slightly red, that may smart a little bit but that should not itch or develop a raw, open, or very crusty top. As with pimples or ingrown hairs anywhere else, it's best not to pick them. If a hair is sticking out of a pustule, you can use tweezers to pull it out, which can alleviate soreness and help it to heal. Hot compresses can also help soothe and heal pimples and ingrown hairs. Generally, just keep the area clean and let it heal on its own; just like with zits on your face, you really want to try not to mess with them.

You should see your sexual healthcare provider—and take a break from any partnered sex until you do—if you notice any of the following:

- Any open, raw, raised, or reddish sores
- Hard lumps that can be seen or felt inside the outer labia or on the mons, testes, scrotum, foreskin, or penis
- Small, white, cauliflower-like growths or warts
- Persistent itching or scratching
- Unusual lumps or bumps that can be felt, but not seen
- Any unusual discomfort with no visible cause

Check Out Your Discharges

Vaginal discharge that is *not* normal but that is a possible signal of infection or illness may

- Be chunky or very heavy, with small curds like cottage cheese

Mouth Matters

Oral herpes (HSV-1) is incredibly common, found in around 50 percent of people in the United States, even in those who have not been sexually active (the majority of herpes cases begin in childhood without any sexual contact at all). It can be sexually transmitted, both orally and genitally. So, be on the lookout for cold sores, which are a symptom of the herpes virus.

There's a lot of confusion as to what cold sores are and where they appear.

Cold sores are *not*:

- Mouth ulcers, which are caused by biting into the mouth or cheek accidentally, by burns or other mouth injuries, or by hormonal changes
- Canker sores

Cold sores *are*:

- "Fever blisters" that appear on the lips or on the skin just around the mouth
- Caused by the herpes virus

If you have cold sores, you have the herpes virus and can transmit it to others, orally or genitally, even when sores are not present.

If you think you've found a cold sore and you haven't seen a healthcare pro about them before, make an appointment as soon as you can: it's best for a provider to see the sore while it's active. Although there is not yet a cure for the herpes virus, medications can help suppress outbreaks and symptoms substantially so that it's usually something pretty easy to live with.

If you have already been diagnosed with oral herpes and find a cold sore or see one cropping up, slow down a little bit and take care of yourself: cold sores are actually a sign that your immune system is stressed out. If you're sexually active (or will be kissing someone or having other oral contact), wait for the sore to be gone before oral partnered activity, or use latex barriers that can **fully** cover your mouth (dams can, but condoms often do not). For more information on herpes, see page 418.

- Be very watery
- Have a strong foul, metallic, or fishy odor
- Be grayish, yellow-greenish, yellow, pinkish, or tinged with bloody spots or streaks
- Cause excessive discomfort, burning, or itching

Penile discharge that is *not* normal but that likely is a signal of infection or illness may

- Be *anything* that is not ejaculate, pre-ejaculate, or urine
- Be any color from clear to yellow or greenish
- Contain blood or appear pinkish
- Appear with pain or burning during urination, a frequent need to urinate, any sort of genital rash, or swollen glands in the groin area

As well, any sort of discharge from the anus—for anyone—that is not clearly fecal matter of some kind should always be investigated.

The above sorts of discharges can be caused by an infection like those listed below or by an STI like gonorrhea or

trichomoniasis. If you have any of the above sorts of abnormal discharge, or related symptoms, please see your sexual healthcare provider.

Urinary Tract, Bacterial, and Yeast Infections

Sexually transmitted infections are called that because they are most often transmitted through sexual contact. But there are common genital infections that straddle the boundaries: they are genital, and sometimes sexually transmitted or exacerbated by sexual activity, but they often can, and do, occur without a person having been part of any sexual contact at all.

Bacterial Vaginosis (BV)

What is it? A bacterial imbalance in the vagina, when the normal healthy bacteria of the vagina are essentially outnumbered by other not-so-nice bacteria.

Who gets it? People who have a vagina, and lots of them (so many vaginas!). BV is very common. It's estimated that as many as two million American people have it at any given time, and it's the most common cause of vaginitis—any irritation of the vagina characterized by discharge, odor, swelling, and/or itching—though many people with BV have no obvious symptoms.

How do you get it? The why and how of BV are not clearly understood, but your chances of developing it are increased by douching, sexual activity (especially with new partners), switching between vaginal and anal sex (either unprotected or by using the same condom for both), sharing sex toys that can't be or weren't boiled or covered with a latex barrier, improper wiping after bowel movements, or antibiotic use.

What are its symptoms? Those with BV may discover a fishy, bad-smelling (especially after sexual activity) vaginal discharge that is creamy and grayish-white.

What do you do to treat it? BV needs to be diagnosed by a healthcare provider and is usually easily treated with antibiotics or nutritional remedies. It is important to get treatment because untreated BV can lead to serious conditions like pelvic inflammatory disease. BV isn't often passed on to partners, though it's common for people who can get BV to get it when they're sexual with new partners, particularly if that partner also has a vagina and BV.

Urinary Tract or Bladder Infections

What are they? Just as BV occurs when "bad" bacteria are introduced to the vagina, a UTI (sometimes called cystitis) or bladder infection occurs when bacteria—from the anus, the external genitals, clothing, hands, sex toys, or partners—get into the lower urinary tract or the bladder.

Who gets them? Everyone, but urinary tract or bladder infections are most common in people with a vulva simply because of the design of that kind of genital structure (the urethral opening on the vulva is just a lot more vulnerable to bacteria getting rubbed up in it).

How do you get them? UTIs or bladder infections can develop from improper toilet wiping, which can bring bacteria from the rectum into the urethra, and from sexual activity (namely, manual, oral, or vaginal sex, though "dry" sex can also cause a UTI). Other culprits can include "holding" urine in too often rather than urinating when you have to, wearing garments or undergarments made of synthetic fibers that don't allow the area to "breathe," spermicide use, kidney stones, and diabetes.

What are its symptoms? Most people with a UTI experience pain or burning with urination, difficulty urinating at all (often coupled with a persistent feeling of having to go), blood in the urine, or very strong-smelling urine. Fever and lower abdominal pain may also occur.

What do you do to treat them? At the *very* first *mild* sign of a UTI—like some very minor discomfort urinating or mild feelings of urinary urgency—you can sometimes fend off UTIs at the pass by drinking a lot of water and taking real (unsweetened) cranberry juice, tablets, or extract (be aware that cranberry juice "cocktails" have very little cranberry juice in them and a whole lot of sugar, which only makes matters worse, so cranberry tablets taken with water or concentrated or partially diluted pure juice, sans sugar, is best: read the ingredients on juice to be sure). There are also over-the-counter medications you can get almost anywhere that help manage the pain of a UTI, but note that these don't treat the infection itself; they just help you deal until you can get treatment.

If, after a day or two of self-treatment, symptoms persist or get worse, it's time to hit the doc's office and be diagnosed and treated, because UTIs can spread and cause real problems for the bladder and kidneys. They also can hurt like hell, which we obviously want to avoid. UTIs are diagnosed with a simple urine test and are treated with antibiotics. They tend to resolve very shortly after treatment begins, usually just a couple of days, and you'll often feel relief the very first day of treatment. (However, even if you feel better, never stop taking an antibiotic until you've used up the whole amount prescribed for you!) Sexual partners don't need to be treated.

For most people, UTIs are temporary and easily managed. However, some people get them chronically. Chronic sufferers are often given stronger antibiotics and sometimes for much longer periods of time. Unfortunately, some people with chronic UTIs find that, after a while, antibiotics don't do the job anymore. If you're having UTIs chronically, your healthcare provider should be evaluating your kidneys and making sure you don't have any abnormalities of the urinary tract that may be causing the condition. If nothing is found, and nothing else seems to help, it's also important to make sure something simple isn't causing the problem, like not drinking enough water regularly, wiping improperly, neglecting proper hygiene, or consuming things known to irritate the bladder, such as alcohol, caffeine, or even citrus.

Yeast Infection (or Thrush)

What is it and who gets it? Everyone can get them. A healthy vagina normally has some amount of yeast within it, but it exists in a delicate and acidic balance

with other vaginal microorganisms. When something occurs to disrupt that balance, and the vagina becomes more alkaline and less acidic, the yeasts proliferate and cause an infection. Genital yeast or fungal infections can also happen with the penis—sometimes it's called *jock itch*—though they are less common than vaginal yeast infections. Anal yeast infections can happen as well, as can yeast infections of the mouth or throat.

How do you get them? Yeast infections can be the result of many things, including an unbalanced diet (especially one high in caffeine, simple carbs, sugars, and processed foods), a food allergy, a preexisting sexually transmitted infection, antibiotics, birth control pills, spermicides, pregnancy, diabetes, or immunosuppression as the result of disease. Douching, feminine "hygiene" sprays or lotions, pantyhose, and synthetic or wet undergarments without breathability are also common accomplices. If you're taking antibiotics for something, be sure to eat plenty of organic, plain yogurt (if you're vegan or dairy-allergic, nondairy yogurt alternatives work, too) or take acidophilus tablets while you're on the medication to help prevent the yeast imbalances that can cause yeast infections. Genital sensitivities can also be a factor: if you're allergic or sensitive to latex, or certain detergents, lubricants, or other substances, use alternatives. It's also possible for yeast infections to be passed from partner to partner.

What are its symptoms? Common symptoms of a yeast infection are itching, burning, chafing, swelling, and/or generalized irritation of the vagina and vulva, or the penis and testes, or anus. The anus, vagina, or vulva may feel uncomfortably dry. It may be painful to urinate or engage in manual sex or vaginal intercourse. Unusual discharge isn't always present, but when it is, it tends to be thick, white, and chunky, sometimes with small cottage-cheese-like curds. A smell may or may not be present (a discharge that smells like baking bread is a sure sign of a yeast infection). Oral yeast infection symptoms generally include a mouth ulcer, usually on the tongue or inside the cheeks, with a creamy, white appearance. A pervasive feeling of dry mouth may also be present.

What do you do to treat them? A healthcare provider can usually diagnose a yeast infection with a visual exam or swab. Most prescribe either oral medications or over-the-counter treatments. You can also be prescribed—or purchase over the counter—external creams designed specifically to relieve soreness or swelling with a genital infection. As with urinary tract infections, you can try some safe at-home treatments at the first sign of a mild yeast infection before hauling out the big guns. Many people find that plain, organic yogurt with active, live cultures is an excellent treatment: acidophilus in the yogurt kills excess yeast by producing hydrogen peroxide. It can be applied on the irritated external genitals and/or inside the vagina by simply spreading it on and in with a finger. Some people fill empty tampon applicators with yogurt and freeze them, inserting them into a genital orifice for use that way (the coolness is also soothing). This is more than a little messy, so it's really only a good remedy for bedtime. It's also not something you can do with rectal yeast infections because those yogurt-tampons don't have a flared base and could get stuck in there. Not fun.

Eating plenty of natural yogurt (especially when on antibiotics) also helps protect and restore the healthy bacteria in your body. Other natural remedies include inserting cloves of garlic as vaginal suppositories (garlic is a natural antifungal) until the infection clears up, and drinking pure cranberry juice or using cranberry supplements can be of help here, though only for very mild infections. If these DIY treatments don't seem to be helping within a few days, see your sexual healthcare provider for more intensive treatment.

It's not advised to self-treat a possible vaginal yeast infection with over-the-counter treatments if you have never been diagnosed with a yeast infection. If you do, and you do *not* actually have a yeast infection, you could either reduce the effectiveness of the medication if and when you do have one later, or you could actually cause a yeast infection by disrupting the acid balance of your vagina. Plus, if you have a different sort of infection—like BV, trichomoniasis, or chlamydia—it's important you get that diagnosed and treated as soon as possible. So, always be sure to see a healthcare provider first to be sure it's even a yeast infection that you've got.

It's best to abstain from partnered sex until you've been diagnosed and treated because yeast infections are contagious, and often sexual activity when you have a yeast infection is seriously uncomfortable anyway (having any kind of sex with genitals that are itchy and raw is not a thing most people experience as anything but ouchy). Informing a partner of a yeast infection is also important; they may have one themselves without knowing it. And to be perfectly plain, yeast infections tend not to look very pretty and they also smell pretty rank, so you probably won't *want* to be sexual with others while you've got one.

As with UTIs, some people experience recurrent or chronic yeast infections. Chronic or recurrent yeast infections should be reported to a healthcare provider and looked into, because they can be a sign of diabetes, HIV infection, or another immunosuppressive disease or disorder. They may also be caused by dietary issues or food allergies, which can be remedied simply with diet changes.

When You Just Can't DIY

Most of the time, you can manage your own health, especially when you're taking smart daily care of yourself and being vigilant about annual sexual and general health checkups. But some things are best managed by your healthcare provider.

Among the reasons to contact your healthcare provider are pain in the abdomen during intercourse or other sexual activity; unusual appearance of genitals or nipples; itching or burning on or in, or unusual discharge from, the genitals or nipples; skipped or missed periods when there is no pregnancy risk; a suspected pregnancy, STI, yeast infection, or UTI; blood in the urine or difficulty or pain when urinating; unusual sores or discharge on or from the genitals or mouth; extended illness (like a cold or flu that

PREVENTING VAGINAL INFECTIONS AND STOPPING THE CYCLE OF CHRONIC INFECTIONS

Because of the way this kind of genital anatomy is "designed," people with vaginas are particularly inclined to infections like UTIs, yeast infections, and BV. But you can do some things to help yourself avoid them:

- Avoid spreading germs from the anus to the vagina. When urinating and after bowel movements, always wipe from front to back—vulva to anus. Wash your hands before and after you masturbate, and if sexual partners are not using latex gloves, have them wash hands before manual sex.
- Practice safer sex, using latex barriers for manual, oral, vaginal, or anal sexual activity. Avoid flavored lubricants for vaginal use, or those with high glycerin content, as well as spermicides or condoms lubricated with spermicides. Spermicides often irritate genital tissue, which heightens the risks for developing infections.
- Use good basic hygiene, making sure to wash the vulva daily with a gentle, unfragranced soap.
- *Don't be a douche.* According to the National Women's Health Information Center (sponsored by the US Department of Health and Human Services), most doctors and the American College of Obstetricians and Gynecologists suggest that people steer way clear of douching. Douches disrupt the delicate pH and bacterial balance of the vagina and the self-cleaning cycle. Some studies show that people who douche at least once a month are over 30 percent more likely to have bacterial vaginosis or a mild vaginal infection than people who never douche, that people who douche have more health problems than those who do not, and that douching can spread vaginal infections into the reproductive organs, which can also cause pelvic inflammatory disease, which often leads to infertility. Recent research also suggests a link between douching and increased risks of HIV, herpes, other STIs, and cervical cancer.
- Avoid or limit too-tight pants *(I'm talking to you, jeggings)*, underwear without a cotton crotch, pantyhose, and other clothing that can trap moisture and that doesn't breathe. Comfortable and loose natural-fiber clothing is always best.
- Do not try to self-medicate with over-the-counter treatments or someone else's medication for a suspected infection. Not only might it not work, while your infection gets worse, but you may end up giving yourself an infection that you didn't even have to begin with.
- Eat as healthy and balanced a diet as you can manage, and avoid processed foods and lots of carbonated sodas. Take good care of yourself.
- If you are being treated for an infection, be sure to take all your medication to the end of its course, as directed, and abstain from sexual activities until you are fully well. In addition, avoid using tampons while infected—if you are menstruating or currently have a genital infection, use cotton pads instead.
- *Do not* let suspected infections go untreated, because they can worsen or spread. Sometimes, symptoms of an infection may go away, but that does not mean the infection itself is necessarily gone. If you suspect an infection, see your healthcare provider as soon as possible.

lasts more than a week or two); unusual tiredness or lethargy; and recurring illness or infections. If you are on hormonal birth control or are using a birth control device like an intrauterine device (IUD) and have changes in your health or habits that may pose increased risks to you while using those methods (such as an STI, smoking, or high blood pressure), consult your healthcare provider. Serious and persistent concerns about nutrition and activity, about body size or shape, about the ability to sleep and rest soundly, about managing stress, or about depression or anxiety should also be directed to them.

[SAFER SEX 101]

STIs can happen to anyone—*anyone*—who is or has been sexually active (and not just those having vaginal or anal intercourse) or who has been sexually abused or assaulted, and they *do* happen to about nineteen million people, in the United States alone, every single year. ***At least one person in every four will contract an STI during their life.*** According to the Guttmacher Institute, over sixty-five million people in the United States currently live with a viral STI. Although teens and emerging adults make up only around 25 percent of the sexually active population, people from fifteen to twenty-five years of age account for nearly *half* of all new STI diagnoses every year. The people with the highest rates of STIs are young people.

By the time you're twenty-four, among you and two of your closest friends, one of you probably will have or have had an STI. Teens and emerging adults also have more of the most common STIs than anyone else: chlamydia, gonorrhea, herpes, and HPV all have higher incidence with young people than older populations. And many teens and emerging adults with STIs don't even know they have an infection because they can't or won't seek annual sexual health care and STI screenings, which are how we find out if we do or don't have STIs in the first place; because of wrong ideas about STIs and how they are transmitted; and because so many STIs don't present visible or obvious symptoms.

As a young person, your STI risks are higher than those of any other age group, and the impacts of some infections can also hit you harder. Adolescents are physically very susceptible to diseases and infections to begin with, and people who have a vagina rather than a penis have increased susceptibility. Young people are also more likely to have greater numbers of new sexual partners, often lack regular sexual health care, and, on top of that, often go without safer sex practices, all of which increase susceptibility and risks for everyone. Some greater risks of complications from sexually transmitted diseases and infection for those with a uterus include PID (pelvic inflammatory disease), reproductive cancers, and complications during pregnancy and childbirth.

STIs can happen to you, whether you've had ten partners or are just starting with your first partner; whether you've had vaginal intercourse or "only" oral sex; whether you're sexually conservative or more freewheeling; whether you're straight or queer, fifteen or fifty, and no matter what your gender is. Viruses and bacteria don't care who is "nice" or who isn't, who is a "virgin" and who's not—they aren't making character judgments; they're just looking for bodies to colonize. If you've got a body, you're a prime candidate.

The good news is that the majority of the time STIs can be easily prevented—ensuring both you and your partner's health as well as the health of all of us worldwide—with a combination of smart risk assessment and reduction, including safer sex practices and regular preventative sexual health care. And when they can't—again, it is very common for someone to acquire or transmit an STI—many of them are curable, and the others can be managed so that having one (or more) in the mix doesn't have to be anything even remotely close to the end of the world.

Some people are now using safer sex throughout their whole sexual lives, right from day one. But for plenty, that isn't the case. Perhaps you started your sexual life without knowing how or feeling able to protect yourself from infection or disease. Or maybe in your relationship, you and your partner started taking risks somewhere along the line, and now you're having some trouble breaking those habits. Some people even think that being responsible when it comes to safer sex—or asking a partner to—is somehow insulting or impolite, even though nobody thinks that about asking someone to please remember to cover their mouth when they cough. No matter the situa-

DID YOU KNOW? . . .

Quick STI Risk Assessment

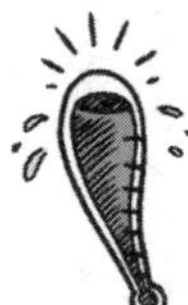

Very high-risk activities:

- Unprotected anal intercourse
- Unprotected vaginal intercourse
- Body fluid or blood play

High-risk activities:

- Unprotected fellatio
- Unprotected analingus

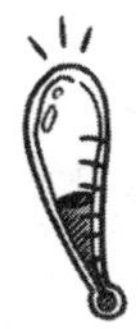

Moderate-risk activities:

- Shared sex toys without a condom or barrier on them (for toys that cannot be boiled)
- Unprotected cunnilingus
- Unprotected manual sex
- Kissing (openmouthed)

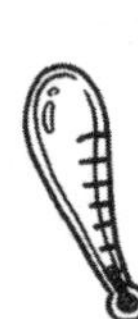

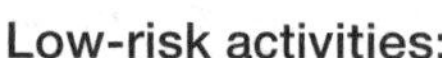

Low-risk activities:

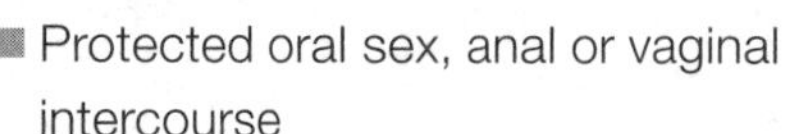

- Protected oral sex, anal or vaginal intercourse
- Unprotected manual sex with handwashing before and after
- Manual sex with latex gloves (or a medical-grade latex alternative)
- Kissing (includes openmouthed and closed-mouth, so long as no wounds or sores are present)
- Oral contact with body parts other than the mouth or genitals
- Dry sex

No-risk activities:

- Kissing (closed-mouth, so long as no wounds or sores are present)
- Massage and petting (nongenital and without fluid sharing)
- Sensation play
- Hugging
- Role-play, sexting, or phone sex
- Mutual masturbation

tion, it can feel awkward at first, and it might seem difficult to settle into healthy practices without feeling like the Sex Decency Brigade. But it doesn't have to be that way.

It's never too late to start having sex as responsibly and safely as possible, and there's no reason it needs to be a drag. If anything, safer sex often makes sex more rather than less enjoyable for people. It has many benefits that support a healthier, happier, and less stressful sex life. Worry and fear about disease, infection, and pregnancy can inhibit our brains from firing off all their sex-happy-making pistons, including the signals that influence things like erection, lubrication, and if things feel good or if they hurt. So, aside from the mental anguish, there are also very real possible negative outcomes or impacts of taking risks we just don't feel good about besides getting or passing on an STI. Safer sex isn't a barrier to the good stuff sex offers, but STIs and feeling like we're at risk can certainly get in the way.

WHAT IS SAFER SEX?

Safer sex is a combination of **three** basic things:

1. Limiting risks during sexual activities through barrier use (condoms, dental dams, latex gloves) and other practices.
2. STI screenings and sexual health exams, usually every year or so, or more often if you have new or multiple partners.

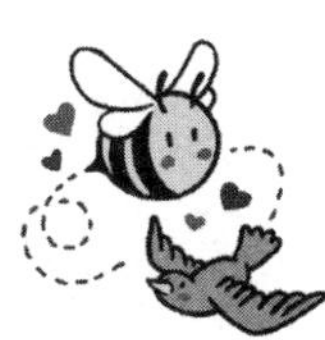

3. Making lifestyle choices that can reduce our risks, like limiting sexual partners, limiting or avoiding very high-risk sexual behaviors, limiting or eliminating nonsexual STI risks in general (intravenous drug use, for instance), using clean needles for body modification work, and taking care of your general health.

The more of those three things you do, and the more consistently you do them, the lower your STI risks will be. What's most important, however, and most effective at preventing infections or the spread of infections, is using barriers with some kinds of sex and regular STI testing.

Practicing Safer Sex: A Lesson in Three Parts

Safer sex practices can't make sex 100 percent safe, even if all of them are used to the letter—they make sex safe*r*. A condom can—especially if not used properly—break or, more commonly, slip off. Some STIs, like HPV, herpes, or pubic lice, can be more difficult to protect from because latex barriers cover only some of the genital area. And even when we practice safer sex guidelines religiously—including barrier use, testing, and lifestyle modifications—we can *still* transmit or contract an STI. We need to accept that STI transmission (passing one around) is always possible. Safer sex practices are a lot like seat belts: even with one, we may still get hurt, but it's a *lot* less likely than if we ditch them altogether.

Safer sex doesn't just make things safer for us, it makes sex, and life, safer for everyone, including better health outcomes. STIs, even the curable/manageable ones, aren't just about us and our partners; they also affect public health as a whole: the more people practice sex safely, the less likely it becomes for any of us to pick up or further spread a sexually transmitted infection. What happens in our bedrooms may be private, but our choices can affect people we'll never even meet, and someone else's choices can have a profound effect on our own lives and health. Whether those effects are negative or positive depends on the choices we all make.

Safer Sex, Part One: Barriers and Other Gear

The use of barriers with sexual activities works just like keeping your front door closed (instead of hanging wide open, for crying out loud, said almost every exasperated parent ever): it helps to keep the bugs out. There are a bunch of different barriers that can be used to reduce STI risks. Which ones you need is about which activities you're part of and which body parts are involved.

Outside or Male Condoms (Latex or Nonlatex)

"Male" or "outside" condoms are the kind of condom most people know about. They're a long sheath made of latex or suitable latex alternatives (like poly-

WHY PRACTICE SAFER SEX?

If you don't practice safer sex, you are at high risk for the following infections and diseases:

Unprotected vaginal or anal intercourse, or vaginal intercourse with a condom that has also been used for anal intercourse, can present risks of contracting (getting) or transmitting (passing on):

- Chlamydia (page 415)
- Gonorrhea (page 416)
- Hepatitis (page 417)
- Herpes simplex (page 418)
- HIV (page 419)
- Human papillomavirus (HPV) and Genital Warts (page 421)
- Mononucleosis (page 423)
- Pelvic inflammatory disease (PID) (page 424)
- Pubic lice (page 424)
- Syphilis (page 425)
- Trichomoniasis (page 426)

Unprotected oral sex presents risks of contracting or transmitting:

- Gonorrhea
- Hepatitis
- Herpes simplex (oral and/or genital)
- Human immunodeficiency virus (HIV)
- Human papillomavirus (HPV, warts)
- Yeast infections/thrush
- Syphilis

Unprotected manual sex can present risks of contracting or transmitting:

- Bacterial vaginosis
- Herpes simplex
- Human papillomavirus (HPV, warts)
- Pubic lice

For more information on each of these infections and diseases, see Appendix A, "Sexually Transmitted Infections: From A to Z."

urethane or polyisoprene) that are put on a penis or toy. Condoms are used as safer sex barriers for vaginal or anal intercourse (with a penis, toy, or other object), for fellatio, and for covering shared sex toys, like dildos or vibrators, especially those that cannot be boiled or sterilized. They can also be used to cover the penis during manual sex, in lieu of latex gloves, or cut lengthwise and opened for use as a barrier for cunnilingus or analingus. For those with latex sensitivity or discomfort, a nonlatex condom should be used; there are a few on the market, and the female condom (see page 292) is polyurethane. Some people can use latex but prefer latex alternatives because they can conduct body heat better and feel a little softer to the touch.

DID YOU KNOW? . . .

Around one in every one thousand people has a latex allergy, according to the Asthma and Allergy Foundation of America (AAFA). Some people aren't allergic, but they are sensitive. People can be tested for latex allergy or sensitivity the same ways they are tested for some other allergies, with a blood test. If you or a partner find that when you use latex condoms or other latex barriers you experience any soreness, itching, or swelling where the barrier is, check in with a healthcare provider. It may just be that you're not using enough lubricant, but it may be that you have a latex allergy or sensitivity. If you do, that doesn't have to mean going without barriers: latex alternatives are available, and within reach, for all kinds of barriers.

How to use a condom:

1. First check the expiration date on the package. You don't want to use an expired condom (though if the choice is expired condom or no condom, expired condom is the better choice. However, not having the kind of sex where you need a condom and holding off until you have condoms to use that aren't expired are better choices still). Always open a condom package carefully—use your fingers, not your teeth, and just tear the edge to open it carefully so that you don't rip the condom by accident. **Don't unroll it until you are putting it on.**

2. To put on the condom, look at it first to be sure to unroll it the right way. The condom should be put on with the edge that's rolled upward, not underneath, facing up: if it were a hat, it'd look more like a fedora or sombrero, not like a skullcap or beanie. Then pinch the tip of the condom with one hand, rolling it out a little bit to leave about an inch of space (if you're using a condom for a toy, not a penis, this part doesn't matter because there won't be fluids going into the condom). To increase comfort and pleasure for someone wearing it, place a couple drops of a latex-safe lubricant inside the tip of the unrolled condom.

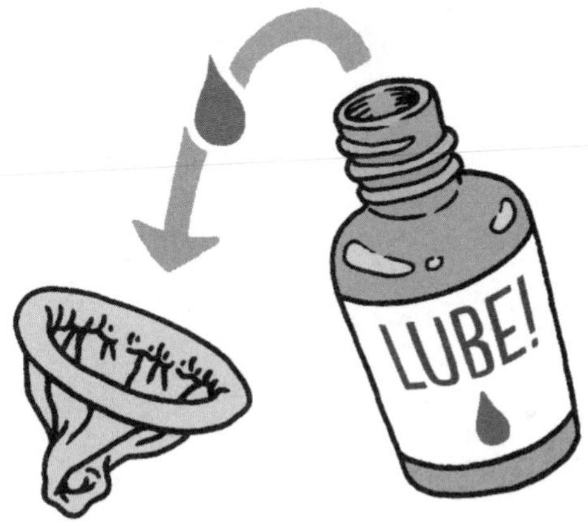

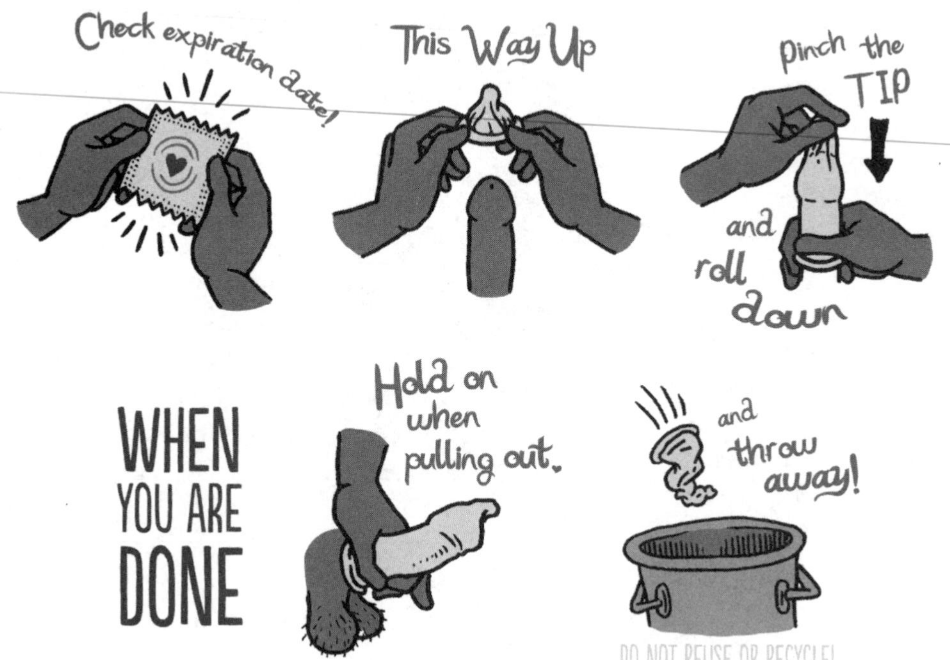
Check expiration date!
This Way Up
Pinch the TIP
and roll down
WHEN YOU ARE DONE
Hold on when pulling out.
and throw away!
DO NOT REUSE OR RECYCLE!

(*Never* use Vaseline [petroleum jelly], cooking or body oils, lotions, or other lubricants not intended for condom use: they can damage the condom or make it more likely to break.) Slowly roll the condom over the shaft of the penis or toy, to the base, gently pushing out any air bubbles inside the condom as you do. To increase the durability of the condom and everyone's pleasure and comfort, apply more latex-safe lubricant to the outside of the condom, as generously as you or a partner would like. Most condoms now come with a little bit of lube already on them, but it is only a very small amount; that is usually enough to get the condom on but won't often be enough for everyone's comfort and pleasure while using it. If you're putting a condom on an uncircumcised penis, push the foreskin back comfortably and hold it back with one hand while unrolling the condom onto the shaft of the penis. When you have the condom rolled down as far as it will go, release the foreskin and let it roll back up naturally. Adjust the base of the condom if you need to so that it's both secure and comfortable.

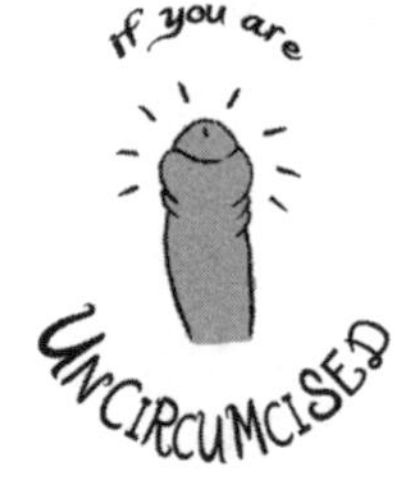
if you are
UNCIRCUMCISED

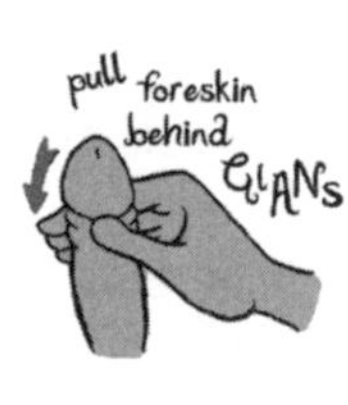

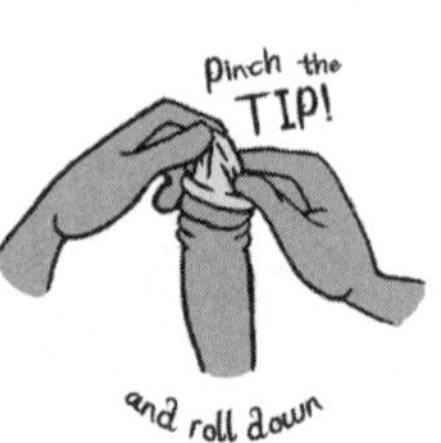
Pinch the TIP!
and roll down

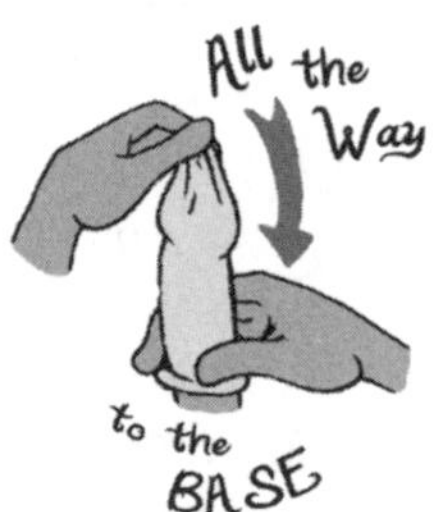

THIS ALLOWS THE FORESKIN TO RETURN TO IT'S NATURAL POSITION AND MOVE COMFORTABLY BENEATH THE CONDOM.

3. After ejaculation, withdraw while the penis is still erect, while holding on to the base of the condom to make sure it doesn't slip off. Roll it off slowly and carefully, knot it at the base to keep any fluids inside it inside, and throw the condom away.

For *every* new or repeated sexual activity, always use a new condom. Do not switch between vaginal, oral, or anal sex without also switching to a new, unused condom. Condoms also cannot be reused: once you've used one, it's toast.

The vast majority of condom failure is due to improper use. A lot of people have heard that condoms break often, but they really don't. Studies on condom breakage reflect a breakage rate of only around 0.4 percent, or only four breaks in every one thousand uses (so, you'd have to have sex every single day for around three years before a break with proper use would happen). Using and storing them properly makes breakage very, very unlikely. Condoms and other safer sex barriers also do not have invisible pores or holes that pathogens (or sperm cells) can pass through; when a condom is used properly, any bacteria or virus that was within the condom (on the surface of what the condom covered) *cannot* be transmitted. It is when a condom breaks, tears, or slips off that it may be ineffective (as birth control and as a barrier to disease). Breaks and tears are pretty easy to avoid: be sure you are using a high-quality condom that has been stored properly (which just means somewhere it doesn't get bumped around a lot, won't get damaged, or isn't exposed to extreme heat or cold), that you use with additional lubricant, and that you put on correctly.

Condoms are easy to obtain in most areas. You can find them at most pharmacies, megastores, and grocers. You can often obtain them at no cost from sexual health clinics and community centers, though in those cases you do not often get to choose the type you get. Condoms can also be ordered online or by mail-order catalog and are generally shipped in plain packages for privacy.

Helpful Hints

▶ **For the most part, most condoms will accommodate nearly all penis sizes, especially lengthwise.** Ring (the condom base) sizes, however, vary more, and are less flexible, so you may need to shop around if the base feels too tight on you or your partner. Condoms termed a "snugger" fit tend to have smaller ring sizes; those with words like "maximum fit" or "larger" on the packaging tend to have larger ring sizes. Some custom-fit condoms are on the market as are several brands of condoms sized with extra room at the head of the condom to provide greater comfort. Most people fit in average-size condoms just fine, so be sure not to purchase larger ones if you don't need them—a condom that's too big can easily slip off.

▶ **Thin is in.** Choose thinner condoms for greater durability, sensation, and comfort. With thinner condoms, less friction occurs, and as a result, thinner condoms tend to be more durable and less likely—not more, as a lot of people believe—to break than thicker ones. And, of course, when condoms feel good, people are more likely to use them in the first place.

▶ **Avoid condoms with nonoxynol-9.** Nonoxynol-9, the spermicide most often used on condoms lubricated with spermicide, is only added to condoms to make users *feel* more secure. Condoms lubricated with spermicide are not more effective than those without spermicide, and they cause genital irritation for many people; inflamed genital tissue makes infection transmission *more* likely.

▶ **Don't double up.** Putting one condom over another increases friction, so *both* are actually more likely to break than one used alone (not to mention that a person wearing two condoms is not likely to feel very much).

▶ **Stay sugar-free.** Flavored condoms are for oral sex, not for anal or vaginal intercourse. The flavored lubricant often contains sugars, which can make yeast infections more likely.

▶ **Be aware of latex sensitivities.** Some people who have a latex allergy experience symptoms with immediate contact; others, after a few hours or even days after contact with latex. So, if you experience any genital swelling, burning, redness, blistering, fissures, scaling, nausea or vomiting, dizziness or faint feeling, or cramps after using latex condoms or other latex barriers, you may be allergic to latex. If you suspect you are, you can try using polyurethane condoms and see whether you have the same symptoms. If not, then you're likely allergic or sensitive to latex, and you can follow up with a test from your healthcare provider to confirm that. Some people just prefer latex alternatives, even when they or their partners aren't allergic or sensitive. The material of most is softer than latex, and latex alternatives also conduct body heat a bit better. Nonlatex condoms work just as well as latex, so you can always try both to see whether you or your partner has a preference.

▶ **Accept no substitutes.** Lambskin condoms do *not* offer protection against STIs. Plastic wrap, plastic bags, or a latex glove *cannot* be used on the penis in place of a condom.

▶ **Don't condoms limit pleasure or make it harder to keep an erection?** That's more something people think than actually experience. Studies, like one published in January 2013 in the *Journal of Sexual Medicine,* haven't found either of those claims to be true at all. In that study, which worked with a nationally representative sample of people ages eighteen to fifty-nine, ratings of sexual satisfaction were high, with few differences based on condom use. No significant differences were found in the ability to have erections with or without condoms. Another study published in the *Journal of Sexual Medicine* in August 2015 found that people who had issues with erection with condom use also most typically had the same issues without condom use. This is often a matter of attitude about condoms, not about condoms themselves. So, change your mind, change your experience with condoms.

Inside or "Female" Condoms

Condoms called "female" condoms, or inside condoms, are nonlatex barriers that can be used for vaginal or anal intercourse. Like male condoms, they're a long sheath, but instead of going on something, they go inside the body, either the vagina or the anus. They're a good option for people with latex allergies or sensitivities and for condom wearers who find the base or shaft of male condoms too tight for their comfort or liking. Unlike outside condoms, they can also be placed well in advance of sexual activity—as early as eight hours before, if you like.

The inside condom has a ring at both ends: one on the inside, at the back of the condom, and then a ring at the shaft like an outside condom but much larger.

1. To use an inside condom, you start the same way you do with an outside condom: by checking the expiration date and opening the package carefully.

2. Next, put a little lubricant on the outside of the closed end (the end with the ring inside of it).

3. Then you'll insert it inside the vagina or anus, depending on what kind of genital sex you want to take part in. Some put the inside condom in while they stand with one foot up on something, or they squat or sit on the edge of a chair or toilet or lay down. You'll find out by experimenting what works best for you. If you know it takes you some time to put an inside condom in, you can always do so in advance of sexual activity. You don't have to do it only at the time of, like with outside condoms.

Squeeze that inner, or back, ring together with your fingers until it basically makes a line, and put it inside the body the way you'd put in a tampon or menstrual cup, pushing it gently back as far as you can until the ring rights itself to be more horizontal than vertical. When it's all the way back, you pull the finger you pushed it inside with out, and let the outer ring of the condom hang about an inch outside the vagina or anus.

4. Then, a partner will insert their penis—or a toy—inside the vagina or anus and the condom inside. The base will not grip them like an outside condom's base does. For those new to sex or to using this kind of condom, do be sure to check that the penis or toy is inserted inside the condom rather than to the side of the condom.

5. To remove the inside condom, just have your partner withdraw—no need to hold anything. Then you twist the outer ring and the part of the condom outside

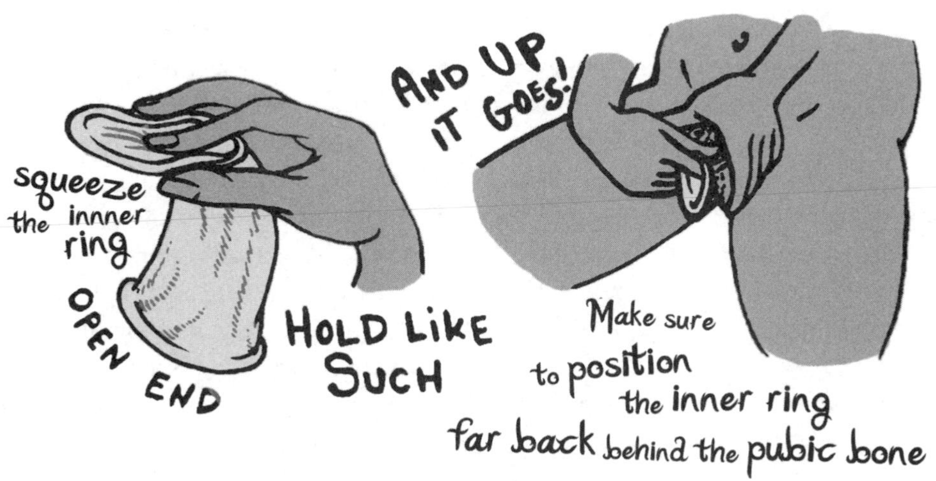
squeeze the inner ring
OPEN END
HOLD LIKE SUCH
AND UP IT GOES!
Make sure to position the inner ring far back behind the pubic bone

your body until it's closed, gently pull it out, and throw it away.

Lubricant

Lubricants are used for any sexual activity, especially with safer sex barriers, or simply for extra pleasure or comfort during vaginal or anal intercourse or manual sex. People using hormonal birth control methods, such as the pill or patch, may also find they need extra lubricant because those methods can cause extra vaginal dryness.

How to use lube:

- To use with a condom, place a couple of drops inside the tip of the condom before putting it on, and then apply lubricant on the outside of the condom when it is fully unrolled and/or on the vulva or anus, if vaginal or anal intercourse will occur. Add more as wanted or needed.
- To use with a dental dam, apply lube on the genitals before the dental dam is placed on them.
- For manual sex, apply lubricant to both the outside of the glove or hands and the other partner's genitals.

How much or how little to use is a matter of preference, but there should be enough lube, at all times, to keep the barrier from becoming dry or tacky and to keep the genitals comfortable and slippery during sexual activities. It's common to find that you need to apply extra lubricant during sex, for both comfort and durability of the barrier.

Lubricant is easily washed off the genitals during regular bathing, though if you are prone to yeast infections, you may want to rinse it off sooner rather than later.

You can purchase lubricants at your local pharmacy (they're usually in the same area as condoms), obtain them at some sexual health clinics, or find them via Internet or mail-order suppliers.

Helpful Hints

- **Accept no substitutes.** Latex-safe lubricant is either water-based or silicone-based and indicates "for sexual/genital use" on the tube or bottle. Body lotions, baby or cooking oils, massage oils or creams, and Vaseline should never be used with condoms, gloves, or dams. Not only do many of these substances erode latex, and thus put it at risk of breaking or tearing, but most of them do not belong inside the internal genitalia, the vagina, or the anus because they can cause infection.
- **Go sugar-free.** Many lubricants contain glycerin, which may create problems for those prone to yeast infections. Glycerin-free or low-glycerin lubes are available. Flavored lubricants should not be used vaginally or anally, because they contain sugars, which can also create or exacerbate yeast infections.
- **Wanting or needing lube isn't weird or a sign something is the matter with someone.** From what we can tell, people have used lubricants for as long as people have been having sex. Lubricants in the way past were often not latex-safe (we didn't have latex through most of history) and sometimes were made of much grosser stuff than lubes are now, like animal blubber (*eew*). Lube isn't something only older people or people who have troubles lubricating on their own need. For consistent pleasure and comfort with sexual activities that involve a lot of

friction—like intercourse, manual sex, or masturbation—most people want or need lubricant and find that it increases their pleasure and sexual enjoyment. Ain't nothing wrong with that!

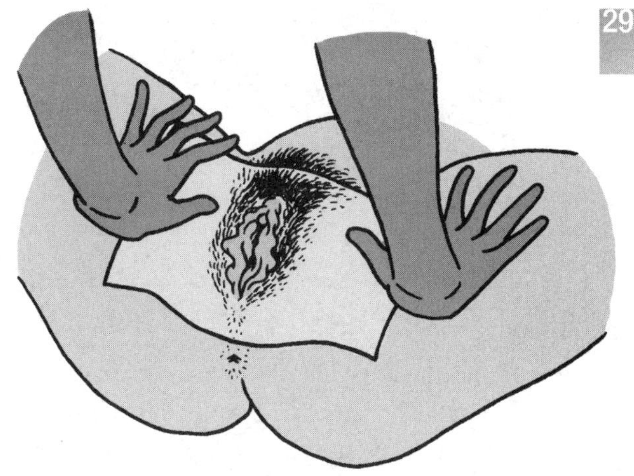

Dental Dams

Dental dams are used for cunnilingus or analingus.

How to use a dental dam:

Most dams have a light talc coating, so first, rinse off the talc with water, because it can cause some irritation. Apply lubricant to the genitals where the dam will be placed. Then, open up the dam—it's like a little sheet of latex when opened—and spread it over the vulva or anus. You or your partner can then hold the dam in place with your hands during the activity.

Dental dams are often harder to find than condoms. Whereas most online safer sex and sex toy suppliers sell them, many pharmacies that sell condoms and lubes do not. You can also obtain them at medical supply stores. If you cannot find a source for dental dams, you may also adapt a condom as directed in the Helpful Hints or use kitchen plastic wrap. You can use the plastic wrap the same way you'd use a dam. For cunnilingus, you can wrap the cling-film dam around the wearer's thighs so no one has to hold the barrier in place with their hands.

Helpful Hints

- **Use one side—once.** Always keep the same side of the dam or cling film against the body. You can't flip-flop dams and have them work effectively—only one side may be used. Dental dams cannot be reused to be effective against the spread of disease or infection.
- **You can make a dam out of a latex condom.** To use a condom as a dental dam for cunnilingus or analingus, simply cut the condom with a clean pair of scissors down the middle, lengthwise, and open it up.
- **You can also make a dam out of a latex glove.** There are a few ways to do this: you can cut off the fingers and base of the glove

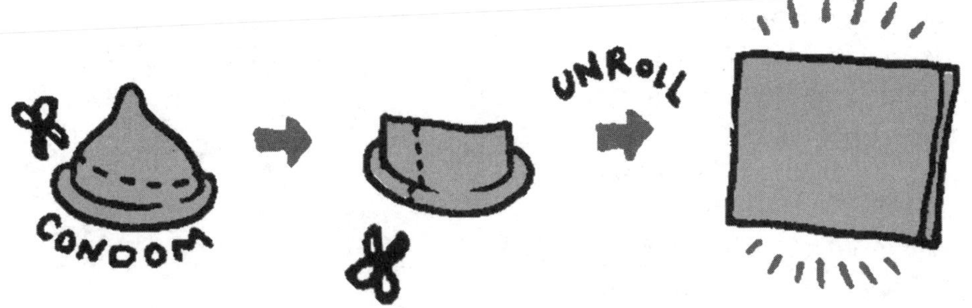

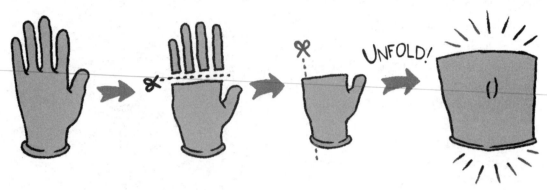

and then cut lengthwise along the thumb and open it up (and you then have four finger cots as well). Or—and this is especially handy if you're performing manual sex and oral sex at the same time—you can put the glove on your hand, then cut a rectangular flap from the base to the fingers, and simply lift that up and cover the vulva while wearing the rest of the glove on your hand or while fingers are inside the vagina already gloved. You can also cut a glove's fingers off, then cut up lengthwise on the side without the thumb, and put your tongue inside the thumb to use the dam.

Latex or Polyurethane (Nonlatex) Gloves

Gloves are used for manual sex. A glove can also be used as a dental dam (see pages 295–296).

How to use gloves:

▶ Be sure to remove any jewelry from your hands before using gloves, and if you have long or sharp nails, it's a good idea to cut them first. Take the gloves out of the box or baggie they're in, and slide your hands into them, just like any other kind of gloves.

▶ For manual sex, the gloves should be lubricated on the outside with latex-safe lubricant. When finished, toss the gloves in the garbage. A new pair of gloves should be used each time, when switching from one set of genitals to another, or from penis or vulva to anus.

▶ To use a glove as a dental dam, see the illustration above.

▶ You can use a whole glove or just the fingers of it to cover shared sex toys, but latex gloves may *not* be used as a condom substitute.

Local pharmacies or megastores should carry latex and polyurethane gloves. They are also available at medical supply stores or via mail order through catalog or Internet sources.

Helpful Hints

▶ **Gloves feel good.** Gloves can be the bomb when it comes to manual sex. It's not just a matter of providing STI protection; ragged fingernails or cuticles and even small calluses can make manual sex less pleasant (and cause abrasions or fis-

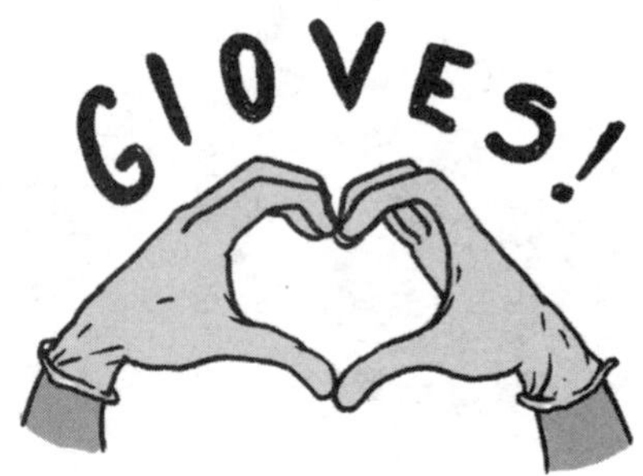

sures of the penis, vagina, or anus), and gloves smooth all that out.

▶ **Pick the right glove.** Again, as with condoms and dams, if either you or your partner is latex-sensitive, nonlatex gloves are also available.

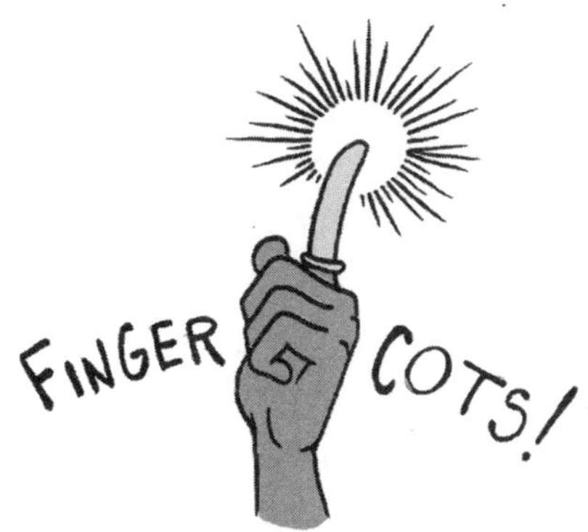

Finger Cots

Finger cots are used for manual sex, when only a finger or fingers are being used, such as for anal play or clitoral stimulation. They can also be used to cover small sex toys (like remote vibrators).

How to use a finger cot: easy-peasy. Just unroll the finger cot onto your finger or a sex toy, like it's a tiny condom. When you're finished with it, dispose of it. Finger cots may not be used as a substitute for condoms.

Finger cots are tougher to find than most other safer sex products but can be obtained by mail order via condom suppliers, medical supply stores, and many sex shops. See page 296 for how to make finger cots out of latex gloves.

Safer Sex, Part Two: Testing and Annual Sexual Health Exams

Because barriers cannot offer complete protection against disease and infection, especially with common STIs like HPV and

ARTS AND CRAFTS, SAFER SEX STYLE

Want another way to use a dam for cunnilingus, hands-free? One of our volunteers at Scarleteen passed on these instructions to make a DIY dam harness:

- Get a packet of garter snaps and any fabric that tickles your fancy (ribbons, silk cord, green monster fur—all available at most craft or fabric stores).
- Take a dental dam (or piece of plastic cling wrap) of the sort/size you will be using. Attach a garter snap to each corner of the dental dam.

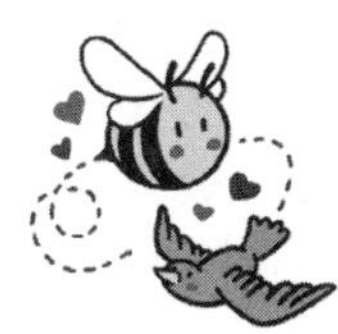

- Position the dental dam over your crotch. Now, the fun bit: attach strips of fabric/ribbon to the other ends of the snaps and tie them around yourself so that they hold the dam in place. You can do this in almost any way you like. Two obvious arrangements are: (1) the bikini type, with just two strips of fabric going from front to back over each hip, or (2) the garter belt type, with a "belt" around the waist and four strips of fabric hanging down, each attaching to a strap. You can get as artsy-craftsy as you like, or not. If you don't know how to sew, you can use fabric glue, or just use ribbons, which you can tie.
- Once you've got it all fixed together to your liking, you can use it, then simply unclip the snaps, toss away the dam, and you're done! You can snap in a new dam with the reusable belt anytime. You can also use existing underpants to make a dam harness by cutting out the crotch area, placing the dam where the crotch once was, and attaching the garter snaps that way.

the herpes virus, it's also important to be regularly tested so that you and your partners know as accurately as possible what your risks are and so that, if either of you does develop an STI, you can get it treated quickly and take extra precautions as needed.

Remember that *sexually transmitted* means that these diseases and infections are *most* often transmitted sexually, not that there is no *other* way they can be transmitted. Oral herpes, for instance, can be contracted by kissing your dad (in fact, most people with oral herpes contract it in childhood from nonsexual contact). Pubic lice can be spread by sharing towels. Hepatitis or HIV can be acquired through a tattoo or piercing done with a shared needle. And *sexually transmitted* doesn't just refer to intercourse but to several kinds of sexual activities. This is why someone who is a "virgin" or who has not had genital intercourse before cannot automatically be assumed to be STI-free.

What Exactly Does STI Screening Involve?

STI testing includes a few simple tests that can be done in your healthcare provid-

SAFER SEX KIT

A basic safer sex kit could contain:

- A variety of outside or inside condoms or both, including a range of sizes
- Latex-safe lubricant
- Latex or nonlatex gloves
- Dental dams (or you can keep a nail scissors in your kit for cutting condoms or gloves to use as dams)

You could supersize it with:

- Finger cots
- Baby wipes (for quick cleanup of genitals, especially after using flavored lubes or condoms or silicone lubricants)
- Cranberry tablets (can be helpful to prevent UTI development)
- An over-the-counter analgesic, such as aspirin, acetaminophen, or ibuprofen (helpful for soreness due to vasocongestion)
- Aloe vera gel (handy for external genital irritation after sexual activities)
- A dose of emergency contraception if you are part of any kind of sex that presents a risk of pregnancy

If you can't access the most basic safer sex supplies, I'd suggest you rethink being sexually active in ways that carry STI risks until you can. Treating STIs also often has a cost, as does testing, and preventing them is usually cheaper than treating or managing them. If paying for these supplies is a strain, check to see whether any of your local sexual health clinics offer some or all of these supplies for free or at low cost: many do. If you have a healthcare plan or national healthcare coverage, some of them may also be covered by your plan, especially if you have contraception coverage (if so, you may be able to have your healthcare provider write a prescription for condoms so your plan covers their cost, even if you're not using them as a contraceptive method). If vaginal or anal dryness or soreness is an issue for you when you don't use a lubricant—as it often is—they may be able to "prescribe" that as well so that you're covered.

er's office or at a general or sexual health clinic. Some may cause slight, brief discomfort. It's important to recognize that when you ask for a full screening, you will get all the tests available to you that will net accurate results. There are some STIs that can't be screened for accurately or that require very specific timing to screen for properly. For instance, without an active sore, it's difficult to test for herpes. Ask your doctor or clinician to tell you which tests they *can* do so you're fully informed.

When you want an STI screening, you'll make an appointment with your healthcare provider by asking for that screening at the time you're making the appointment. If you want to be tested for everything that you can, what you'll ask for is a "full STI panel." You can also ask for STI screenings during annual check-ups or exams if you prefer. If you've come in for a screening because you know or suspect that you have been exposed to a specific STI or you have symptoms that lead you to believe you may have contracted one, give that information to clinical staff during this time.

The healthcare provider will first do a visual examination of your body and genitals, looking for evidence of sores or lesions, abnormal discharges, or unusual tissue texture or color. If you have a vulva, this may include a pelvic exam. The provider performing the exam will take a small sample of cells and fluids called a smear or swab. This is similar to a Pap smear (see page 269), except that in this case, when the lab technician looks at the cells through a microscope, they will be looking for signs of the various microorganisms, antibodies, or cell changes that can indicate specific STIs.

If you have a penis and are given a swab test (page 271), it will involve the insertion of a long cotton-tipped swab into the urethra to get a sample of cells. The cells gathered on the swab will then be examined under a microscope.

Depending on your sexual history, your health concerns, or any concerns your healthcare provider has, the healthcare provider may also take a sample of cells from your throat (to check for STIs that can be present in the mouth or throat, such as gonorrhea) and/or your rectum, by swabbing the same way your genitals

DID YOU KNOW? . . .

Many people feel they don't need STI screenings. Plenty more think they *have* been screened when they haven't: many people assume annual pelvic exams involve STI screenings, when they often do not unless a patient asks for them. Some people think that, if someone went into the military, their health screenings include a full STI screening (nope). Some folks who may have been tested for HIV think that test screens for all STIs; it doesn't. Unless someone has asked for STI screening explicitly or has exhibited symptoms that made a healthcare provider suspect they might have an STI and run some tests, assume screenings haven't happened. Most STIs, most of the time, are asymptomatic: they don't cause any noticeable symptoms or anything a person or their partners can tell just by looking at them or their body parts. So, if someone hasn't been screened and *has* an STI, they usually will have no idea they have one.

were swabbed. If you are being tested for HIV, it will usually involve a cheek swab.

For a full screening, your healthcare provider will likely also take saliva, blood, and urine samples for screenings that require those.

Your healthcare professionals may be able to tell you immediately if you do or do not have some STIs; for most, you have to wait a few days or weeks for complete results of your tests. How long depends on the lab and how busy they are at a given time, not your healthcare provider. Waiting for test results is never fun for anyone—it's normal to feel very nervous, scared, or anxious. But because you have had your screenings done, so long as you are not taking additional risks while you wait, you should know that you've done all you can currently do. So, try to relax. Take care of yourself. And give yourself mad props for taking steps to take care of your sexual health.

For more on testing for specific STIs, see Appendix A.

Safer Sex, Part Three: Lifestyle Issues

Although anyone who is sexually active can contract STIs, the following lifestyle issues can present greater risks:

▶ **Multiple partners:** Of any sex, gender, or orientation, simultaneously (such as in threesomes) or sequentially (having a string of partners one after the other). Think about it this way: someone who crosses a busy street a few times a day is more likely to get hit by a car than is someone who crosses the same street once a month. Same goes with multiple partners: the more partners we have, the more possibilities there are for us to transmit or contract an STI. That's simple math. This isn't about value judgments; it's just about mathematical probability.

▶ **Drug and alcohol abuse:** Because of shared needles, paraphernalia, or bottles (most folks know that shared needles create HIV and hepatitis risks, but did you ever think about oral herpes being passed around with that bottle?) and increased risk taking that often occurs while under the influence of drugs or alcohol. One reason many people enjoy alcohol or drugs is the feelings of reduced inhibition they can produce, but that same effect can also lead to sex with unknown partners, ditching safer sex practices and precautions, and engaging in other risky sexual activities that a person might otherwise have avoided. In addition, it is common for date or acquaintance rape to occur when one or all parties are intoxicated. Being sober helps keep you safer, and not just from STIs.

▶ **Denial or secrecy:** People in denial about having sex tend to have sex less safely. For example, refusing to admit that you *are* sexually active (by staying "technically" a virgin); hiding from friends or family that you are sexually active in general; or being secretive about dating someone whose age, sexual orientation, race, behavior, and so on, may be seen as unacceptable can incline you to also be in denial about sexual responsibility and safety. The whole world doesn't need to know about everything that happens in your bedroom. However, if you can't be honest about it with yourself, your partner or partners, and those closest to you, your sexual health may be at a greater risk.

▶ **Poverty:** Because sexual health care and safer sex tools cost money, poverty and/or homelessness increase STI risks when the basics to make sex safe are not affordable or available.

▶ **General poor health or poor self-image:** When you're unhealthy, malnourished, stressed out, worn out, or battling off existing infections or conditions, your body is at a greater risk. When you don't feel well physically or don't hold yourself in high regard, you're more likely to make poor choices than when you're well and self-respecting.

Gender, Orientation, and STIs

No one sex, gender, or orientation is immune to sexually transmitted infection and disease, and no one gender or orientation is responsible for the spread of STIs. However, there are some specific differences and concerns with STIs that are worth knowing about.

People with penises are the most common transmitters of sexual infections and diseases. There is also a far greater chance of someone with a vagina contracting an STI from a partner. Because of the construction of the vulva and vagina, and because cervical cell maturation isn't complete until the mid-twenties, young people with a vagina

SEX AND DRUGS AND NOT-SO-MUCH

A lot of people have the idea that alcohol or recreational drugs (including prescription drugs used recreationally) are sexual enhancers. Although some people have that experience with some recreational substances, and many people feel less emotionally inhibited when using many of them, *most* recreational substances actually get in the way of human sexual response. Many inhibit erection or lubrication, make abrasion and bleeding more likely, increase anxiety, and slow the nervous system's and brain's responses (the bits that do the most when it comes to experiencing pleasure and sexual responses like orgasm). Many increase health risks with sex, either directly (like by increasing the risk of genital injury, and thus, STI transmission) or indirectly (like being strongly associated with reduced or improper condom use).

Alcohol happens to be the most commonly used substance mixed with sex. It also happens to be one of the substances *most* associated with all those response and enjoyment inhibitors *and* with sexual violence. At least one-half of all violent crimes, including sexual assault, involve alcohol consumption by the perpetrator, the victim, or both. From both legal and practical perspectives, hooch and other recreational substances in the mix make sex anything from consensually-iffy-at-best to not-consensual-at-all, but instead assault.

Chances are good that when you look back on your life, you'll feel that most of your best sexual decisions were made sober, or mighty close to it, all around, not when drugs or alcohol were involved. If something seems like it's a good thing when you or anyone else is wasted, it will still be a good thing—and also be much, much more likely to actually turn out to *be* a good thing—when you and everyone else involved are clear-headed.

are more susceptible to infection. As well, fewer people who have a penis seek out or receive preventative sexual health care than people with vaginas do.

People whose sex lives don't involve and haven't involved partners with a penis—most often, lesbians—are currently known to be at the least risk of STI transmission. However, because of biases and some data collection problems, we can only be so sure about this. For instance, it's likely that lesbians' risks are greater than are typically stated because in much STI data *lesbian* is defined as someone who has *never* had a partner with a penis, which excludes the majority of lesbians. Too, plenty of research and reporting is still biased in placing the greatest burden of STI transmission on gay men, even when that isn't factually so. Right now, the people with the highest global rates of HIV are cisgender, heterosexual women who acquire the virus from cisgender, heterosexual male partners.

Easy Ways to Incorporate Safer Sex into Your Sex Life

Safe can be just as (or more) sexy. Knowing you're responsible, educated, and safe is empowering, and when you are sexually empowered, you're in the driver's seat of your sexuality. And being in charge of your sexual self is about as sexy as it gets. Having the sexual confidence to set limits, like by insisting on safer sex practices, and to communicate openly with partners about safer sex tends to increase sexual confidence overall.

Accentuate the positive. Condoms can help to maintain erection and delay ejaculation in a way that's often desired. Manual sex or anal play with a glove and lube usually feels a whole lot better and more comfortable. Vaginal intercourse using condoms and lubricant can even feel *better* than without because latex provides a smoother texture and lubricant keeps everything from drying out and getting sore. And that's just the tip of the iceberg. Most people find that when they make an attitude adjustment about safer sex, they discover great things about it they never suspected.

Use safer sex as a tool to strengthen your relationships. Taking the initiative and sharing the responsibility for safer sex can really solidify the emotional bond between you and your partner. Take turns putting on the condom or holding the dam. Create a joint budget for safer sex supplies, and do the shopping and choosing together. Make a safer sex kit that is just for the two of you: create a cool case or container for it that's personalized, special, and fun. (Finally, a use for that Bedazzler you found in the basement!) By all means, talk about it. Get tested for STIs together. It doesn't have to be torture if you make a date of it. Go have a nice breakfast, go get tested, support one another while you wait for results, and when the results come in, do something fun together. Sex with each other is about partnership and mutuality. Learning to communicate and cooperate when it comes to safer sex also helps us to communicate and cooperate in our relationship and in our general sexuality.

Make it fun. On the day you want to introduce condoms into your partnership, blow up a bunch of them like balloons.

Or buy some glow-in-the-dark ones and don't tell your partner what they do until the lights go out. To introduce latex gloves and lube, you could borrow a stethoscope and play doctor. To start using a vaginal barrier, make an oh-so-stylish bikini out of the plastic wrap. If things get awkward as you're learning to use these items, let yourselves laugh about it—there *is* something very funny about a glove that shoots across the room or a neon green condom, and sex is *supposed* to be fun.

"Don't You Trust Me?"

One of the biggest obstacles to sound safer sex practice is the issue of trust and the assumptions some people make about trust and sex. Some people feel that being asked to use safer sex practices means that their partner doesn't trust them. Some people are of the mind that because they trust their partners, they don't have to be concerned about STIs.

Many STIs can be present, even for years, without a person knowing they're there. **Most STIs, for most people, most of the time, are asymptomatic.** People often have no noticeable symptoms or may not know that certain symptoms they're experiencing are due to an STI—especially if they don't get regular sexual health care and screenings. Some STIs, such as HPV and herpes, are still difficult to test for when they're asymptomatic, especially in men. Many people haven't ever had screenings. They might think that since an ex-partner was a "good" girl, there wasn't a risk, even with unprotected sex. An ex-partner of theirs may have lied about their sexual history or said that they had tests done when they hadn't. Someone might not know that activities other than vaginal or anal intercourse carry disease or infection risks. And many people are so terribly afraid of having an STI that they don't get screenings at all, even when they know they should; they just don't want to know, even though they may be endangering themselves and their partners with that avoidance and denial.

When we ask for safer sex practices, it's in the interest of protecting ourselves *and* our partners as best we can, ensuring our health and well-being, and having sex in an environment of safety and smarts. Trust doesn't provide health protections, and trust also can't do an STI test. So, "*Yes, I trust you. I also trust science and what it can do that just trusting each other can't.*"

Anyone who is profoundly hurt or offended by requests for safer sex or testing perhaps doesn't know or accept the facts about STIs; is scared to deal with all that partnered sex entails; is embarrassed to admit that they don't know how to use safer sex tools, like condoms or dams; or may well *not* be trustworthy. Trying to make a partner feel guilty about asking for safer sex practices is unfortunately something that works all too well for a lot of people—people we really *shouldn't* trust or be sleeping with. By making you feel bad about not trusting them, they're trying to make you forget that you have good reason not to.

Before you become sexually active with a partner, you hopefully both already trust one another a good deal and know that trust is present and bona fide without much doubt. When that's the case, and when people are accurately informed about STIs and sexual health in general, trust really shouldn't be an issue or an obstacle, because taking care of one another is *part* of trust.

What If Your Partner Won't Practice Safer Sex?

A partner who absolutely refuses to practice safer sex is refusing to be responsible and care for your health and well-being and their own. (Sadly, over the years at Scarleteen, many people have asked whether *they* could contract something from a partner, yet they don't express any concern about whether a partner could contract an STI from *them*.) In short, a partner who will not practice sex safely and responsibly is a partner I think it's best to say no way to until or unless they change their tune. Someone like that may likely be equally irresponsible, unsafe, and inconsiderate when it comes to other issues that affect you greatly: about having other partners or not, about caring for your feelings and emotional needs, about respecting your right to say no to certain sexual activities—the works.

Sometimes, partners may say no to safer sex because they just don't understand that unsafe sex is just that—unsafe—and that that lack of safety can't be fixed by just trust.

Someone who says no to safer sex the first time around may be someone worth talking to plainly about safer sex, about the risks involved with sexual activity. Now and then, a partner who says no can turn into a partner who says yes easily and gladly once they're furnished with accurate, honest, and compassionate information. But what if that person maintains their position of "no" to safety after you or someone else has supplied accurate information and they know your rules for being safe? Time for you to say no, too: no to sex with them. That way, they get to have their no respected, but you also get to stay safe.

Sex that is safe on all levels involves sane limits and boundaries. We could give all sorts of witty, smart answers to possible partner comments like "But it doesn't

IS SAFETY SLUTTY?

We're all too aware of the profound double standard that sends the message that it's more okay for men to be sexually experienced than women: sexually active men are studs or "players," whereas sexually active women are sluts or easy lays. That double standard makes some young women reluctant to keep safer sex supplies on hand or to ask partners to use them, for fear of seeming more sexually experienced than they really are or want to appear. In *Slut! Growing Up Female with a Bad Reputation,* Leora Tanenbaum points out that the slut label is affixed more arbitrarily than most of us would think: not only to girls who are self-possessed sexually or are known to have been sexually active but also to girls who merely dress differently or don't fit into traditional roles, who have different social circles than others, or who have been victims of sexual assault. We can all agree that labels and double standards like this really suck. But not having what you need on hand to keep yourself safe and well isn't an effective counter to them or a smart way to avoid them. Put your health first—without it, you'll be in no shape to tackle your daily life let alone pervasive social problems.

feel as good with a condom," or "I don't like condoms," or "You don't trust me," but the fact of the matter is that your best bet is to walk into any sexual situation with clearly communicated limits about safer sex, and not waver on them or get pulled into arguments about practicing safer sex. More times than not, if you let a partner know, kindly and diplomatically, that you're just **not willing** to risk their health or yours for sex and that, if they want to have sex with you, they are going to need to do so safely, you'll find that people who are trustworthy, mature, and caring partners aren't going to balk at all.

Sure, that's not always as easy to do as it sounds. Someone you've got a major jones for sexually and/or romantically may make it hard to make or keep those limits. It can be a struggle even to keep your head intact when you've got a bad case of the super-duper in-love woozies. Someone's arguments may sway you from doing what you know is best for yourself. If others in your peer circle are vocal about not practicing safer sex, or about thinking it's stupid, it can be hard to be the only one being safe and smart, and harder to be the first person to lay down the law to your partner. It's all too easy to give in, every now and then, if a partner whom you do trust and who is normally safe and smart, suggests trying unsafe sex "just once to know how it feels." It can also be difficult to resist the emotional manipulation of someone who believes they're healthy and insists that you want to practice safer sex because you don't trust them. Remember, you can trust them all you want, but if they're walking around with chlamydia, unaware, trust isn't going to keep you safe.

Most people don't need to practice safer sex or all portions of safer sex with a given partner forever if they don't want to and can still be safe. If you've been with a partner exclusively for at least six months, and the same is true of them; if you have practiced safer sex during that time for all moderate- to high-risk activities; and if each of you have two full and negative screenings at the end of that six-month period, your risks are usually very minimal.

What If You *Do* Get an STI?

Discovering you have an STI can be rough, especially when you're young. It's hard enough to find out you're ill in any way, but with sexually transmitted diseases it can be even more difficult. Because of social stigma and ignorance about STIs and sexuality, you may feel ashamed, dirty, stupid, or naive (even though you are none of those things). Because some STIs can have long-term effects and even change your life completely in some ways, and because of how daunting it can seem to inform current and future partners about it, it can all feel really scary. Although it's okay to feel however you do, there really is no need to feel any of those ways.

We're only human: we get sick and can get infections of or through any site on our bodies. STIs are infections just like the cold or flu virus: people don't get them because they're good or bad people; people get them because they have a body that's vulnerable to those pathogens, as all bodies are. Most illnesses can be treated or managed these days. We make mistakes, and sometimes mistakes carry consequences we have to deal with—and sometimes, things just happen. You may have contracted an STI even while being careful and practicing safer sex. Getting an STI doesn't mean you're a bad person, doesn't mean you're dirty, and doesn't mean you have to live the rest of your life like a leper or a monk.

If and when you're diagnosed with an STI, the very first person to talk with is your healthcare provider. Be sure to ask all the questions you have about:

▶ **Healing:** If a treatment is available, what are the directions? Are there any special cautions? Do partners also need to be treated at the same time? Do you need to abstain from protected sex while being treated? When should you start seeing improvements in symptoms with treatment? If you don't see improvements within a certain time, what should you do? Will you need more than one treatment? If so, when?

▶ **Dealing:** What are all the specifics about your particular STI? Are there long-term effects or risks you need to be aware of and on the lookout for? Do you need to make, or might you benefit from making, any lifestyle changes in terms of your environment, diet and nutrition, exercise, or other elements? Will you need any extra health care in the future? Is there a counselor or support group in your area available to you? Are there high-quality resources for managing or finding out more about your specific disease or infection—books, brochures, or websites—that your healthcare provider can refer you to?

▶ **Revealing:** Which partners do you need to inform besides your current partner: how many partners back? What should they be told? How might they have gotten or passed on the STI? Once treated, what extra precautions do you need to take with partners in the future? Do your parents need to be informed? If so, how do you want to do that with your healthcare provider? What might you need to tell any new partners *before* being sexual with them?

TECH TIP

You can use online tools or mobile applications to notify partners about an STI if doing so in person is impossible, difficult, or just something that adds more stress to an already stressful situation, like having to talk to an ex when a breakup went horribly or when an ex-partner was abusive. Those tools—like inSPOT or dontspreadit, to name a couple—allow you to notify partners anonymously about an STI they may have been exposed to through you or may have already had and passed on to you. Notifying partners is something where just making sure people know is what matters; how you tell them (presuming you're not being abusive or cruel in any way) isn't what matters here. So, if an online tool or mobile app is what feels like the best way or the only way you feel comfortable disclosing an STI, by all means, do it that way.

Our society has often made STIs sound like the worst thing in the world to get. STI panic and stigma are caused by a lot of different cultural ideas and situations: some STIs are or have been transmitted by infidelity; sex and the genitals are considered shameful or sinful in certain traditions or communities; and, more than anything, most people aren't well informed about STIs—they believe that most STIs are far worse than they actually are, or they believe that only "dirty" people or people of low moral character contract sexually transmitted diseases or infections.

Part of dealing with life with an STI involves dealing with those attitudes, which is unfortunate and sometimes difficult. The best approach to take is to furnish anyone putting that sort of thing on you with the real facts, with accurate, up-to-date information. And if that doesn't change their tune, then remind yourself that those messages and attitudes are coming from ignorance and have little or nothing to do with you personally at all.

How to Make Disclosing an STI Easier

▶ Remember that, despite how some people or cultures treat STIs, transmitting or acquiring an STI really isn't that different from transmitting or acquiring a cold or the flu. Just like with those kinds of illnesses, transmission usually happens because people didn't know they had an illness, because they didn't know how to properly prevent the illness from spreading (or didn't feel able to ask for prevention behaviors), or because prevention behaviors just didn't work. Try not to get caught up in shame or blame—it only makes everyone feel worse and makes disclosing or talking about an STI harder on everyone. This is just about sharing health information, not some kind of moral indictment.

▶ No one wants to be sick, and people don't tend to want to make other people sick either. Talking about STIs also usually means talking about sex and drums up a ton of fears, including those many people have as a result of ignorance. Anyone involved in the exchange of an STI may also be angry or upset, especially if an STI appears to have been—or by all means was—the result of any kind of intentional dishonesty, like having sex with others outside an exclusive relationship or someone saying they'd been tested when they hadn't been. Do your best, whatever "side" of this conversation you're on, to take the high road. This is so loaded and, thus, so potentially volatile. Do your best to talk about it with the kind of care and sensitivity we give other loaded disclosures, like disclosing sexual abuse or assault or talking about something we did that we feel very ashamed of. Use conflict resolution skills (see page 169), and keep your cool.

▶ Just like with a breakup, however you *can* give the information to someone else is the way to do it. If you don't feel able to disclose in person or over the phone, although things like e-mail and text messaging are certainly a bit less sensitive ways to share, if they make the difference between telling someone and not telling them—not telling them leaves their health at risk—these tech methods sure beat the alternative of not telling at all.

▶ If you're the one being told, remember that the person telling you probably feels very scared, very ashamed (even though they likely have no reason to be), and very vulnerable, but they're most likely telling you anyway out of care, concern, and respect for you and in the interest of doing what they can to protect your health. It's not fun or easy to hear someone tell us we might have contracted an STI from them or been the person to initially transmit the infection to them—but it's a lot harder to say than hear. Do your best to be a sensitive, kind listener and to thank the person telling you. They're doing you a solid, in a potentially big way.

Breaking the News

Telling current and recent partners, which needs be done when you discover you have contracted an STI, is rarely easy. If you care deeply about your partners, you may be upset with yourself for potentially getting them sick. If you've been in a relationship for a while and develop an STI, you may have to battle trust issues: Did your partner cheat? Did you? Was someone dishonest about their sexual history or about testing? If so, what now? If they deny it, can you fully believe them and get past your doubt?

With partners you've had for a while, the best bet is to be honest and to supply as much complete information about the STI as you can. Give yourselves plenty of time to talk, to process, to deal with emotional and physical consequences. Either or all of you may find that sex isn't all that appealing after a diagnosis or that it's difficult to connect sexually for a little while. All of those things are normal. If you need help dealing with them, you can ask your healthcare provider for resources or referrals.

It's hopefully obvious, but if you're diagnosed with an STI, it's something you should tell someone about before you're sexual with them in ways that can transmit that STI. Part of informed consent is telling people considerations—especially when they involve big risks—that you know about but that they won't unless you tell them. Otherwise, you make their choices for them, and that's no kind of consent at all. If they do want to go ahead and have sex with you, knowing about increased STI risks, you'll just decide together what you want to do to reduce those risks.

If you acquired an STI from a partner you don't know very well or haven't been involved with that long, telling them can be especially awkward. Sometimes, even tracking them down can be problematic, so just do what you can. If this was a very casual sex situation, you may feel angry at yourself, especially if the sex was unprotected, or if you chose to have sex when your judgment was impaired in any way.

It's important to recognize that an STI is no more a divine punishment for having sex than a runny nose is a punishment from G-d-on-high for going outside in the winter. **STIs are just natural consequences of being in close, intimate contact with other people, like any other kind of human infection.** They happen to all kinds of people, in all sorts of situations: married, single, monogamous, nonmonogamous, young, old, rich, poor, straight, queer—the works.

If you chose not to take preventative measures, then you made a mistake. We all will make mistakes sometimes. Beating yourself up over it doesn't make you well again. It's nonproductive and isn't likely to help you do what you need to, which is to stay well and simply make better choices for yourself next time. If you're angry at yourself, go ahead and entertain that for a bit, but be sure to take care of the practical things you need to do, however awkward, and then put your energy into forgiving yourself, managing the consequences, and moving on, smarter and safer.

Continuing sexual partnership can be a hurdle when you have an STI. With something temporary and treatable, like chlamydia or BV, it's pretty easy in the long run, because it'll be gone completely before too long. Other infections and diseases that are not fully curable and that might or will stick around—such as herpes, HPV, and HIV—are more of a challenge because you need to inform every new partner about the infection before you become sexually active with them, and you may need to take extra precautions you aren't accustomed to and may even have to radically change how you live your daily life.

You may even find that some potential partners won't want to have sex with you once they learn about the risk. That's their right, and logically you can probably understand it, but rejection, however sound or fair, still hurts. Fear of that rejection may keep you from being upfront, but it's a whole lot easier to deal with that rejection than it is to deal with a person who contracted an STI from you, when you *knew* you were putting them at risk for it and didn't inform them. Living with rejection is easier than living with yourself for doing that (see page 140).

Long-Term Dealing

Despite the prevalence of STIs, there aren't simple road maps for dealing with one. For the most part, it's very individual and involves some trial and error. But informed, honest communication can really serve you, and those involved with you, well. Taking care of yourself—physically and emotionally, presently and preventatively—is key. Seeking out and finding the emotional support you need, via friends, partners, family, or support groups for STI sufferers, is incredibly important, especially if you have an STI like HIV or hepatitis that may make you severely ill, present ongoing health issues, or involve long-term treatment.

TOP TEN BITS OF B.S. ABOUT STIS

1. "Virgins" can't transmit or contract STIs.
2. Only vaginal intercourse is risky.
3. Most infections will clear up on their own.
4. Only people with more than one partner can get an STI.
5. HIV is the most common STI.
6. Only semen can transmit STIs.
7. You can always tell when you or someone else has an STI.
8. Lesbians don't pass on or get STIs.
9. STIs are most prevalent in gay men or men with male partners.
10. If you love and trust your partner, it's safe to have unprotected sex.

If you have more than one STI at a time—which is common enough, especially as any one STI often makes the acquisition of others more likely—make sure your healthcare provider is working closely with you to be sure you're getting treated properly for all of your infections and doing what you need to do to deal with the ways in which any one might make another you have more dangerous for you.

Remember that you aren't anything close to alone: again, over nineteen million people each year develop an STI, and more young people contract STIs than people of other ages.

Whether we like it or not, or accept it or not, STIs are common, normal, and prevalent, just like lots of other kinds of illness and injury. They aren't any better or worse for being sexually transmitted, and *you* aren't any better or worse a person for having an STI.

11

Harm's Way: Abuse and Assault (and What You Can Do About Them)

I hope you have never been, and won't ever be, abused in any way. I also hope you have not chosen, and never choose, ever, to abuse anyone. We all deserve to be and should be physically and emotionally safe—safe in how others behave with us, and safe in how *we* behave with other people—in all of our interpersonal interactions and relationships.

But if abuse is or has been part of your life, please know that you aren't alone. We may all deserve to be safe in our relationships, but for many of us—myself included—that just hasn't always been or won't always be our reality.

More children and adolescents experience some form of abuse or assault than those who do not: over 50 percent of all children and adolescents have experienced some form of physical assault, relational aggression (bullying), or both. Almost 25 percent have been victims of physical bullying, and around 10 percent have been victims of assault with a weapon. Of fourteen- to seventeen-year-olds in the United States, almost *70 percent have been assaulted in some way,* with almost 30 percent being sexually assaulted, and just over 40 percent having been maltreated—abused or neglected by a parent, caregiver, or another person in a custodial role, like a teacher or a religious leader. (This information comes from "Violence, Crime, and Abuse Exposure in a National Sample of Children and Youth: An Update," by David Finkelhor et al., and was published in *Pediatrics* in 2013.) Abuse and assault are unfortunately very common, for people of all ages, but particularly for young people.

Abuse and assault of any kind are, at the very least, emotionally and psychologically dangerous and traumatizing while they are happening or we're in them, let alone the other ways they can be physically dangerous, even deadly. But even when we can survive any kind of abuse or assault and get away, we're still left hurting and with a lot of wounds, wounds that can be very challenging to heal and to go through our lives with.

Before we dig in, I want to make three big things oh-so crystal clear:

1. If you have been assaulted or abused or are being abused in any way now, it is not your fault. IT IS NOT YOUR FAULT. (Got it? **Not. Your. Fault.**) Abuse and assault are things someone *intentionally* chooses to do to someone else, not accidents, misunderstandings, or something that just "happens" without the person or people doing it making it happen. We can't be assaulted and abused if someone isn't assaulting or abusing us. Just like a robbery doesn't happen because someone has something to steal but because someone else *chooses* to steal from that person; a cake gets baked not because all the ingredients were just sitting around but only because someone made a cake with them—the same goes here: abuse and assault happen because someone chooses to abuse someone else, and when no one chooses to do those things, they don't *just happen*. No one ever "earns" or deserves abuse or "gets themselves abused." The person whose fault abuse is is the person or people who choose to abuse, not who they choose to victimize.

2. If you have been abused or assaulted or are in abuse now, you *can* get away from it so that it stops for you, even if the person doing the abuse or assault won't stop (and they most often won't). You can get help to get to safety, to stay safe, and to make it as likely as possible that abuse won't happen any more in your life. However hurt you are or have been by it, you can heal in time and live a life of quality with healthy relationships in which you are safe. No abuse or assault ever "ruins" people or makes it so that all we can ever have in our lives is abuse. **We are hurt and wounded by abuse, by all means, but we are not forever broken or ruined**. Just like we can break a bone and do things so that it heals, we can heal and again feel whole after any kind of abuse.

3. All of us can do things to prevent or help prevent or stop abuse and assault. What's most helpful—and much easier—is what we tend to hear the least about. What's most helpful and most effective isn't about what anyone can do to get away from abuse or keep themselves from being abused—it's about what everyone can do to stop abuse from happening in the first place by not abusing anyone and by refusing to enable abuse or be passive bystanders to abuse or things that enable abuse. We all can, and should, make a choice and a strong commitment not to abuse or enable abuse and to intervene with abuse or danger when we can, rather than being passive bystanders, especially when we aren't the ones most vulnerable to it or in danger ourselves. **That** is what best prevents or stops abuse.

Healthy, beneficial, and consensual sex and relationships are democracies, not dictatorships. Everyone involved always gets an equal vote and an equal voice. When anyone is refused that kind of equality and instead someone in a relationship or interaction is seeking power and control over another person, that is abuse. If someone intentionally doesn't treat someone else with respect and at least basic care and regard for their physical, emotional, and sexual well-being, the relationship is not healthy, beneficial, or consensual anymore, it is abuse. Abuse, reduced to its most simple definition, is about power and control and someone wanting and trying to get more than their share of both; someone who's abusing someone else doesn't want interpersonal equality or to share power and control: they want power and control all for themselves. Someone being abusive is robbing another person of security, safety, and joint ownership of and active participation in their relationship and full ownership of their own heart, mind, body, or life.

[THE UGLY TRUTH: STATISTICS]

I mentioned some stats above. As awful as those are, there are more. As I said, abuse and assault are unfortunately very common, for people of all ages, and particularly for young people:

▶ One in three adolescents in the United States is a victim of physical, sexual, emotional, or verbal abuse from a dating partner, and that figure is much higher than rates of all other types of violence for adolescents.

▶ A 2013 CDC survey found approximately 10 percent of high school students reported physical victimization and 10 percent reported sexual victimization from a dating partner in the twelve months before they were surveyed.

▶ Another CDC survey from 2011 found that 23 percent of women and 14 percent of men who ever experienced rape, physical violence, or stalking by an intimate partner first experienced some form of partner violence between eleven and seventeen years of age.

A lot of people think about sexual abuse, specifically, as being only something that happens with or is most commonly forced receptive intercourse, but a 2010 survey found that approximately one in twenty women and men have experienced sexual violence other than forced receptive intercourse, such as being made to penetrate someone else, sexual coercion, unwanted sexual contact, or noncontact unwanted sexual experiences, in the last twelve months (*National Intimate Partner and Sexual Violence Survey [NISVS]: 2010 Summary Report*). Those kinds of sexual abuse are as potentially dangerous and damaging as forced receptive intercourse, even though they're more often downplayed or denied by people.

More Vulnerable = More Vulnerable to Abuse

The more marginalized people are, the more vulnerable they are, including to some or all kinds of abuse, and the greater the rates of abuse in that population tend to be. For example:

▶ Transgender people are 1.7 times more likely to be the victims of sexual violence than cisgender people are (*2013 Report from the National Coalition of Anti-Violence Programs*)

▶ A survey of over seven thousand people with disabilities (*2012 National Survey on*

Abuse of People with Disabilities) found that more than 7 in 10 with disabilities have been abused: over half experienced physical abuse, around 40 percent reported sexual abuse, and nearly 90 percent indicated they were verbally or emotionally harmed. Fifty-seven percent indicated they had experienced mistreatment *more than twenty times* in their lives so far. And, of course, if the abuse is coming from a caregiver someone needs to do some of those most basic things in life, getting away from abuse is far harder than usual.

▶ Statistics from the US Bureau of Justice in 2001 show that African American women experience intimate partner violence at a whopping rate that is 35 percent higher than white women do.

[TYPES OF ABUSE]

From a literal standpoint, to abuse is to harm or injure. From a broader viewpoint, the most common categories of abuse are:

Emotional and/or verbal abuse: Behaviors that are used to emotionally control, dominate, manipulate, or intimidate a person. Emotional abuse can be threats, name-calling, belittling, criticizing, or using words or actions in an attempt to make another person feel stupid, small, ashamed, worthless, or like they're crazy. Other aspects of emotional abuse can include isolating a person by keeping them from friends or family; dismissing or refusing a person's limits and boundaries; intentionally withholding general

THE BIG PICTURE AND HOW MUCH IT REALLY, REALLY SUCKS

Sometimes abuse is taken seriously in our culture and our communities, but it's still very common for abuse to instead be denied, dismissed, or shrugged off as unimportant or "just the way things are." Victim blaming runs amok: all too often, a victim is held most—or even completely, in an epic display of how stupid and cruel people can be—responsible for rape or abuse instead of the person who chose to abuse them and did the abusing. Many forms of abuse are based on socially accepted or supported inequities between genders, ages, races, or social strata, like the idea that men are "supposed to" dominate or control women sexually and sex is something women are supposed to submit to, not be an equal part of. "Outcasts" or anyone generally seen or thought of as "other" are often viewed as somehow asking for abuse by not conforming to social norms. Some kinds of abuse or warning signs of abusive behavior—like possessiveness or cyberstalking—are even thought of and idealized as romantic!

When people say we are "living in a culture of abuse" or "living in a rape culture," this is what they mean: that we all live in an overall culture that supports and normalizes abuse, whether that's a little or a lot, no matter where on the planet we are. And when abuse is so prevalent, common, and both culturally supported and denied, it's not surprising that often a person who is abused may not even feel sure or know they've been or are being abused or know that it is never okay. ■■

care, approval, or support; constantly laying false blame on a partner (often for the things the person being abusive themselves is actually responsible for); attempting to control someone's appearance, like how they dress, or their physical freedom through threats or belittling; profound possessiveness; stalking or cyberstalking; or a pattern of harming someone and then begging for their forgiveness or their sympathy, or shifting the blame for abuse onto them. Emotional abuse is often thought to be the most benign form of abuse; however, it has the capacity to harm just as deeply as any other type of abuse, and for many people who have suffered a range of different abuses, emotional abuse can carry the deepest scars, especially if it occurred during childhood or adolescence.

Emotional abuse also can be the hardest kind of abuse to see and identify. Pair that with the fact that it's a kind of abuse most often strongly culturally enabled *and* denied and you can see how particularly sneaky and dangerous emotional abuse is, how easy it can be for people to get away with it, and how it can have a really big, harmful impact.

Physical abuse: Intentional bodily harm or injury. Hitting, slapping, punching, pushing, biting, kicking, choking, or burning someone purposefully are all examples of physical abuse. Throwing things at another person or physically restraining someone against their will is also physical abuse. Not everyone who is physically abused will have obvious injuries; you cannot always tell who is physically abused merely by looking, nor does a lack of scars, bruises, or broken bones mean that a person has not been physically abused.

Sexual assault and abuse: Forcing someone to engage in any sexual activity or response they do not want, have not actively and freely consented to, and/or are not in a position to be able to consent to (see page 192) is *rape* or *sexual assault.* Those two terms are mostly words for the same things. Sometimes *rape,* as a term, is used to describe only forced receptive intercourse, and *sexual assault* is used to mean other kinds of sexual violence; sometimes those terms are used interchangeably to mean all kinds of sexual violence. Sex that involves physical abuse is sexual assault. Forcing a person to view, create, or share sexual media (like pornography), to wear certain clothes for sexual purposes or go without the clothes they wish to, to look at the genitals of someone else against their will, or to watch certain sex acts (like masturbation) against their will can also be classed as sexual assault, as can name-calling or other forms of emotional, verbal, or physical abuse during sexual activity.

Force may be physical, verbal, or emotional, including coercion. When a person who sexually abuses or assaults someone is known to their victim, it is often called acquaintance, partner/spouse, or date rape. It is rape or sexual assault if a person consents to a sexual activity at one point and then later rescinds that consent—changes their mind and says no—and another person continues with sexual activity, dismissing or ignoring that person's limit. It is sexual assault *any* time one person does not want to be engaging in sex and someone else chooses to make them engage or be engaged in sex because it's what *they* want.

Sexual abuse or assault also occurs when someone engages in something sexual with a person unable to give meaningful consent, like someone who is in a position of considerably less power, who doesn't understand what they're being asked to be part of, who is asleep, who is intoxicated, or who is in serious distress of some kind.

Coercion: Coercion, when it is part of any kind of sexual activity, is a way of committing sexual abuse or assault—for example, arguing incessantly for or initiating a sexual activity so often that another person gives in because their will to disagree has been intentionally and effectively worn down. If someone pushes, pressures, argues, or in any other way manipulates someone else into doing what that person doesn't want to do, they've taken part in coercion. The other person has not meaningfully consented just because they finally gave in. Consent must be freely and gladly given to be meaningful.

Consensual activity, sexual or otherwise, **never** involves pushing or coercion or anyone being part of something they don't very much want to be part of. Consent is not "I really don't want to, but whatever, just do it" or "Oh, all right, already!" It also isn't saying yes after someone has refused your no's or not-right-nows until you just gave up. Consent is a **yes** when a no would be an equally acceptable and accept*ed* answer. For more on consent, see page 192.

If you want to do something someone else doesn't want to do or isn't sure about yet, all you need to do is to let them know that if they ever change their mind or want to do that thing but in a different way or situation, they can just let you know. Then you drop it. Asking again and again isn't okay—it's coercion. Don't argue or try to change their minds. Someone saying no to

DID YOU KNOW? . . .

Roofies, ketamine, GHB, or prescription drugs like sleep or antianxiety medications are drugs some people use to facilitate sexual assault, but alcohol, all by itself, is also a date rape drug, and it's the one most commonly used. It's way easier to get than something like GHB and can be just as effective at impairing people's judgment and mobility. Want an easy hard-and-fast rule to do what you can to keep yourself safe? Drink only with friends you are 300 percent sure are safe for you, take a pass on booze at big parties or clubs, and just keep it in moderation as a habit.

In the event where alcohol is concerned that the dangerous person could be you, check yourself about any drinking you're trying to pair with sex. Booze is not liquid courage. If that's what you think, *put the drink down,* step away from sex (and the drink, for that matter) for now, and start doing some work for and with yourself to become more at home in your sexuality, gain sexual confidence, and learn social skills that don't have any alcohol content. If you have established a pattern of any kind of alcohol abuse, including integrating it with your sex life, it's a good idea to seek help with substance abuse.

something in any way is a red light, and it's not okay to try to drive through it just like it isn't okay to drive through an actual red light. Ultimately, the only right answer when someone says "no," "not this way," "not today," or "not with you" is some version of "Okay, no problem."

Child abuse: Physical, sexual, verbal, or emotional abuse that occurs to a child or minor. Although teens and young adults are not children from a developmental standpoint, they are often legally considered so in instances of abuse when they are younger than the age of majority.

ABUSE: NOT SOMETHING ONLY MEN DO TO WOMEN

Although the overwhelming majority of people who abuse are men, **that does not mean that abusers are only men and victims are only women.** They're not. Abuse is something people of all genders can and do do: no gender or any other group of people is magically immune to abusing others. People of every gender can be and have been victims of abuse.

Because of this statistical gender divide it's also often assumed that abuse doesn't exist within queer relationships. Statistically, rates of domestic abuse in queer partnerships are equal to those in relationships between heterosexual people.

Invisibility when it comes to that reality can make finding support even more difficult for queer victims and survivors of abuse than for their straight counterparts. There are also challenges specific to or more prevalent for queer people within abusive relationships: social isolation may be greater, the abuse may not be believed, or it may be assumed that it must be "mutual." People who are not yet out may have to come out in the process of reporting abuse and getting help. Because queer communities are often very small, reporting abuse may mean that everyone in the community will know about the abuse and "take sides." For lesbians, as with heterosexual men who have been or are being abused by women, reporting abuse can be difficult because some women's organizations are unfortunately reluctant to acknowledge that women can be abusive. Queer people often have to face homophobia in the process of reporting and seeking help with abuse, and queer women, specifically, may also have to face sexism; for gay men and lesbians of color, racism as well.

Transgender people often have to deal with transphobia. If a queer person in abuse is marginalized in more ways than by just being queer—like being an ethnic or racial minority or poor—the challenges when it comes to seeking and finding help and support often get bigger and bigger.

If you're a victim or survivor of abuse that is less likely to be recognized or acknowledged (and that goes for within your family as well), please do *not* let that stop you from seeking help and/or reporting the abuse. Although it can certainly be extra-challenging to get help and support in these situations, it's always going to be better to deal with those challenges to get yourself safe and sound than to remain trapped in abuse. Check the Resources section of this book for organizations that help men who are being or have been abused or LGBTQA victims or survivors as well as anyone else in abuse.

Incest: Incest is sexual abuse within a family—like rape or fondling, voyeurism, sexual comments, forcing a family member to masturbate, and exploitation such as child sexual trafficking—usually by an adult who is a family member: parents or guardians, grandparents, uncles or aunts, but also siblings or extended family members. Incest is a particularly damaging form of abuse because it most often begins when victims are very young, it happens with the people and in the places (home) where a victim should be the most safe, and it is perpetrated by people often responsible for the care of a victim and in whom victims and other family members have placed the most trust. It is also a kind of abuse that is most often very deeply denied in families where it is occurring or has occurred.

Sexual harassment: Sexual harassment can be sexual and emotional and verbal abuse. *Bullying* is another word for harassment, and it is frequently sexual in nature. Sexual harassment is uninvited and unwanted sexual behavior, like being touched when you don't want to be, being the target of sexual name-calling or jokes, slut shaming or gay bashing, or continued sexual propositions or sexual attention after you've already said no. Sexual harassment is incredibly prevalent online and in schools and sometimes even comes from school staff, not just fellow students. *Street harassment* is a term used to describe behavior like catcalling or eve teasing, where passersby sexually harass someone who is just walking down the street.

Hate crimes: Hate crimes are physical, verbal, emotional, or sexual abuse based on and motivated by intolerance of or bias toward people of a given group, like those of a certain sexual orientation, race, gender, nationality, religion, age, or disability. Violence that specifically targets queer or gender-nonconforming people is one kind of hate crime. Given the frequently gendered nature of sexual abuse and assault, it's also sound sometimes to talk or think about rape as a hate crime.

Domestic, partner, or dating abuse: Emotional, verbal, physical, and/or sexual abuse that occurs within a family or between sexual or romantic partners, spouses, or people who live together. The abuse may also include threats or injury to property, pets, children, or other family members. *Battering* is a term sometimes used to describe domestic emotional abuse.

Cyberstalking and other technology abuse: Using technology to stalk (like by putting GPS on their phone without someone's knowledge or permission or stalking someone's social media sites), harass (like by texting someone over and over to gain control over their time and lives), bully, and otherwise endanger someone or violate their safety or privacy (like doxxing—publishing private information about someone publicly with malicious intent—or revenge porn, publicly posting private images of someone to intentionally hurt them) are all forms of technology abuse.

A 2014 study by the National Network to End Domestic Violence (NNEDV) found that nearly 90 percent of victim services agencies reported that survivors came to them for help after abusers intimidated and made threats via cell phone, text messages, and e-mail, and 75 percent of programs noted that abusers accessed victims' accounts (e-mail, social media, etc.) without the victim's consent and often without their knowledge. Seventy-two percent of agencies reported a survivor's location being tracked by smartphones or other devices; more than half of the programs reported that survivors said that people abuse spoof caller ID

ABUSE DOES ALL THIS

Beyond physical injuries (like a broken arm) and other physical health issues (like insomnia, an STI, or a pregnancy) that people sustain or develop from or because of physical or sexual abuse, abuse is also associated with many common psychological, cognitive, and social impacts, such as the following:

- Low self-esteem and feelings of worthlessness
- Suicidal thoughts or behaviors, depression, phobias, or anxiety
- Self-harming behaviors, like eating disorders or cutting
- Self-doubt, including questioning even the reality of the abuse ("Did that really happen to me, or did I make it up?")
- Addiction or substance abuse
- Inability to set healthy boundaries and other difficulties in maintaining or creating healthy relationships
- Feelings of isolation
- Difficulty concentrating or staying motivated with goals and dreams
- Dissociation (experiences of severe detachment from oneself)
- Fear of intimacy
- Loss of trust and difficulty building trust
- Shame and guilt
- Fearfulness
- Difficulty feeling or expressing a full range of emotions or doing so in healthy ways

Abuse also often results in PTSD (post-traumatic stress disorder). PTSD is a mental health condition triggered by experiencing or witnessing something traumatic. PTSD can create a pretty wide a range of symptoms. Recurring flashbacks or dreams of the abuse that just won't let up or getting "triggered" by things that remind someone of the abuse and having severe and often debilitating emotional reactions is one common way PTSD manifests. It can also create avoidance, dissociation, or feelings of emotional numbness, memory problems, feelings of anger, guilt, shame, or hopelessness that just feel totally unmanageable. Sometimes, someone develops PTSD right after abuse or assault; others develop PTSD months or even many years later.

Victims' advocates and counselors for any kind of abuse can help with PTSD, and it is best to get help when it's within reach. General healthcare providers can sometimes play a part in helping, too, including with temporary medications like a sleep or antianxiety medication to help a person cope with PTSD and some of the impacts it can have. PTSD is a lot to manage on your own and awfully hard to find your way through without help from someone who knows how to help with it.

(manipulate caller ID so that it appears as though someone other than the abusive person is calling); and nearly 70 percent of programs report that abusers post pictures or videos of victims online for the purpose of distressing or harming the victim.

Although it is ultimately up to the person who attempts or does the abusing whether abuse or assault happens, we can do some basic things to protect ourselves and have a better chance of keeping ourselves safe. Self-defense classes are very helpful for learning physical and other protections and responses, and they're also great self-confidence boosters. When we feel safer and more able to protect ourselves, as learning self-defense often results in, we tend to carry ourselves differently and respond in subtle ways that can give harmful people the message that we are *not* who they want to mess with.

We can do our best to limit our vulnerability with people we're not totally sure about yet, like by building trust over time, being more vulnerable with them only when they've given us plenty of evidence they're safe, and being alone-alone with people only selectively. This can include creating a good buddy system with friends or family so that we have someone else keeping an eye out for us who is ready and willing to step in and up if we need help getting or staying safe.

Personal safety is *not* about things like not wearing a short skirt or not being sexual with people unless you're married—we know very well that things like that don't actually protect anyone and are, instead, usually just things people think or say based on ignorance or victim blaming. Personal safety isn't about limiting our freedom; it's about doing what we can to keep ourselves for-real safe from harm—including harmful people—so that we can enjoy it.

"But I Love Them"

Sometimes we want to deny, excuse, or write off abuse from people we are close to. We might tell ourselves that maybe they just like "rough sex." Or that maybe they were confused; forgot ways you're

THE LIE OF STRANGER DANGER

The most prevalent risk of abuse or assault isn't from strangers but is from people we know: friends and acquaintances, neighbors, family, boyfriends or girlfriends, and the partners of other friends.

As reported in a 2010 survey (the *National Intimate Partner and Sexual Violence Survey 2010 Summary Report*), for women who were rape victims, 51.1 percent of perpetrators were reported to be intimate partners, 12.5 percent were family members, and 40.8 percent were acquaintances. Only 13.8 percent were strangers. Among men who were victims of forced receptive intercourse, the statistics are similar: 52.4 percent of perpetrators were reported to be acquaintances, and only 15.1 percent were strangers. Among men who were made to penetrate someone else, 44.8 percent of perpetrators were reported to be intimate partners, 44.7 percent were acquaintances, and only 8.2 percent were strangers.

insecure, vulnerable, or just plain human; or just don't understand that what they're doing is wrong because they're not smart enough to understand. Maybe you think you did something wrong to "make" them act that way. It's common to feel (and to want to think) that being raped by a person close to you—like a boyfriend or girlfriend—isn't "real" rape. There are plenty of ways you can try to deny or rationalize abuse from someone you care about; it is incredibly hard for anyone to swap the title of *boyfriend* or *girlfriend* with *rapist* or *attacker,* and we don't ever want to think that the people we have trusted the most have intentionally done us harm. It's just one of the most terrible truths in life there can be, and one of the hardest to accept.

It's typical for loyalties to feel divided when a friend, family member, or other person you know abuses or assaults you. It's typical for victims of abuse by people close to them, who are also probably close to others in their lives, not to report the abuse or to seek support or to even ever tell anyone else, because they don't want to hurt, divide, or lose those they love.

But the only sound way to deal with someone close to you who sexually abuses

DID YOU KNOW . . . ?

The Cycle of Abuse

There's a constant and ongoing pattern nearly all abusive relationships follow:

1. A **honeymoon** (or **seduction,** if you prefer) **stage,** which is a state when everyone involved appears to be or feels happy in the relationship and seems to be experiencing the relationship as loving and enjoyable.
2. The **tension phase,** when small arguments or conflicts start, and someone who is abusive starts feeling frustrated or unhappy with their partner and may also start up with smaller attempts to control them.
3. The last stage is the **abuse stage** (or **explosion stage**), where one specific incident or the piling up of all those little tensions leads to an explosion of anger through one or more kinds of abuse: emotional, verbal, sexual, or physical.
4. The abusive person then usually reverts to the honeymoon stage to try to "make up for" their behavior and to keep the other person around and in their control, and the whole cycle begins again. How long each of those stages lasts and how frequently people go through them vary a lot, but that basic pattern is nearly universal.

So, "being really sweet sometimes" or someone not always engaging in explosions of abuse doesn't mean abuse isn't happening. In fact, in an abusive relationship, that "being sweet" is rarely about actual sweetness but instead is about how someone has learned they have to behave so the other person doesn't leave and so they can keep the person under control. It's an act, basically. When "being sweet" is what happens before and after abuse, it's not sweet at all: it's another part of the cycle of abuse, a part that is unfortunately very effective at keeping someone being abused from leaving.

or assaults you is just as you would deal with any other type of abuse: tell someone the truth, get help, and do what you can to get away and stay away from that person and the relationship. You know they're not safe: they showed you that very clearly when they abused you.

Survivors of partner sexual assault, specifically, are statistically more likely to be assaulted or abused multiple times than are stranger and acquaintance rape survivors, and partner rape survivors are more likely to suffer severe and long-lasting physical and psychological injuries. That's not surprising because abuse or assault from people we know and are close to is a huge betrayal of our trust and can really shake up our worldview in some tough and terrible ways. Like any other kind of person who engages in abuse, a partner, friend, or family member who sexually assaults or abuses is also not likely to stop, no matter how you behave or how much you love them. Like any other kind of person who engages in abuse, this is about *their* behavior and *their* lack of love for you, not the other way around.

Taking the Blinders Off: Identifying and Coping with Interpersonal Violence and Abuse

When sexual or romantic relationships or sexual activity are new in our lives, it all usually feels risky to some degree, even if you feel ready and very much want to be part of that. It can be tougher to know when those feelings are happening when things are okay and when they're happening because we are in danger. If any kind of abuse or control feels normal—if you've grown up with or around it, it often does feel normal because it's *been* your normal—or inevitable or is something you've gotten the idea is romantic or a demonstration of love or passion, it can be awfully hard to see coming or recognize when you're all the way in it. Growing up in abuse often teaches us to dismiss our own feelings of fear and our sense of danger, making it harder to access our intuition and to trust it.

The feeling of being in danger or of being harmed is never a good one, but it's a lot harder to live with the idea that we can be at the highest risk of harm from the people we may trust the most. It can also be really confusing: whether abuse is coming from family members, someone we're dating, or friends, it's tough to wrap our brains around how we can love someone who is abusing us. But we can, and in fact, the very fact that so many people do love the people who abuse them is something that is easy to get trapped in.

Maybe you have no doubt that what you're dealing with or have lived through is or was abuse. Maybe you're not sure. For many people who have been or are being abused, it can become difficult to know, especially because many aspects of abuse are manipulative, unexpected, or even considered to be normal behavior; because our experiences or people who abuse us may not resemble what we've been told about abuse or assault; or because we're just in denial.

But some things can tip you off to potentially abusive patterns or abuse that's already happened or is happening.

Are You in a Relationship or Partnership That May Be Emotionally Unsafe or Unhealthy for You or Others?

Give yourself a checkup. Are you:

▶ Suffering from anxiety, stress, depression, or low self-esteem or having ongoing physical symptoms like stomachaches, insomnia, changes in energy levels or appetite, a sudden drastic increase or decrease in sexual desire, or other physical symptoms that are not caused by an existing condition, illness, or outside situation?

▶ Putting other important relationships or goals of yours at risk or aside because of your relationship when you really don't want to?

▶ Taking chances for that relationship that put you in a position of sexual, physical, or emotional risk (not the positive kind), or feeling like you must make sacrifices to have or maintain the relationship?

▶ Feeling isolated from everyone or everything *but* your partner and your relationship with them, or having trouble thinking of others or your life outside yourself and your partner's?

▶ Discovering that other important parts of your life you care about are taking a backseat to your relationship or are really suffering (your grades, your job, your friends, etc.)?

▶ Feeling scared, anxious, sad, frustrated, or upset about or with sexual relationships or encounters, far more than you find yourself feeling happy, excited, and comfortable?

▶ Feeling you must keep sexual activity, tension, or emotional issues high and intense to maintain the relationship, using sexual activity or other behavior to avoid or defuse relationship conflicts, "zoning out" during sexual activity, or feeling like you have to be predominantly passive or dominating during sex with your partner?

▶ Becoming unable to be autonomous and have a life and sense of self independent of your partner or a sexual relationship?

▶ Feeling bad about yourself in general or specifically in regard to your sexual relationship or behavior?

▶ Doing things you really don't want to do but feel you have to, or pressing a partner to do so?

▶ Having trouble discussing, making, or enforcing limits and boundaries (sexual or otherwise), or respecting those of your partner?

▶ Feeling followed or highly monitored or controlled in person, online, or through other tech tools, like your mobile phone, or following or highly monitoring or controlling someone else in any of these ways?

▶ Making a lot of excuses for yourself or a partner?

If you're experiencing any of these things, abuse may be or is why.

It's *Already* Really Bad

Don't wait until it gets "really bad" or until you're as sure as sure can be that abuse is happening or on the horizon to do what you can to help yourself. If there's a "might be" in your head or a "sure is" when it comes to abuse, talk to someone. If you're saying you'll wait until it gets *really* bad, it's clearly bad already: talk to someone now, not when it's even more dangerous for you and you're even more unsafe than you already are.

Find someone who isn't abusive and who's also trustworthy, wise, and outside your partnership to talk to: someone you feel is objective and also cares a lot about you, like a parent, friend, or sibling; a community leader or teacher; a healthcare provider or counselor. Be honest and real, even if you feel ashamed (and although you have no reason to be, those feelings are common). Ask for help, whether that is their feedback and emotional support, help getting away or staying away, help getting physical or mental health care, help getting information, or all of those things and more.

Sometimes concerns about being a burden can keep a person from asking for help or talking to someone they trust. But as any of us who care deeply about anyone know, someone we care about asking us for help and support when they need it, help and support that gets them out of danger and makes it most likely they'll be able to be safe and healthy is usually something we *want* to be asked for. We don't want someone we care about to suffer, and we want to do what we can to stop that suffering. It's okay to ask people who love you to help you carry your burdens; when they can, they will usually want to.

If you don't have any sense or worry it will compromise your safety, you can talk to the person you're in this relationship with, as well. If you suspect or know you *can't* do that without risking your emotional or physical safety, then there's no question you're in something unhealthy or abusive, and it's safest to figure that talking about abuse to someone abusing you without any kind of mediator and by yourself just isn't a good idea. In that case, stick with your other helpers and supports.

If it does feel safe for you and you want to talk to this person, you can voice your concerns. Point out what things on that list up there have been going on and make clear they need to stop or change. Things like those listed may be a signal that your sexual relationship or behavior isn't healthy and balanced, may be doing you or a partner harm now, or may be part of a relationship that could easily become abusive if it isn't already.

To identify and step away from abuse:

▶ **Listen.** Sometimes, it can be difficult to accept that a parent is really concerned, not just overprotective or too rigid, or that a friend is earnestly worried about your safety, not jealous that you have a boyfriend or girlfriend and they don't. Often, when the people who care about you most, and know you best, voice concerns, it's for good reason. And if and when everyone around you is voicing the same or similar concerns, they're probably right to be concerned. Listen to what the people who care about you have to say. As always, trust your own instincts, and in cases of abuse, give your head more clout than your heart. Because all abuse includes emotional factors and confusing someone emotionally is one of the biggest parts of abuse, it's typical for people's emotions to be confused and convoluted when they've been abused.

▶ **Tell.** If no one else notices what is going on—with so much abuse so normalized in our world, and so many people bystanding rather than stepping in, that's not unusual—you can tell what's going on and ask for help. Keep your eyes peeled for good opportunities. For example, a speaker who comes to your school to talk about teen relationship abuse could be a great person to tell. Speak to someone you know you can trust: friends or your friend's parent, immediate or extended family, a teacher, a coach, a school counselor, or a neighbor. Talk to someone who has said something that makes it clear they have survived abuse or are strongly opposed to it. You can also call a hotline or a community service for victims of abuse; your local phone book will have listings, or you can use a search engine: put in your zip code and a keyword phrase like "abuse help" or "crisis center." There are Internet communities where you can post, chat, or get other kinds of help anonymously. You can also go directly to local community centers, shelters, police stations, or social service agencies. It can feel very scary to tell, especially if any of your abuse or assault has involved threats to you or those you care about if you do. But telling is also usually the first step we have to take to do what we can to make abuse stop, and it is also the first step that can move you away from danger so that silence doesn't keep you trapped.

▶ **Leave.** Once you get some help, you can make a safety plan to start taking action. That may include making sure you have other people around to help keep you safe when you leave the relationship; making places where you may see your partner, like your school, safe for you; filing charges or requesting a restraining order

To Report or Not to Report, That's the Question

Whether to report any crime done to you to the justice system—to the police—should be (and usually is) up to you and mostly about you, your safety, and what you feel you need to be safe, supported, and helped. If you're a minor, sometimes crimes are reported when you don't want them to be as part of mandatory reporting laws. But more times than not, reporting or pressing charges is up to you when one or both are options. Reporting, and related things, like getting orders of protection, or pressing charges often help you get or stay safe. They also can help others stay away from the dangers of the person or people who harmed you. But however much it might benefit others for someone who has been victimized to take legal action of some kind, the person who has been hurt and harmed is the person who needs to matter most. Going through any of the justice system as a victim is rarely easy, especially with dating, domestic, or sexual violence or when the victim is in any way marginalized, and sometimes it is outright terrible and traumatizing on its own. So, it's got to be something you want to do, something you feel strong enough to do, and something that feels like it helps you, not just other people. There's no right or wrong choices with reporting: there's just whatever you feel as sure as you can is the best choice for you. This choice should be about you, most of all. (For more on this, see page 337.)

against someone; and getting yourself the emotional support you need via friends and family, counseling, or support groups. With any sort of abuse, it's easy to get stuck in a pattern of feeling at fault when your partner is abusive or angry and taking to heart what they say. But every now and then there may be moments where your head says, "Bullshit," or "Wrong!" to an abusive partner. Use the strength those moments of awareness can give you and make those moments the ones to get out and get away. Leaving abuse of any kind can be precarious and create dangers, particularly if the abusive person is physically violent, so unless you just find a window of opportunity out of the blue, one that you know is as safe as it gets, you're going to need a solid plan to ensure that leaving makes you safer rather than puts you in greater danger. Sexual abuse and assault, domestic and dating violence, and other crisis care organizations can help you make a safety plan that will help you leave safely.

You may have doubts throughout this process, miss the person who was abusing you, or try to convince yourself that what happened wasn't really abuse or that you asked for or deserved it in some way. There's often a lot of one-step-forward, two-steps-back stuff in dealing with abuse. You may have a confusing range of emotions, from anger to apathy, sorrow to relief. Do your best to honor and explore all of those emotions and seek outside help and support. Support groups specifically for abuse survivors can be especially helpful, because the people in them know exactly what you're going through. Healing from abuse is often a long process, and abuse leaves traces all over your psyche that you have to learn to navigate. The help and support of those who have been there is often priceless.

Some people are reluctant to seek therapy, counseling, or support groups for abuse (or assault) because they aren't ready to really face up to having been abused, don't want to talk to people they don't yet know well, don't want to share what seems very private to them with someone else, or don't want to deal with the stigma still attached to therapy and counseling. You might also be concerned that a therapist or counselor is going to blame you for the abuse or tell you how to live your life or even bash a partner to whom you still feel loyal despite the abuse. Almost always, those are misplaced concerns. A good, qualified abuse counselor will never do those things. What they do is listen, ask questions to try to help you come to your own realizations and truths, and help you to make your own choices and do your own healing, at your own pace, rather than trying to do it for you or trying to force it. You also don't have to work with just any counselor, support group, or therapist; shop around and wait to start therapy until you find someone who feels best for you.

You might also be reluctant to enter therapy or counseling because it feels like a statement that there's something profoundly wrong with *you*. But therapy isn't about "fixing" people or about being "crazy." It's about having someone who is objective and fully present who listens to you, who has experience with and education and training about all the things

Exit plan

Those in abusive partnerships are often advised to have vital items at hand as part of an exit plan so that when they have an opportunity to leave they can do so quickly and efficiently, without having to leave behind birth records, clothing, pets, or other essentials. Because most young adults in abusive relationships do not live with their abusers, your preparation for leaving may be less extensive. Just be sure, if you're not yet ready or able to leave, that when you see your partner, you have the following items with you on your person at all times: your basic identification (such as a driver's license or state ID), your house or car keys, your cell phone or address book, any medications you take, and your debit card, credit card, checkbook, and/or cash. If you don't already have a taxi number or app on your mobile phone, put one on there. That way, if and as soon as the opportunity or necessity of getting out presents itself, you'll be ready and able to go immediately.

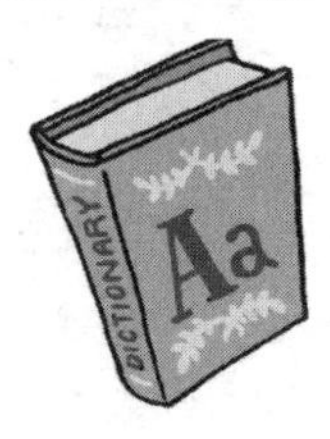

you're dealing with, and who knows and can share good tools for managing them and for getting stronger as a person so you can move forward. Common impacts of abuse or assault like depression, post-traumatic stress disorder (PTSD), anxiety and/or panic attacks, self-injury, low self-esteem, substance abuse, and a host of other disorders or issues also often create a need for additional support and qualified help (see box on page 318). The point of therapy isn't to fix you because you're broken but to help you deal with the impacts of someone else who is or was part of your life and who *tried* to break you. You're still here, seeking out help and care for yourself, no less, so we can know they didn't succeed. Qualified mental health care helps us start healing and moving forward toward a life of real quality, without abuse.

Breaking the Cycle

It's true that someone who is abusive is a troubled person. An abuse victim may feel that by remaining with or going back to the person who abuses them, they can fix that person or save them from themselves. You may feel that if you just love them enough or stick around long enough, the person who abuses you will miraculously get better and stop the abuse. **Unfortunately, that's just not true.**

No abusive person is helped by being enabled or allowed to continue abusing by being provided the opportunity to abuse. Thinking that is akin to saying that someone who has a problem with alcohol is best served by living in a bar or that someone with an eating disorder will get better if you just let them starve themselves to death. No one can love abuse away, and continuing to give someone opportunities to abuse doesn't help them, it only hurts everyone involved and ensures that abuse will continue and escalate.

Writer, artist, and all-around amazing person Lynda Barry said something pretty to-the-point once in an interview: "There are rotten people in the world that cannot be cured by magical hippy love. They will always be the way they are and if they are friends/romantic partners/parents/co-workers/dude who just cut you off in his Acura, GET AWAY FROM THEM! DO NOT LINGER! You cannot fix Dracula by trying to convince him to just party in the sun with you. This is what I wish I knew earlier. Bad people, jerks, sociopaths, and narcissists are always among us. Do not try and help them with your loyal love. RUN! NOW! GO!"

We can't fix people's issues for them, and if we're doing anything to give them opportunities to harm us because they can't or don't want to work on those issues themselves, not only are we doing the opposite of helping them but we're also risking our own well-being and sometimes even our lives. If and when someone abusive does want to change and seeks the right kind of help to do that, one of the very first things they'll usually be told is that they can't change if they are still involved in anything where there's an established pattern of abuse; so, they first need to get and keep themselves away from anyone they have been abusing or have abused. If we stick around, not only will they likely get worse instead of better but we also don't give them any reason to have to try to change.

It really is best for *everyone* involved—especially anyone in danger—to get away from abuse and stay away. Doing that isn't about not loving anyone or abandoning them; it's about holding a line for everyone that says safety is utmost, which it always is for love. We can't fix people's problems for them, but we can do things that help them to help themselves if they're going to make positive changes. Not allowing anyone the opportunity to abuse us anymore is one of those things that helps someone who wants to change help themselves, and it happens to be what moves us out of danger as well.

Study after study has shown very clearly that until the *cycle of abuse* is broken, a person who abuses will continue to do so. The cycle is most often stopped when a victim leaves the abuser or when the abuser is imprisoned, or, more rarely, when an abuser is given long-term anger management classes or therapy.

Someone who abuses someone else isn't the victim; the person being abused is, and that's whose needs must always come first, because that is the person in the most acute danger and in the most need of help. If you've been abused, it is *not your* responsibility to get help for the person who abuses you—it's their responsibility to get help for themselves. It's your responsibility to do what you can to get yourself to safety and away from abuse.

Fair or not, the only person in an abusive relationship who usually can and does effectively interrupt the cycle of abuse is the person being victimized, and they do that by getting and staying away from the person or people abusing them.

Check Yourself: Does This Ever Sound Like You?

- Do you feel the need to control people around you, especially those close to you?
- Does letting others take the wheel or share power, control, or decisions make you feel very uncomfortable, angry, afraid, or insecure?
- Do you betray the trust of others by sharing very private information or secrets or by emotionally blackmailing in some way?

- Do you find it hard to be patient with or empathetic to the troubles of others?
- Do you have a hard time handling variance in opinion? When someone thinks something different from what you think, do you belittle, dismiss, or attack them?
- Are you prone to making fun of or teasing people?
- Do you often feel very jealous or possessive?
- Do you feel your partners must be cheating, lying, or betraying your trust? Do you accuse them?
- Do you use technology to keep an eye on your partner or to keep them responding to you?
- Have you ever hit or pushed a partner? Have you grabbed their arm or held them tight while you were arguing? Are you prone to do or want to do things like that when you're angry or frustrated rather than talking or walking away?
- Do you ever throw things, slam doors, or threaten your partner when you're angry? Do you feel unable to manage your anger in any way?
- Have you ever forced or coerced a partner into having sex with you or made it difficult for them to say no? Do you ever do this now?
- Do you ever call people you're close to names that hurt them or use your words to make someone feel insecure, small, or worthless? Do you ever say negative things you know have a big emotional impact on a partner because they're a way to make your partner feel vulnerable or unsure?
- Have you ever threatened to harm yourself, your partner, or those he or she cares for if your partner leaves you or breaks up with you?

If any of that looks familiar to you, I need to tell you that *you* are or may already be engaging in abuse or other unhealthy and unsafe interpersonal behavior.

Even if you were reared in an abusive environment yourself and some abusive behaviors seem normal to you, or even if you've started to exhibit abusive behaviors, you are *not* obliged to become or stay abusive: you *can* head it off at the pass or change how you're behaving now and for the future. If you're concerned about being abusive now or in the future, do all you can to get away and stay away from anyone you have abused or are abusing—rather than leaving it to them to do the harder work of getting away from you—and seek out counseling and support **now.** Learning different patterns of behavior isn't easy, but it is doable when you really commit to it and get the right kind of help. The earlier in life someone does that work, the more likely they are to grow into healthy people who don't abuse others or who can stop doing it. You can ask your family doctor or a school guidance counselor to point you toward help and resources.

Even if you've never exhibited abusive behaviors but are just concerned you might, perhaps because you grew up around them yourself, you can ask for help and seek support. There's absolutely no reason to feel ashamed about those concerns. If everyone were that concerned and aware, far fewer people would be abused.

PROTECTING YOURSELF FROM ABUSIVE PARTNERS AND RELATIONSHIPS

The hardest part of recognizing signals of an abusive relationship is that often people mistake the earliest signs of abuse for aspects of romantic love. Intense jealousy, possessiveness, and claims of ownership; defending your "honor" with bullying or verbal or physical intimidation; very traditional ideas about gender and the "place" of men and women or other groups; and extreme codependency or neediness are all strong indicators of a possibly abusive person, not someone in love in a healthy way.

Some other common early signs or symptoms can include a history of violence or a criminal record, existing violence within someone's family, abuse of or dependence on drugs or alcohol, a fascination with weapons or with acts of violence, or extreme mood swings. Someone moving very, very fast in a new relationship—like saying they love you and want to be with you forever when they only just learned your middle name last week, or insisting on sex or big commitment right from the front—is another common flag in abusive relationships.

A big part of being able to protect yourself is being aware not just of someone else's behavior or issues but also your own. Whereas people who are abused come from all walks of life, people who find themselves in abusive relationships often have some things in common: low self-esteem; emotional, social, or economic dependency; social isolation; depression; and stress or anxiety disorders. Many victims of abuse have been abused before or grew up with abuse. That's not about any of us being perennially unlucky or deserving it; it's about the fact that experiencing any abuse makes it seem more normal so that it can be harder to see or know when we're in it. It's also harder to know that it's *not* something we have to live with.

Many abuse victims falsely believe that abuse is something they deserve. They may blame themselves for the abuses they suffer; they may defend or excuse the person who is abusing them. So, in many ways, only entering relationships when you and your partner are both really able to handle them—when you already feel okay with yourself, when you feel 100 percent able to stand up for yourself and be independent, when you're not in a crisis, when you want to be with someone else rather than "have" someone else—is a big help when it comes to prevention. If you face issues like these, seeking help through friends, family, or counseling rather than in romantic or sexual relationships is also helpful.

Can't Happen to You?

The shame of being abused or staying with someone abusive can run very deep. It's sometimes hard to really see abuse coming, so it's not that uncommon to truly just wake up one day and suddenly realize you are in the thick of an abusive relationship without really knowing how on earth you wound up there. Some people also have it in their heads that abuse shouldn't be happening to them because they're too smart, too good, or too something to be "that" kind of person. But there is no "that" kind of person:

nothing makes any of us magically immune to abuse, just like nothing makes anyone deserving of abuse.

For others, accepting that their partner is anything other than a wonderful person who loves them is very hard. Some abused people feel that if they acknowledge or address abuse, they'll only be hurt even more, or they worry that their partner will be harmed. Plenty are convinced that, miraculously, their abusive partner will get better, possibly though their love.

Sadly, it's also not uncommon for friends or family to defend people who abuse or certain types of abuse, especially if they are survivors of abuse or abusers themselves and they perceive abuse to be normal or acceptable. Denial of abuse is very common, from many different perspectives.

Protecting Each Other from Abuse

People who abuse, sexually and otherwise, are very opportunistic: they tend to choose victims not by what they look like or how they're dressed but by who is available, who seems less resistant, who can be overpowered and harmed. Again, everything we know to date about rape confirms that, like all forms of abuse, it is about power and control of another person, first and foremost.

People who abuse also tend to choose people or situations where they feel someone else is unlikely to intervene. And that's pretty easy to do because so many people won't intervene, because they feel certain someone else will do something (which is usually what that someone else is also thinking), because they don't feel any sense of personal responsibility for their greater world, because they are afraid, whether it's valid or not, to behave differently from everyone else, or because of their own safety, even when it isn't actually at risk. Abusive people can unfortunately count on bystanders to be passive instead of intervening, and in that way, bystanders—whether they mean to or not—often help people to abuse.

▶ **DO:** What you can to dial *down* conflict. To successfully intervene, you usually have to be calmer than anyone involved, not just as or even more aggressive or agitated.

▶ **DON'T:** Escalate any kind of explosion, like by intervening in someone else's violence with your own—physical, verbal, or any other kind—or threatening violence.

▶ **DO:** Trust your own sense of danger or abuse. If you aren't certain something you're seeing isn't abuse or isn't a prelude to it, it probably is abuse. Rather than assuming something must not be, assume the opposite. It's not like asking someone if they're okay or distracting someone is going to do anyone harm; at worst, it'll be a momentary social gaffe that hurts nobody. At best, it can save someone's life or well-being.

It should go without saying that intervening isn't helpful if it just puts more people in danger or harms both the intended victim and anyone trying to help. If intervening in abuse makes it so you and the person being abused are *both* in danger, that doesn't help anyone. Trust your gut, and if you know or strongly suspect it isn't safe for you, yourself, to intervene, find someone to ask for help who can do it safely. That's still you intervening and doing what's probably the safest thing for everyone.

How Can Everyone Prevent Abuse or Assault in One Easy Step?

By not abusing or assaulting anyone. If no one abuses or assaults someone else, abuse and assault don't happen. So much of what we hear about preventing abuse is about people who are or may be victims doing things to try not to *be* abused. By all means, whatever any of us can do to protect ourselves is important and can help to keep abuse and assault from our lives or get us away from it. But that actually isn't preventing abuse because it's not something that prevents people who are abusive from abusing. People who would abuse or assault must not do either in the first place. Or they must stop and seek qualified help and intervention when they are. Just like sex isn't something that just happens but is something people choose to do, and the media don't exist outside of the people who make it, the same goes here. Abuse and assault aren't objects or things that exist outside of people or outside people's control: they are things people choose to do, and things people can choose not to do.

▶ **DON'T:** Just figure that because no one else seems to be doing anything that means nothing needs to be done or that you shouldn't do something. It's often precisely because everyone thinks that the abuse or assault that could have been prevented by intervention isn't.

▶ **DO:** Step in when someone is saying something that enables abuse. Don't let statements that blame victims, voice ignorance about what is or isn't abuse, or dismiss abuse stand. You can help change the social environment to send a message to people who are or may be abusive that it isn't okay—and that you know what abuse is, so they can't hide it from you easily. Shooting down false statements about abuse also gives anyone in an abusive situation or who might be at risk of it later an idea that you're someone they could ask for help. It also makes your own social circles places where abuse is less likely to happen or continue.

▶ **DON'T:** Let those statements stand or, worse still, laugh or otherwise reinforce them. Abuse isn't funny, nor are all the things—like *–isms* and other biases, violence of any kind, and control or interpersonal aggression—that create a perfect place for it. If you ever don't feel safe or able to take an active stand, you still can passively refuse to enable by simply walking away from conversations like that—you don't even have to say anything about it if you don't feel able to safely—and refusing to take any part in them.

If You or Someone You Know Has Just Been Sexually Abused or Assaulted

Dealing with the aftermath of sexual abuse or assault is hard enough. It's much, much harder without any sense of what you can do and how you can do it. It's also helpful to know what we can expect

Text continues on page 336

HERE ARE SOME THINGS TO KEEP IN MIND:

DON'T BE ANTAGONISTIC. YOU DONT WANT TO ESCALATE A SITUATION BY CREATING MORE CONFLICT AND POTENTIALLY PUTTING YOURSELF IN DANGER.

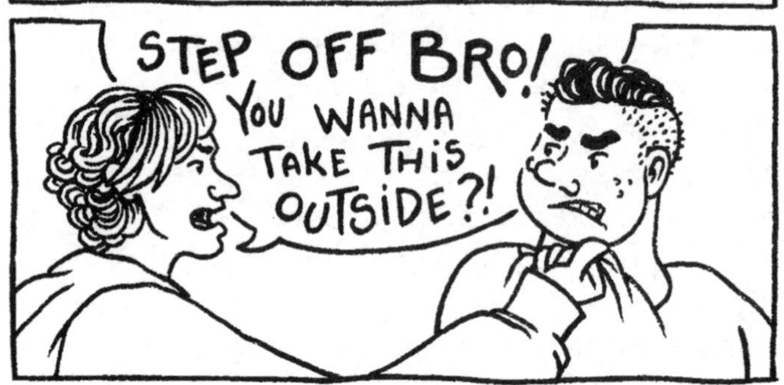
BAD IDEA EXAMPLE #1
STEP OFF BRO! YOU WANNA TAKE THIS OUTSIDE?!

IN MOST SITUATIONS, THE MOST IMPORTANT THING IS TO SEPARATE THE PEOPLE IN QUESTION. CONVERSATIONS ABOUT RESPECT AND CONSENT CAN WAIT UNTIL THE IMMEDIATE DANGER HAS PASSED.

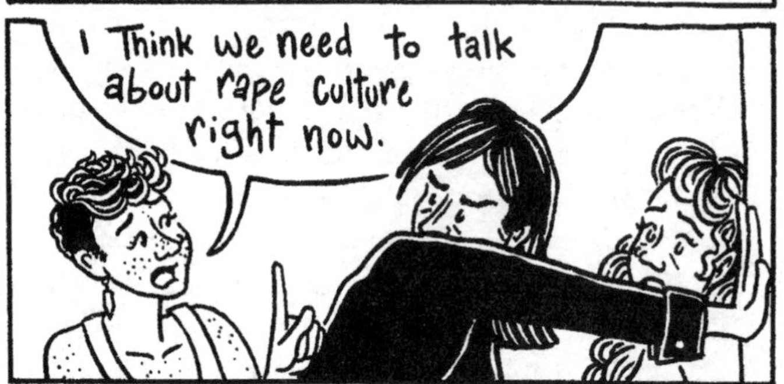
BAD IDEA EXAMPLE #2
I Think we need to talk about rape culture right now.

RECRUIT HELP IF NECESSARY. NEVER ENTER A SITUATION ALONE IF YOU FEEL YOU WOULD BE PUTTING YOURSELF IN DANGER.

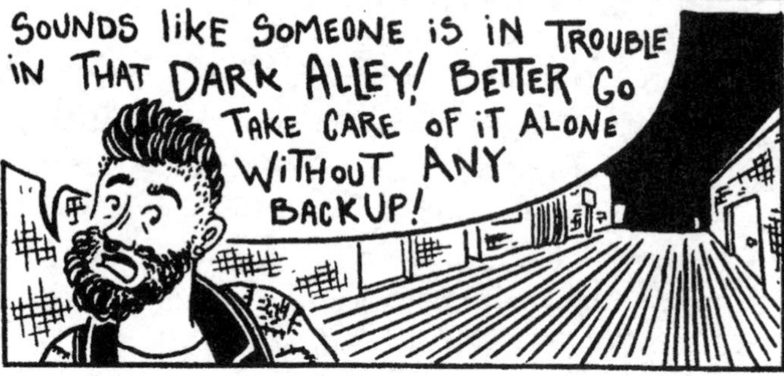
BAD IDEA EXAMPLE #3
SOUNDS LIKE SOMEONE IS IN TROUBLE IN THAT DARK ALLEY! BETTER GO TAKE CARE OF IT ALONE WITHOUT ANY BACKUP!

THE SPLIT

SEPARATE THE TWO PEOPLE. THIS TECHNIQUE WORKS BEST WHEN YOU MAKE IT APPEAR THAT YOU ARE REMOVING SOMEONE FOR REASONS OTHER THAN AVOIDING POTENTIAL ABUSE. CONVERSATIONS ABOUT THE TOPIC CAN HAPPEN LATER, WHEN THE IMMEDIATE THREAT HAS BEEN REMOVED.

MAYBE YOU KNOW THE VICTIM

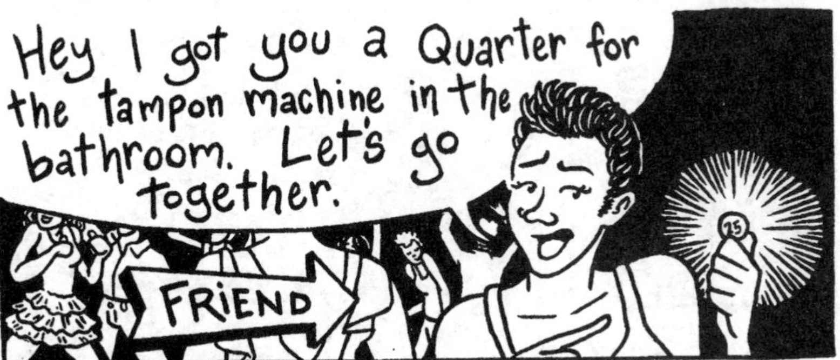
Hey I got you a Quarter for the tampon machine in the bathroom. Let's go together.
FRIEND

MAYBE YOU KNOW THE PERPETRATOR

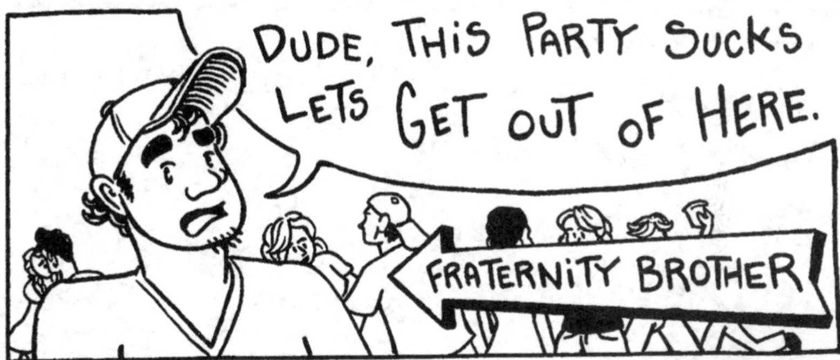
DUDE, THIS PARTY SUCKS LETS GET OUT OF HERE.
FRATERNITY BROTHER

PERHAPS YOU ARE A COMPLETE STRANGER

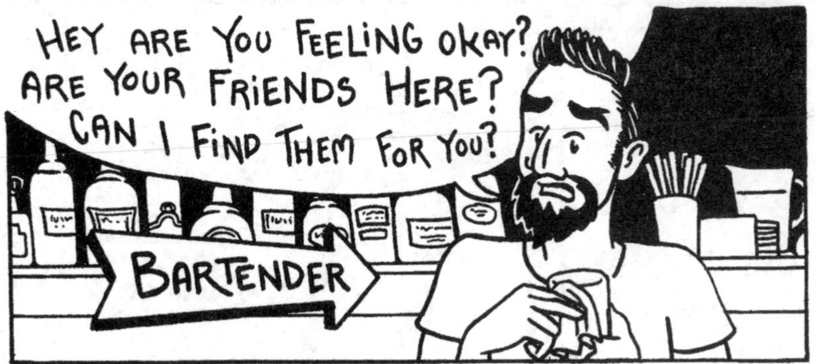
HEY ARE YOU FEELING OKAY? ARE YOUR FRIENDS HERE? CAN I FIND THEM FOR YOU?
BARTENDER

THE DISTRACTION

DIVERT THE ATTENTION OF ONE PERSON FROM THE OTHER BY REDIRECTING THEIR FOCUS, OFTEN FOR THE PURPOSE OF ALLOWING THE INTENDED TARGET AN OPPORTUNITY TO LEAVE THE SITUATION SAFELY.

YOU COULD CREATE A REASON TO CALL THE INTENDED TARGET AWAY.

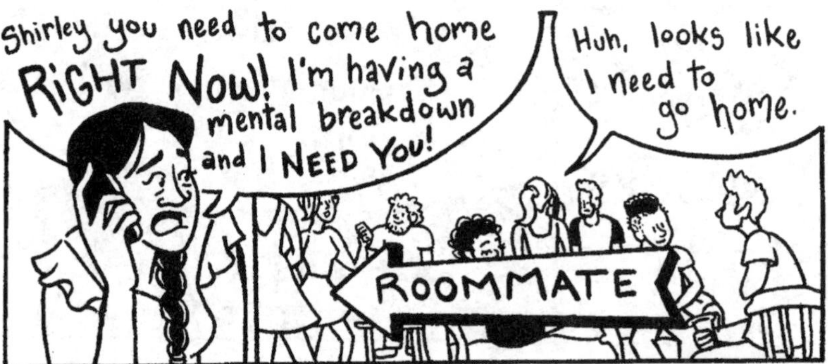
Shirley you need to come home RIGHT NOW! I'm having a mental breakdown and I NEED YOU!
Huh, looks like I need to go home.
ROOMMATE

OR FIND A WAY TO TAKE UP THE POTENTIAL PERPETRATOR'S TIME.

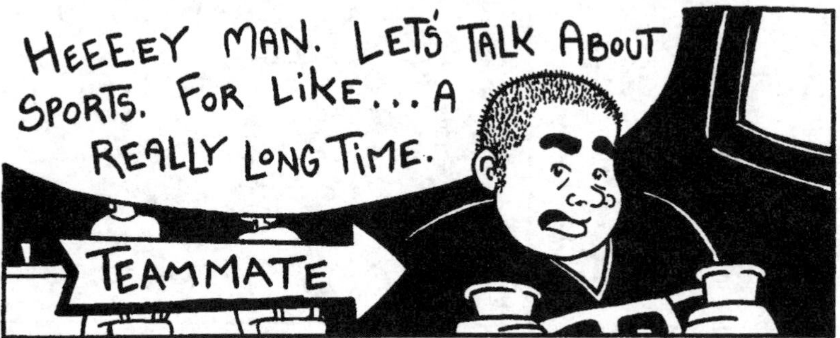
HEEEEY MAN. LET'S TALK ABOUT SPORTS. FOR LIKE... A REALLY LONG TIME.
TEAMMATE

YOU COULD EVEN PULL A DIVERSION OUT OF THIN AIR.

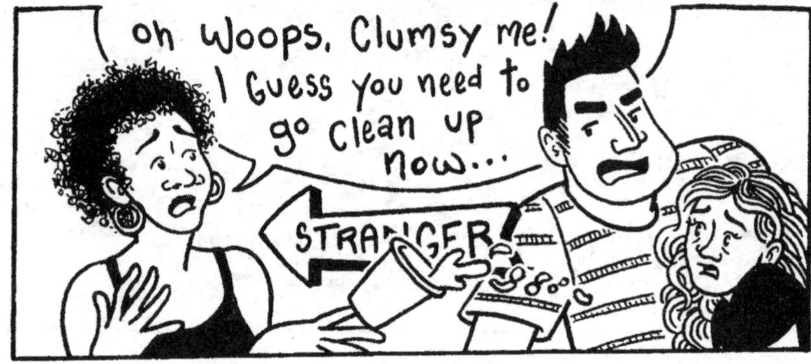
oh Woops. Clumsy me! I Guess you need to go clean up now...
STRANGER

CALL IN THE TROOPS

IF A SITUATION IS TOO POTENTIALLY DANGEROUS TO INTERVENE ON YOUR OWN, REACH OUT FOR HELP. THERE IS STRENGTH IN NUMBERS, AND USUALLY IF ONE BYSTANDER MAKES STEPS TO INTERVENE, OTHERS WILL AS WELL.

THIS COULD BE ASKING YOUR FRIENDS TO INTERVENE WITH YOU,

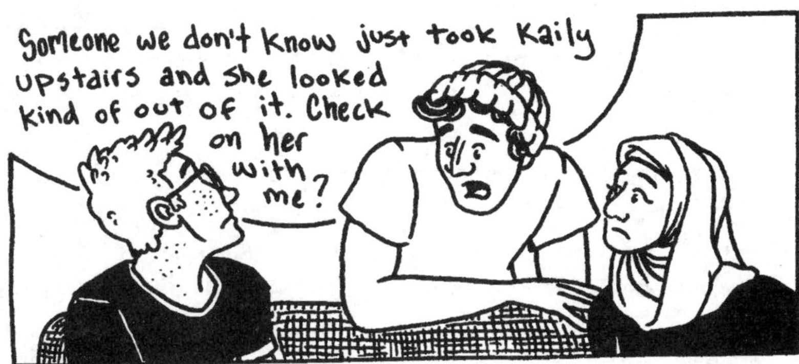
Someone we don't know just took Kaily upstairs and she looked kind of out of it. Check on her with me?

RECRUITING A POTENTIAL ALLY,

* SUCH AS AN EMPLOYEE OF THE ESTABLISHMENT YOU ARE IN.

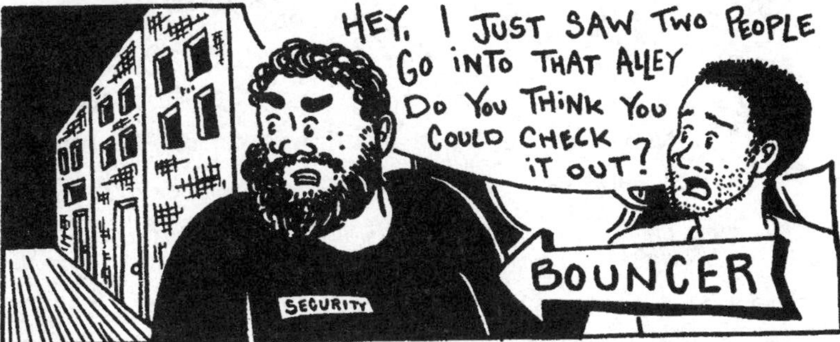
HEY, I JUST SAW TWO PEOPLE GO INTO THAT ALLEY DO YOU THINK YOU COULD CHECK IT OUT?
BOUNCER
SECURITY

OR ALERTING AN AUTHORITY FIGURE.

* SUCH AS PUBLIC SAFETY OR THE POLICE

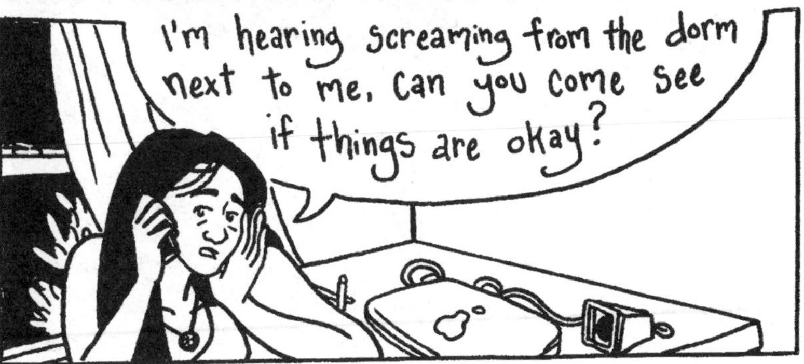
I'm hearing screaming from the dorm next to me, can you come see if things are okay?

from anyone supporting us and what they should—and shouldn't—be doing. I so hope you never need this information, but if you do, I want you to have it.

Sometimes a person knows very clearly that they've been sexually abused or assaulted. But if abuse or assault has come from someone known to you or someone you've been consensually sexual with in the past, or if the force involved was verbal or emotional rather than physical, it's common to feel uncertain or to not even know what happened wasn't perfectly acceptable. If you have the idea that you can't be raped or sexually assaulted because you belong to a certain group or are a certain type of person—maybe because you're a guy, because you're careful, or because you feel you're unattractive—it may be harder to believe. As well, it's very typical during and after rape to be in shock, to want to deny it happened, or to feel very confused about what exactly did happen and how. But if you feel or know that what happened was something you did *not* enthusiastically want or agree to, that you withdrew agreement at any point, or that you expressly said no to, know you're dealing with sexual abuse or assault, not consensual sex.

The most important thing to do right after assault is to get to a safe place, away from your attacker(s) or the place of the assault and out of any danger. The very next best step is to contact someone who can help and provide emotional support immediately, be it a friend or family or a rape or crisis hotline or other advocate. For hotlines, see the Resources section.

After sexual abuse or assault, it's best not to shower or wash your clothes. If you want to press charges, very important evidence can often be found on your body or clothing. Even if you do not know right away whether you want to press charges or don't want to make that decision right away, it's important to keep your options open and do what you can for the best chance of prosecution if you do press charges, which includes doing what you can to make it possible for physical evidence to be collected and preserved.

If possible, it's best to get to or call a hospital or urgent care center, regardless of whether you do or don't have healthcare coverage; someone who has been sexually assaulted will not be refused care. The hospital can handle calling the police and can call any wanted friends or family. If you're somewhere unfamiliar and without a phone, look or yell for help and ask someone to call the police for you.

In many cases, a rape counselor or rape crisis worker will also be available throughout the process of reporting. Some hospitals have what are called *SANEs—sexual assault nurse examiners*—who are trained expressly to deal with rape and assault. If a SANE or rape counselor is not present, you can ask for one and wait until one is available before proceeding with the rest of your exam. That person is a powerful advocate and ally. They can help a victim deal with the initial emotions, talk them through the process, and give important and accurate information about options for reporting, pressing charges, getting counseling, and joining support groups. If someone is a member of a group that faces discrimination even from people or in places that are supposed to be safe—like if you are transgender, undocumented, or of size—it's always appropriate and okay to ask for an additional advocate for that extra vulnerability or marginalization.

Pressing Charges

Reporting and pressing charges are usually choices, and ones with pros and cons, like all choices in life. Bringing abuse or assault to the justice system can often help a survivor obtain medical care and counseling; protective measures to prevent more abuse (a restraining order, for example), which are of particular concern when a rapist is known to the victim; and a sense of justice and emotional closure.

As noted on page 324, though, pressing charges isn't easy, and because someone is already struggling so much after abuse or assault, it's just not something that's the right thing for everyone. Going through the justice system as the victim of any kind of abuse or violence, especially sexual abuse or assault, often involves a lot of vulnerability, some loss of privacy, and a few risks. For someone who reports, it can be a very hard pill to swallow when an attacker or abuser is not charged or prosecuted, and they often won't be because most of our justice system still has very strong biases about some kinds of abuse or assault.

Having more people than your immediate circle know you've been raped or abused can make you feel even more vulnerable than you already do. Abuse or assault trials are not easy on the victim in a lot of ways, and they are an arduous, emotionally trying process. Many people still hold the outdated and ignorant notion that, in some way, rape is the victim's fault, especially if that victim is part of a stigmatized group—like sex workers or transgender women—or the circumstances of an assault involve anything that's part and parcel of victim blaming, like alcohol or a victim having had an active sexual life before their assault. Trials take time, as well, sometimes even taking a year or longer.

WHAT HAPPENS DURING A RAPE EXAM?

Once someone is admitted into the emergency room or care center:

- Any overt general injuries (such as cuts or broken bones) will be tended to, and medical staff may ask some basic questions, primarily to determine what immediate healthcare is needed.
- An overall examination is done, including a genital exam and STI and HIV testing. A healthcare provider will use a "rape kit," a (terribly unfortunate) term for a collection of materials expressly designed for gathering evidence from a rape victim and their clothing. They will probably also ask if it's known or possible that drugs or alcohol were used to facilitate assault so they can do the appropriate urine or blood tests and give the proper health care. Photographs may be taken. An examination after a rape can feel invasive and additionally traumatic, so if any of it feels like too much or not okay, it's always okay to ask for stops, pauses, or anything needed to make it easier to get through.
- Preventative medications for some STIs (like PEP for HIV) and emergency contraception should be offered. If either is needed and not offered, they can be requested.

Know that a person, especially a minor, can also report or press charges after the fact. If you were raped or abused some years ago and wish you'd reported it, chances are good that you can still do so. Because physical evidence is probably missing, those cases aren't as likely to result in convictions, but they *can* offer you some resolution and acknowledgment, help support someone else's case against the same person, as well as get a report on file to help protect others from the same person in the future. If you can report down the road and need more time to make up your mind and figure out what's best for you, you get to take that time.

In deciding whether to press charges, what's most important is *you* and your needs. This is about *your* safety and well-being, and who you're responsible for caring for and protecting most is yourself, not the rest of the world. It's up to you to decide to press charges or not, and it should ultimately be about what's truly in your best interest—there are no rights or wrongs here.

Talk about this with someone supportive you can trust, and who you know will honor your choices with this, whatever they are. You can get particularly sound advice and quality support from a rape hotline, local rape crisis center, or legal advocacy service. Help from people whose job is to work with and for survivors can include everything from accurate information about your options to direct connections to people in the justice system they know are strong survivor advocates (they might go with you to legal appointments so someone has your back), help filing orders of protection and understanding how to use them, safe housing or safe school help, and even help with how (and whether) to talk to people in your life about whatever legal choices you're making so they honor and respect them.

[HEALING AND DEALING]

One of the toughest things about surviving abuse is finding resolution and closure. Reporting and pressing charges are things that can help with that (see page 337), but they're not always helpful, and there are also other ways of finding and feeling resolution and closure.

Emotional support is crucial to healing and moving forward. Counseling or even talking about the abuse or assault may seem like the last thing you'd want. However, it's often the most important thing you need.

Although friends and partners can be very sympathetic, someone who hasn't been through it or who isn't experienced with or knowledgeable about the issues involved in healing from abuse or assault is unlikely to be of great help to you. And, sometimes, the people close to us are, unfortunately, jackasses about abuse or assault and do the very opposite of supporting us. Braving it out on your own can seem more appealing than talking about it with others, and sometimes it takes a while to find people who are safe for us and who are supportive to tell and talk to. Just know there is never a deadline on getting counseling or support. Even if you don't want it right now, or looking for it feels like too much, at any point you decide you need or want it you can seek it out.

But when you've been raped or abused and don't deal with it or put off dealing with it for a very long time, your life can suffer pretty greatly. You may struggle with post-traumatic stress disorder. You may struggle with triggers and not learn how to manage them, so you wind up having your life and the joy you can find in it considerably limited. It may be difficult to ever feel completely safe or to fully trust others again. Your own sexuality, sexual partnerships, or other relationships may elicit feelings of shame, anxiety, or fear rather than comfort or pleasure. Enjoying relationships of all types and even living a normal daily life can be really inhibited by denial of a rape or failing to deal with it. When the rapist is someone known to you, especially someone who was close to you, silence may give that person more opportunities to abuse you again or in different ways.

Learning what you need to feel safe—with others and even just in your own skin—what you're ready for at any given time, where you're at in your healing process, how to manage a whirlwind of different emotions, what are and are not healthy ways of dealing with sexual abuse and assault are all vital to your well-being. If your ways of coping are essentially just replacing one trauma or injury with another—for instance, via reckless or harmful sexual relationships, cutting, or other self-injury—you can find yourself in a never-ending cycle of agony.

As Buddhist writer and teacher Thich Nhat Hanh says, if we don't untie knots when they happen, over time they tighten and get harder to undo: the sooner you can do whatever you can to start your own healing process, the better.

To work through assault and come out whole and healthy, you've got to not only accept that it did happen but also do the work—however unfair it seems—to heal.

Healing 101

There are some things we know help nearly everyone in processing and healing from any kind of abuse or assault. Some help more with one kind of abuse than another, but all are positive things you can do for yourself as a survivor of abuse that are likely to help you come out feeling more whole and stronger:

1. Tell your truth. Just the telling of what happened to you, in whatever way it works for you to tell it, is very powerful. Any kind of abuse is silencing in one way or another, and some kinds of abuse or assault are more silenc*ed* in our lives and our world. Getting what was done to you out of your head and heart and saying (or writing) it out loud can feel scary but usually is ultimately something that can lift a great deal of your burden. At first, the only way you might feel safe speaking the truth is somewhere that's out of your head but still private, like writing it all out for yourself. Hopefully, you can also or soon find one other person—then more as you go—who will listen to you, hear you, and be willing and able to provide you some good support. The more we do this, the more we let it out and lift some of our burden, the more we're also usually helped in letting go of the shame that survivors of any kind of interpersonal violence, especially sexual violence, so often struggle with.

2. Don't feed the brain weasels. One of the bigger impacts of abuse is that survivors are often inclined to believe what someone who abused or assaulted them told them about themselves, either with words or by how they treated them. Because so many big cultural messages from so many influential sources, like mainstream media, also blame survivors for many kinds of violence, it's easy to believe those messages, too. Our heads are pretty inevitably going to go to those dark places until we start learning how and being supported to crawl out of them. Do what you can to intercept any messages that blame you or further hurt you and replace them with messages or logical thought patterns that support you and do you good. It can help to write the positive messages on index cards or put them in a notes or journal

IF YOU'RE CLOSE WITH SOMEONE WHO HAS BEEN ASSAULTED OR ABUSED IN ANY WAY

You can help them in some or all of these ways:

- Helping them to find safe emotional space by asking what *they* need and doing your best to provide what, of that, you can: Don't decide for them what they need or just do things without asking. Someone who has been abused or assaulted has had someone make decisions for them already, and it was a terrible thing. Don't do things for an abuse survivor without asking their permission first, and don't dismiss what they are saying they need because you feel you know better. **You don't.** Respect their right to their own choices and decisions, and ask, don't tell.
- Believing and supporting them: The behavior of abuse or assault victims varies widely from person to person; being emotionally controlled or calm is just as common as weeping openly. If your friend has told you they were raped or otherwise abused, believe them, and let them know that however they are feeling is okay and valid.
- Listening without judgment or correction: Allow them to express their feelings, even the ones that make you uncomfortable or that don't seem appropriate to you or how you think *you* would be feeling. If you know you have any biases or preconceived notions about rape, be self-aware and do not bring them to the table. If you need some limits and boundaries, that's okay and even good: limits and boundaries are healthy—and any kind of abuse or assault is all about a lack of healthy boundaries—as no one person can do or be everything for someone. Just set them gently and, if you can, offer to help find additional support or help that you don't feel able to give.
- Offering to be an advocate: In reporting, the legal process, or telling others, they may want and need an ally. Rather than giving advice, share options and resources for help, such as hotline or support group numbers, offer to be with them for medical appointments, or volunteer to talk to parents and other friends.
- **Remembering that this is about them, not you:** It's normal to feel upset or angry when someone we care about has been hurt or even to want to go out and actively do something

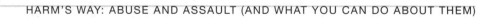

app on your phone for easy access when you need them. Counseling, especially with counselors or therapists qualified to work with abuse or assault survivors, can be really helpful in preventing you from getting all tangled up in ways of thinking that keep you in pain.

3. Find safe people and places where you don't have to hide. These may or may not be people you have told or even will tell your whole story. You don't have to. What you need are people and places where you can at least acknowledge you have survived abuse and are healing and be absolutely assured of support, care, and, with some, qualified help for survivors. Many areas have free counseling or support groups available for survivors of sexual or other interpersonal abuse as well as other crimes. These built-as-

on their behalf, but we need to manage those feelings ourselves or with support and counseling elsewhere, not with our friend or partner who has been harmed. If we know the person who committed the abuse or assault or, harder still, they're someone we're close to, we'll have our own intense feelings about that, too. But anything we do with this needs to come from a place of help and support for the person who was victimized based on what they're asking us for and what they need, not our own emotional reactions. Helping someone who has been harmed needs to be about them. You may feel you know what someone needs to heal, but that's not helpful (and often not correct); instead, follow *their* lead and listen to what they are expressing they need. By all means, do *not* threaten any kind of violence with or about the person or people who abused them. Someone who has been abused has already experienced violence, and threatening—or, even worse, doing—more only ensures they'll keep feeling unsafe. More violence also never solves any problem of violence: it only adds to it.

- Being patient with them, even over months or years: It takes time—sometimes a very long time—to process and recover from abuse or assault.
- Reminding them as many times as they need to hear it: this is ***not their fault.*** They didn't do this to themselves; someone else did this to them.

If you have a sexual or romantic partner who is a survivor of abuse, you'll also often need to take into consideration and work with certain sexual and intimacy issues or needs they may and often will have.

Your partner may have *triggers*—things that make them experience emotional impacts of the abuse very acutely—that you need to become aware of and work to avoid or help them manage when they do happen. There may be certain types of intimacy or sex or certain interpersonal dynamics with either that are off-limits for your partner, temporarily or permanently, and/or it may take them a longer time to feel comfortable with certain types of intimacy than it can for people who haven't been through abuse or assault. Forming trust may be more difficult for your partner. In many areas, you can find support groups or counseling for the partners of survivors to help you best manage these issues for your partner as well as yourself. For books about abuse for survivors and/or their partners, see the Resources section.

support services, from people trained in providing this kind of help, are also great to have because sometimes friends or family just won't be able to provide the kind of help we need or they lack the emotional bandwidth or time to help when we need it. Hopefully, you can also find some support and care from people already in your life. See if you can't start by identifying at least one safe person to fill in on the situation and then lean on as you heal. If you're having trouble figuring out who that is, see if you can think of any conversations you've ever had with anyone about victims and abuse before in which someone clearly was supportive of victims rather than shame-y, blame-y, or just otherwise unsupportive or ignorant.

4. Be patient with yourself, and remember the process of healing from abuse is in many ways lifelong, and nothing anyone can do in hours, days, months, or even years. Anyone who has been through abuse or assault of course wants to be as far away from it as possible, to "get past it" and be all better. But it just doesn't work that way, no matter how much we might wish it did. The process of healing is long term, and we usually have many times when we move forward, and then feel like we slid back. It's hard, and it asks a lot of us, including requiring a lot of love and care for ourselves, something that can sometimes be hard to do whatever our life circumstances but that any kind of abuse or assault makes more challenging. So, be patient with you: you really do have your whole life to heal, and whatever your pace is, is whatever your pace is, and it's okay. Give yourself credit for all your steps and any of your healing, not just big milestones. See all of this as really powerful self-care you might not be doing otherwise that has some serious side benefits, like getting to know yourself better and seeing your own strengths more clearly.

5. Honor your needs and your limitations. We just can't do some things in some ways after abuse or assault, whether that's having a certain kind of sex, building trust with people quickly, or being able to be around certain people, places, or things that remind us too much of the abuse or assault or that create post-traumatic triggers we're not yet able to cope with. It really, really sucks to be limited in our lives because of something someone else did to us, not because of something we chose for ourselves. It feels unfair because it *is* unfair. But it's also our reality: abuse usually has serious and lasting impacts. Just like getting better after a serious illness, healing is gradual, not instant, which means we might want to do some things, but can't, or we might want to be ready for or get back to some things, but aren't.

When someone abuses or assaults someone else, they are doing so to take power and control. If that's been something someone has done to us, it's because, for any number of reasons, we just couldn't stop them from doing it. But we can survive, and we can get that power back and be even stronger after abuse than we were before it. When we survive and we reclaim our lives and power, we put an end to that person continuing to hurt us or taking over us or our lives. We get back everything that should only have been ours to begin with.

The process of healing—and even just acknowledging you have a need to heal and a right to—reclaims your absolute and inarguable right to physical and emotional safety, autonomy, your life, and power within and for yourself, power you can share, if you want, but that isn't for someone else to take. It's coming to and always holding up the truth that you didn't do this to yourself, someone else did; that you aren't to blame, they are; that you aren't broken, they are.

Survivors with a capital *S* give themselves credit, care, and love—and require others to do the same—for all they are and all they've done to survive and thrive. Rather than blaming yourself for the abuse and taking responsibility for a harm you didn't do, healing gives you something to take responsibility for that *is* all yours, something that is positive and amazing, not harmful and terrible. It also can give you your life back so that abuse or assault doesn't stop you from living it.

Someone who abuses or assaults someone else is, very literally, a terrorist. Someone who survives abuse and goes through the process of healing and reclaiming their lives and selves from a place of love and compassion—and that's what real care for yourself always is—is a revolutionary rebel peacemaker, and that's something that doesn't just benefit that person, but all of us.

Surviving, healing, and reclaiming yourself and your life after abuse or assault take a great deal of time, energy, strength, courage, and love and care for yourself, probably more than you've ever given yourself before or might ever again. To believe that we are worthy of great love and care, and that we are worth everything we've got to give, isn't easy in the best of circumstances, but it's often exceptionally difficult after we've been through something that attempts to convince us of the opposite. Surviving and healing from abuse ask so much of anyone, and it can give us a lot, too—it's worth all we have to give it.

Being abused or assaulted is terrible, and healing is hard, but coming through to that other side feels more amazing than almost anything. And when we do get there, even just when we start to take steps on that journey, it's always going to be much, much harder for anyone to make us doubt our own worth, value, and strength ever again.

12

To Be or Not to Be . . . Pregnant: Contraception

We've got evidence of contraception—birth control—dating back thousands of years, but never in history have we had so many effective, safe, and widely accessible options as we do now. Hooray!

Until fairly recently, most forms of family planning weren't an option for many people, either because they didn't have access to methods or because sex, reproduction, or both weren't choices for them in the first place. (Sadly, this is still the case in some places, communities, and relationships.) Even as recently as a little over a century ago, a bill was passed in the United States—the Comstock Law—that defined birth control information as *obscene.* No joke: OBSCENE!

Many people were and still are pressured to reproduce, and are unsupported in effectively preventing pregnancy, regardless of their own wishes or circumstances. These scenarios, and a lack of safe, reliable, and accessible birth control, sometimes led to or enabled (and again, sadly, still does) abuse, abandonment, and other harms to unwanted children; unsafe or fatal abortions; and poor overall health and life outcomes for pregnant people and their children, and they compounded—and still compound today—overall oppression, especially of women. Today, some lobbies, communities, and cultures—often the same ones who bemoan the "epidemic" of teen pregnancy—still seek to block or reduce access to birth control and other forms of reproductive choice. The people who are most vulnerable to and most deeply affected by unwanted or unplanned pregnancy—such as people living in poverty, people without adequate health care, and young people—currently still have the *least* access to the most effective means of preventing pregnancy.

Unwanted pregnancy and childbearing can result in private and public problems. From a global standpoint, we face real problems with lethal malnutrition and poor health in infants and children—even here in the richest nation in the world, which also just happens to have the highest infant mortality and childhood poverty rates of any developed nation. Those problems increase with poverty, lack of education, unprepared or unwanted parenting, and the stigmas affixed to teen, young, or single parents and their children. Unwanted pregnancy can seriously undermine someone's health and well-being, physical and emotional, especially if they are not already in good physical or mental health. Viewing partnered sex as a gamble tends to create crummy relationships, crummy feelings about ourselves, and crummy parents. For much of history, refusing to allow them to have reproductive rights and control was one of the most common and most effective means of controlling women: women's rights are and have always been deeply linked to freedom of reproductive choice and the ability to control births. Whether it's done by a government, a culture, or a partner, keeping people from the power to choose whether and when to become pregnant keeps them from having sexual and personal agency and freedom.

Becoming pregnant—not just parenting—should be a *choice,* and one that has real bearing on the rights and well-being of all people, especially of women and children. When reliable birth control methods are used properly and consistently, and sex for both parties is fully consensual, few people will become pregnant before they are ready.

According to the US Department of Health and Human Services, in the United States there are currently 26.5 births for every 1,000 adolescents classified as female between the ages of fifteen and nineteen years. And that's just births; about as many people become pregnant and miscarry or choose abortion as people who choose to remain pregnant and deliver live births. Between 1990 and 2010, pregnancy among teens in the United States declined by 51

Obviously, most of this chapter is directed toward people who are themselves at risk of pregnancy. However, if you can't get pregnant but are having sex with someone who can, especially the kinds of sex that present pregnancy risk—or are thinking about it—**read up!** This is about you, too. Even if the possibility of pregnancy doesn't and will never have anything to do with our own sex life, we all have friends or family members for whom this matters. Everyone could always use more folks around them in the know about birth control. So much sexuality information is shared by peers, rather than between people and professional educators or healthcare providers, that the more accurate information anyone knows, the better. It's good for everyone to know about this stuff.

---

percent—from 116.9 to 57.4 pregnancies per 1,000 teens classified as female. The Department of Health and Human Services attributes this decline in part to the combination of an increased number of adolescents engaging in intercourse at a later age than those of previous generations did *and* increased access to and use of contraception.

But despite big developments in birth control methods and widely increased accessibility, the majority of pregnancies for young people *are* still unplanned or accidental. Unplanned or mistimed pregnancy is very common for people of **all** ages: around half of people who become pregnant usually report their pregnancies as unplanned. For people in their teens, the current rates in developed nations for unplanned pregnancy among teens are usually between 75 and 90 percent..

People become pregnant unintentionally or accidentally for several reasons. The biggest reason is simple: *birth control methods weren't used at all or were not used consistently and correctly, sometimes by choice, sometimes not.* With major health organizations like the CDC and the Guttmacher Institute releasing data that still show only about 30 percent of sexually active young adults using contraception regularly and many young people having intercourse for a year or more before even seeking out contraception, it's pretty obvious how unplanned pregnancies can often occur. There are many reasons birth control may not be used: because of lack of information about birth control methods, how to obtain them, and when they are needed; lack of access; reproductive coercion; sexual abuse or assault; concerns about privacy and discovery; embarrassment or shame; denial (of being sexually active and at risk, for instance); and the epidemic malady "it-can't-happen-to-me-itis."

Many young people who do use birth control use their methods inconsistently (sometimes because they don't have consistent access to them) or incorrectly; failure rates for birth control methods that allow for a lot of user error (like condoms or the birth control pill) are far higher for young people than for older people, and most methods' typical use and failure rates are far higher than they would be if methods were more often used correctly and consistently.

PREGNANCY RISKS, PLAINLY WRAPPED

Direct genital-to-genital contact between someone with a penis and someone with a vulva and/or direct contact between semen and the genitals of someone with a uterus is what produces a risk of pregnancy. It doesn't matter how long (or not) that kind of contact goes on for or what someone calls it. Sparing in vitro fertilization technologies, when none of that kind of contact is happening, pregnancy isn't going to be happening either.

MYTH BUSTING

When people use reliable methods of contraception for those kinds of contact, consistently and correctly, pregnancy risks are reduced at the specific rate of effectiveness a given method or methods can offer.

People of any age choosing to be sexually active with partners *are* responsible for their own choices, and your reproductive choices are—or should be—just that: *all yours.* You choose not only to be sexually active in the first place (or not) but also—as a result—to have to live with and be accountable for those choices and any of their outcomes. If you're someone who can become pregnant, the ability to choose when and whether you want a pregnancy is—and when it isn't, should be—**your right.**

Unwanted or unplanned pregnancy is not a "punishment" for sexual activity. It's just a basic and common physiological outcome of some kinds of sexual activity, just like catching a cold is a common physiological outcome of having a friend who's got one and coughs in your face.

NO BIRDS, NO BEES, NO BULL: HOW CONCEPTION REALLY HAPPENS

If how pregnancy happens seems simple, know that it's not. It's way more complex than two different kinds of cells happening to be in the same place at the same time or a single, heroic sperm cell just taking the right turn and—*voila!*—baby. How pregnancy happens, when it happens, is actually pretty complex.

What you've probably heard about most when it comes to how pregnancy happens are gametes: a special kind of cell that can fuse with another gamete to potentially create a pregnancy in organisms, like people, that reproduce in this way. Sperm cells are one kind of gamete; ovum (egg) cells are another. When those two kinds of cells come into contact with each other at a specific time and in a very specific way, a pregnancy can potentially result.

In most people of reproductive age (who've had a first period and haven't reached menopause) who have a vagina and a uterus, their ovaries—tiny sacs just outside the ends of the fallopian tubes—contain ovarian follicles, or ova, that are immature (as in, not ready yet, not meaning they are acting like jerks). People younger than age forty usually have millions of them.

During each fertility or menstrual cycle, one of those ova usually develops, is released by the ovaries, and is pulled into one of the fallopian tubes. (For more about the fertility or menstrual cycle and its particular timing, see page 33.)

When an egg is released, it moves slowly through the fallopian tube (it is always moving gradually and bit by bit along the way to the uterus; it's not just sitting around waiting for a sperm cell to call and ask it out). When an ovum is in the fallopian tube or one is soon headed that way, a couple other things are also usually going on. For one, cervical mucus, the fluid around the cervix, tends to become very watery and stretchy. The os, the opening of the cervix, softens and opens. For sperm cells to even have a chance of getting to the egg, both of these other things *must* be happening or they must happen within a few days. And both of these things, as well as the available ovum, are limited time offers: all of this usually takes place over only a few days in each cycle.

While all of this is going on, should someone with a penis ejaculate ("come") inside the vaginal opening or very directly, and without barriers, onto the vulva, then we've got some of the other things needed for a potential pregnancy: semen and sperm cells.

A lot of people don't get that semen and sperm aren't the same thing. Semen (seminal fluid or plasma) is a fluid deriving from the seminal vesicles, prostate gland, Cowper's gland, and bulbourethral glands, which comes through the urethra and out of the opening of the penis during ejaculation. Ejaculation most typically happens right around or nanoseconds after orgasm, but not always: sometimes people ejaculate without any orgasm. You can see semen when it's ejaculated outside the body.

Semen almost always contains sperm cells, but it is not, itself, made up of only sperm cells. Sperm cells make up less than 5 percent of semen. The rest is a whole bunch of essential constituents that enable sperm to do anything: proteins, enzymes, acids, and a good deal of fructose (a sugar). The fluid of semen is the medium in which sperm cells can move out of the penis and through the vagina. Just like a fish can't swim out of water, same goes for sperm without the fluid they're ejaculated with. But semen does more than that. It supplies nutrients and energy sperm cells need to be able to function, and it also neutralizes other elements that create problems for sperm like traces of urine and the vaginal environment. The squirty push an ejaculation gives seminal fluid also plays a part in the viability of sperm.

Someone with testicles usually produces millions of sperm every day. They're microscopically small; we can't see them without a powerful microscope. When ejaculation occurs—and this is something a person with a penis almost always knows has happened, not something they can't know or have to guess at—there's usually around a teaspoon or so of semen, which can contain hundreds of millions of sperm. Sperm cells are very fragile and super-duper sensitive. They are not resilient to things like being moved around from place to place—like from penis to hand, then hand to vulva—to changes in temperature, or to environments besides the testes and special lab conditions designed to protect them. They are not powerful, almighty superheroes; they are damsels in distress.

Let's say we have an available ovum, and all the other conditions within that person's body to make pregnancy even possible, and someone with a penis has also ejaculated inside the vagina or very nearby (and by nearby, I mean on the genitals, not on someone's thighs, chest, or a few feet away). For the next step to happen, sperm cells need to get through the vaginal canal and then into the cervix. But they often can't do one or both of those things.

During some parts of the fertility cycle, cervical mucus is too thick and pasty for sperm cells to be able to move, and sometimes the opening of the cervix isn't open or soft enough for them to get inside of it. Sometimes, sperm cells have to, and can, wait within parts of the reproductive system because they arrived too soon: an egg and the other conditions needed weren't there for them yet. Sperm cells can potentially live within the vaginal environment for a few days—they're the ones waiting for the phone to ring, as it were. Other times, there's just not enough semen or viable sperm cells in that semen for the next steps to pregnancy to occur. Weird as it sounds, in a lot of ways the vagina, cervix, and uterus aren't friendly to sperm cells: that reproductive system even "attacks" *(hee-ya!)* some sperm cells to try to counteract them similar to the way our bodies try to counteract unhealthy bacteria or other potentially harmful visitors.

Even in perfect conditions, less than a thousand sperm cells—of those initial millions!—make it to the fallopian tubes, and only a few dozen sperm cells may wind up reaching the outer membrane of the egg cell if any do. That's one reason the body produces so many sperm.

When they can get through the vagina and through the cervical opening, the sperm cells that remain go both directions, some to one fallopian tube, some to the other. Once in the fallopian tubes, contractions of the uterus and by the cilia, supertiny organelles (a specialized subunit within a cell) in the fallopian tube, push the sperm cells toward the egg cell. (The fallopian tubes do quite a lot of pulling and waving through: no wonder they look like small arms and fingers!) Some get kind of tangled up and stuck in the cilia instead. Chemicals inside the reproductive system also help out, charging the sperm cells to give them more energy.

Those that make it to the fallopian tube that contains the live egg—at this point, usually fewer than fifty sperm cells are left—surround the egg and try to enter the sac. If the ovum is healthy, sperm push into the protective layers around it, and into sperm receptors that are part of the membrane around the egg cell. Then it's just a matter of which one of the few remaining sperm cells can enter the egg first and fertilize it. The egg also takes part by pulling that sperm cell inside. When the egg does that, it also secretes some special enzymes that lock out any of the other sperm cells left trying to get in.

That's when we've got what's called fertilization of the egg. But we *still* don't have a pregnancy yet.

If the process continues, about a day or so after fertilization the egg cell and the sperm cell together become something new, a zygote. It contains forty-six chromosomes (the carriers of hereditary characteristics, like hair and eye color, body size, and genetic health conditions): twenty-three from the egg and twenty-three from the sperm. The zygote's DNA structure is new and different from the structure of either the sperm or the ovum.

That zygote remains in the fallopian tube and starts to divide into many cells. Over the next few days, as the zygote—called the *morula* at this stage of the game—progresses down the fallopian tube, it divides several times, until it becomes a hollow, sixteen-celled structure called a *blastocyst*. *That's* what may—or may not—implant in the uterine wall, attaching to the endometrium (the uterine lining, the same lining that sheds during a menstrual period) and the developing *placenta* (a temporary organ formed by the outer cells of the blastocyst that grows over time to nourish a developing embryo and fetus via the mother's bloodstream), and then becoming an embryo. *Conception* and *implantation* are the terms used most often for this stage of the process.

Many times, without any interference from anyone, fertilized eggs don't divide or implant, and a pregnancy does not occur. It's estimated that as many as 50 percent of fertilizations do not complete (and this isn't something anyone is ever likely to notice or know happened to them because when a blastocyst fails to implant, menstrual periods tend to occur as usual, and a person doesn't feel anything different with just a fertilization).

But if and when *all* of that up there does happen? **That's** when we've got ourselves a pregnancy. (To find out what happens next, when a pregnancy is sustained, see Chapter 13.)

All in all, the process from the moment ejaculate enters the vagina to the stage that's medically recognized as a pregnancy takes anywhere between around five days and two weeks. This is one of the reasons emergency contraception can work even though it's taken after intercourse, and this is also why, if someone is freaking about feeling pregnancy "symptoms" just a couple hours or days after a possible risk, we can know that whatever they're feeling is not from a pregnancy because pregnancy and its physical impacts just can't happen that fast.

Pregnancy Risk Q and A

Can Someone Get Pregnant If Their Partner Ejaculates While Someone Has Pants on, Is in the Bathtub, or Is Across an International Border?

The *most* likely way—the way pregnancy almost exclusively happens—to become pregnant is through direct vaginal contact with semen. Sperm cells in semen can live for about twenty minutes in an environment that is unfriendly to them, but that's about it. So, for instance, having unprotected anal sex where sperm can dribble right down into the vagina may pose some possible pregnancy risk, but pregnancy from this isn't even remotely as close to likely as it is with unprotected vaginal intercourse.

Scenarios like giving a partner unprotected oral sex in which you have oral contact with their semen, then kiss them, and then your partner engages in cunnilingus presents STI risks, but not pregnancy risks. Sitting in a tub with someone who ejaculates in the water without actual genital contact? No way. If there is a distinct barrier between a vagina and a penis, such as thick or impermeable clothing (like a few layers of denim or polyester), water, or an international border, there is not a risk of pregnancy.

In addition, pregnancy cannot occur by swallowing semen from oral sex or from manual sex with no vulvar contact with fresh semen. The digestive system isn't directly connected to the reproductive system: sperm trying to get to the fallopian tubes through the digestive tract would be like you trying to get to class on time by running through a brick wall.

What If My Partner Says They're Infertile?

It's very rare for a young person to know their fertility status because, barring certain medical conditions or diseases (such as PID, polycystic ovary syndrome [PCOS], eating disorders, some ways of being intersex, or profound testicle injuries) or the impact of certain medical treatments, most people have not had tests done to determine their fertility. A young person claiming to be infertile who also happens to suggest that one or both people don't use any birth control is probably either lying, uneducated, or confused about something their doctor told them. Unless you hear it from the doctor diagnosing infertility, assume you and your partners are fertile.

I've Heard That the Chances of Becoming Pregnant Are the Same as the Chances of Winning the Lottery. True or False?

The chance of winning a state lottery jackpot is a mere 1 in just under 14 million, or a 0.0000000716 percent chance. Most accidental pregnancies that occur for young people do so within the first six months of having intercourse, and teens or emerging adults who do not use contraceptives for penis-in-vagina intercourse have around an **85 percent chance (0.85)** of becoming pregnant within just one year. If only the chances of winning the lottery were that good!

[THE BIRTH CONTROL BREAKDOWN]

Different people have different birth control needs. There's no one "best kind" of birth control for everyone: which kind or kinds turn out to be best for someone is very individual.

For many people, what's most important is that a method is affordable, easy to use and obtain, effective, and allows them to enjoy their sexual lives. Some people are comfortable with hormonal methods, like the pill, whereas others don't like or can't have synthetic chemicals or hormones. Some people need a constant birth control method or want benefits some constant methods can offer, such as decreasing menstrual cramps or clearing acne; others need or want something they can use only occasionally.

Effectiveness and ease of use, including access—after all, if we can't get or can't always get a method, it's not going to be of any real use to us—are generally the biggest factors in most people's birth control choices. Most barrier and hormonal methods are highly effective and easy to use. **Using methods incorrectly or using them inconsistently are the big factors in contraceptive failure.**

Also, two methods—like condoms used with the pill or a Depo-Provera injection, or a diaphragm used with fertility charting—are usually better than one. Health organizations have found that using two methods, called ***dual contraception***—at Scarleteen, we like to call it "The Buddy System"—is the most effective way of preventing pregnancy.

You have options. If and when it's time to consider birth control, it's wise not to leap at a method just because it's what everyone else seems to be using or to assume it must be best because you've heard of it often or seen ads for it.

Which birth control method is best for you is a very individual choice, and it may change a few times during your life (and involve some trial and error). Have a look at what's out there now, and then talk with your healthcare provider to figure out what's most likely right for you. If your provider is choosing a method for you rather than asking what you want and need and exploring all your options with you, then either advocate for yourself directly or find a different provider who will take more time and help you choose more effectively. What's best for them or what they think is best for a patient may not always be what the patient knows will work. A good healthcare provider is going to be doing more listening to you and paying more attention to your unique needs and health history than talking or paying attention to their own preferences. Because developments are always taking place, you should also always ask a healthcare provider to tell you about anything new rather than assuming you already know what all of your options are.

On the following pages, you'll find brief descriptions of all currently available and effective methods, including approximate cost, where and how to get them, ease of use, common side effects, pros and cons, special concerns, and effectiveness.

Effectiveness data come from a wide sample of people, not from younger people specifically.

According to Family Planning Perspectives, the failure rate of oral contraceptives (aka, the pill) for adolescents may be as high as 15 percent just based on inconsistent use alone. For all contraceptive methods, young people experience a failure rate of about 47 percent in the first year of contraceptive use, whereas the overall failure rate for people over thirty is only 8 percent. That's a giant difference. Because younger people more frequently make mistakes with methods—no judgment; that's just the reality—and have less reliable access, backing up any method with a second method is always an especially good idea.

With any method you use, listen to your healthcare provider's instructions carefully, ask any questions about how to use a method that you have, and be sure to take time to read the patient literature that comes with your method. When you're new to a method that asks you to do something—like a pill or condom, rather than something like an IUD or implant—backing up with a second method leaves you room for mistakes you might make while you learn how to use a method.

Specifics of many methods are not listed here, and birth control data, methods, and information tend to change or be updated pretty regularly, so it's always smart to ask or check for the most current information and data with any method of contraception. Patient leaflets and prescribing information are updated more frequently than reference books.

COST RATINGS

$: Cheapedy-cheap (under $200 per year)

$$: In the middle ($200–$600 per year)

$$$: Big bucks (over $600 per year)

How much or how little a method of contraception costs depends on its base cost and whether someone has healthcare coverage for contraception—through insurance or public health services—and how much of the cost that coverage covers. Sometimes even the most expensive of methods can wind up being free with certain types of insurance plans or public health programs! If you're a minor and don't have insurance, don't have a plan that covers contraception, or don't want to use your family insurance, be sure to check into any national, state, or county health programs that may be available to you to cover your contraception costs, even if you have insurance under a family plan.

Cost estimates also are not merely for single use: the estimates posted are for use over one year, assuming a user has sex around a hundred times in that year (according to the Kinsey Institute, the average eighteen-year-old reports—self-reporting about sex may be inflated—having sex 112 times per year). Take note that, for instance, whereas an IUD costs much more at the onset, in less than a year it can cost about the same or even less than the pill. And in just two or three years, it will cost considerably less than the pill.

The average rate of effectiveness is listed both for perfect use (these are clinical trial rates for one full year) and for typical use (how people actually use it in real life, which includes common mistakes like occasionally taking a pill late or spacing out a condom every now and then).

Those statistics figure for *one full year* of use—they're not rates for a single use—and are come by based on how many people using a given method alone simply did or didn't become pregnant during that year.

Perfect and *typical* use can be tricky terms and frameworks, so you may find it easier to think of effectiveness rates for methods as being about how well a method is or isn't used. If someone is using it as well as anyone can for a full year, they're probably getting very close to that perfect use rate. Once any errors and mistakes occur in that year, we're sliding into the typical use rate. Not using a method at all puts you totally out of this range altogether: no method = no protection from pregnancy.

Abstinence

Refraining from the kinds of contact or sex that present risks of pregnancy—or from partnered sex altogether—is something people can do to expressly avoid pregnancy. Abstinence may be a good choice of method for people who don't feel a strong desire or readiness to have sex with partners, who have religious beliefs or convictions against engaging in sex, or who do not have access to any other methods.

We may often hear that abstinence is the most effective and foolproof method of birth control. However, that's not exactly true. By all means, if someone isn't part of any of the kinds of contact or sex that can present risks of pregnancy, then they are 100 percent protected from pregnancy. But, as noted in *Contraceptive Technology,* **about 26 percent of young adults who report they are "practicing abstinence" become pregnant within one year,** which would make abstinence only about 74 percent effective in typical use and, thus, one of the *least* effective methods of contraception, not the most. That low rate of effectiveness most likely reflects people who may intend to be abstinent, want to be, or say that's what they are but who have, in reality, engaged in some kind of sex that could create a pregnancy. So, like other methods, it certainly isn't 100 percent, and it can work more or less well depending on how—and if—someone is using it.

If you're planning to use abstinence as your method of birth control, you also have to at least be honest about engaging in sex. Your body, after all, doesn't care whether or not you call something sex: what you call it makes no difference. A study of high school students published in 1999 in the *Journal of the American Medical Association* found that around 30 percent of students who identified themselves as people who hadn't had sex *had* engaged in penis-in-vagina intercourse. So, if you're not going to have sex because you don't want to take pregnancy risks, you need to *not have sex* that presents those risks regardless of what you call it.

Being realistic is also important. If you're with a partner and are physically intimate at all—or are in any way half-hearted about abstinence—do yourself a solid and have a backup method of birth control (and safer sex) around, just in case you change your minds impulsively. Talk about pregnancy prevention in advance of any sexual activity, even if you don't plan to engage in intercourse. And talk together about how you're going to support each other in abstaining from sex. Like any method of contraception (if that's your aim with abstinence or a benefit you want from it), abstinence involves actively doing things, not just *not* doing something. That can mean doing things like creating strategies to employ together when you feel strong desires to be physically sexual, establishing and reestablishing boundaries, providing emotional support, or learning and exploring ways to be intimate or sexual without doing activities that present pregnancy risks.

Barrier Methods

Barrier methods—condoms and cervical barriers (see pages 288–297)—work by preventing sperm from reaching or entering the vagina or cervix: by creating a barrier to sperm cells. Many people like barrier methods because they're easy to get and use, affordable, noninvasive, effective, and convenient. They don't change the fertility or menstrual cycle, don't change body chemistry, and don't carry any likely serious or long-term side effects. For people who can't remember to take pills on time every day, who feel something like an IUD is just not where they're at yet or what they can afford right now, or who cannot abide with any hormonal methods or intrauterine devices, barriers are just the thing. Condoms also offer protection from STIs that other methods can't offer. Some studies have suggested that other barrier methods, such as the diaphragm, may also provide *some* extra STI prevention, including protection from HIV, by protecting cervical cells from infection (though these should not be considered a sound method of safer sex).

Barrier methods may not work well for those who feel uncomfortable touching their genitals; who have a hard time communicating with partners; or who don't want to "interrupt" sexual activity to insert a device or ask partners whether sex is on the menu for later so as to insert the device in advance (for people in those situations, partnered sex isn't usually real smart, either). Barrier methods made of latex are not good choices for people who are latex-sensitive or allergic, but most of these devices do have latex alternatives.

Condoms

Effectiveness with perfect use: 95–98% effective

Effectiveness with typical use: 79–85% effective (Lower rates are for inside, or female, condoms; higher for male, or outside, condoms)

Cost: $

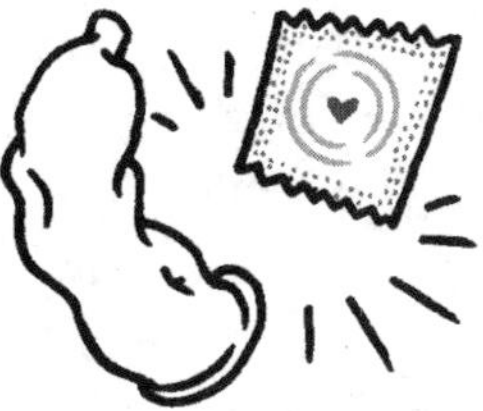

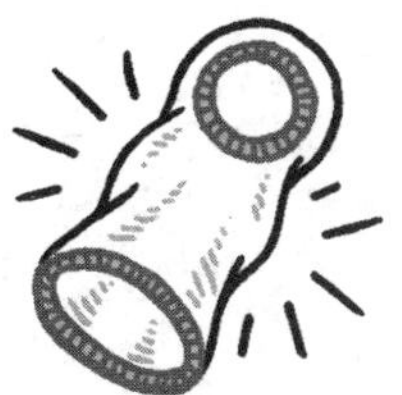

What are they, and how do they work?

Condoms—latex or nonlatex sheaths—either rolled onto the penis or, when using inside or female condoms, inserted into the vagina work by preventing sperm cells from having any contact with the vagina or vulva, because any fluids are contained within the condom. For detailed instructions on how to use condoms and more information on condoms, see pages 288–297. Condoms fail if they are not used for all genital contact from start to finish and if they break, tear, or slip off; they most often fail because they're simply not being used for all genital contact or used at all. If a condom fails, it will be fairly obvious—either because it's slid off and into the vagina, in the case of a male condom, or because it's broken, in which case it'll usually look like a popped balloon does—and a method of emergency contraception (see page 368) can be used.

How and where do you get them?

A doctor's visit or prescription isn't required to get condoms, nor must a person be of a certain age. Condoms can be found all over the place: pharmacies, grocers, megastores, online vendors, student and community health centers, and clinics (where they can often be found at no cost). When buying condoms, try to avoid places where they may have sat on shelves or in hot or cold areas for a long time (such as in gas station windows). Then store them properly yourself, away from heat or cold or places where they might get torn inside the wrapper.

Pros and Cons, Risks and Benefits

Hundreds of different styles or brands of condoms are now available, and condoms are also thinner and better designed than ever before, so it's usually easy to find condoms that everyone likes. Condoms are a method most often worn by people who themselves can't become pregnant, so unlike methods like the IUD, birth control pill, or injection, negotiation about condom use is often part of using them. One big benefit of condoms is that they are the **only** birth control method that also provides STI protection (and protection against cervical cancer by helping to

"The Water Test"

Ah, the Internet, providing us such widely believed and inaccurate (though entertaining) myths and urban legends as giant camel spiders in Iraq, "blue waffle disease" (nope, not a real STI and never was), and an apparent zombie nibbling shoppers in Tennessee. Then there's what some people call "the water test," the idea that to find out whether a condom has failed, you have to fill it up with water after sexual activity. When condoms tear, it really is obvious: no one needs a microscope to find a tear. Or to fill a condom with water. Testing condoms with water—and then with other ways, like with an air-burst test—was already done when they were manufactured. Each condom is put through testing so rigorous before it's ever distributed, you couldn't do it better yourself if you tried. If you or a partner feel like you don't trust condoms alone, the answer is to do something sexual where you don't need them or to add or swap out for another method—not to add a running-to-the-sink-after-sex panicky test to the mix that doesn't actually tell you anything but where the bathroom is.

prevent HPV, the virus most associated with cervical cancer). It's a very good idea to back up *any* other method of birth control with condom use for that reason. Also, condoms are one of the few self-directed methods of contraception available for people with penises.

Some people have a harder time learning to use inside, outside, or both kinds of condom. Sometimes, when someone is trying to wiggle their way out of using them, it's because they don't know how or don't feel confident and feel embarrassed to say so. It's ideal for everyone to know how to put a condom on; that way, if a partner needs help—or finds it's sexy when their partner puts on the condom for them as part of sex!—help can be, literally, at hand. It's much more low-pressure to learn to put a condom on without somebody else around, so someone can always learn and practice on their own.

Some people expect condoms to get in the way of intimacy or sensation. We know from both anecdotal evidence and study that neither is rarely true unless someone convinces themselves it is. Some people have only experienced condom use, so far, as a drag or uncomfortable. If either of those is the case, more experimenting with different styles of condoms as well as with different ways of using them (like always adding lube on the inside or having partners put them on as part of sexual activity, not as an interruption to sexy-times) often takes care of these issues.

Diaphragms and Cervical Caps

Effectiveness with perfect use:
90–94% effective
Effectiveness with typical use:
84% effective
Usual cost: $, including exam and fitting, when needed

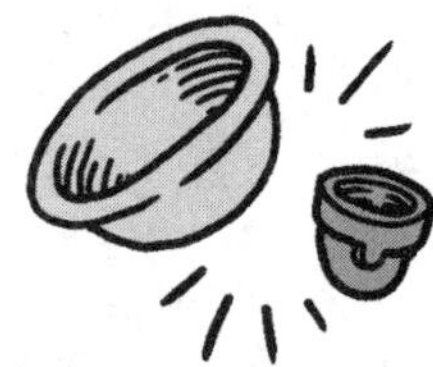

What are they, and how do they work?

A *diaphragm* is a latex, silicone, or rubber cup, about the size of your palm, that is inserted into the vagina before intercourse (even a few hours before, if you like) and used with spermicidal jelly. It is held in place behind the pubic bone, and it covers the cervix to prevent sperm from entering; the spermicide kills any sperm that may wind up squiggling their way around the cup. Diaphragms are reusable and can be used for a couple of years before they need to be replaced. The diaphragm needs to be left in after sex for at least six hours or up to twenty-four hours (but no longer than that) before it is removed. That's because the sperm can remain viable for that amount of time inside the vagina, so if you took it out right away, rather than leaving it in to keep those sperm out of the cervix with the help of the spermicide, it could fail. It can be used for multiple acts of intercourse so long as extra spermicide is inserted into the vagina before each additional act.

A *cervical cap* is a reusable soft latex or rubber cup with a round rim that fits snugly around the cervix. The cap currently available does not require a fitting. It comes in three sizes: one for people who have never been pregnant, one for people who have but didn't have a vaginal delivery, and one for people who have had a vaginal delivery. You do need a prescription for it from a healthcare provider, however. Like the diaphragm, it is used with spermicide. A cervical cap protects for forty-eight hours and can be used for multiple acts of intercourse within that time.

How and where do you get them?

A diaphragm most often currently requires a fitting, prescription, or both from a gynecologist or other sexual healthcare provider. But a new diaphragm, the SILCS diaphragm, is becoming available and does not require either of those things. It will be available over the counter. It may be that, soon, diaphragms that require fittings from a healthcare provider are replaced by this kind of barrier that doesn't.

Current cervical caps do not require a fitting but do require a prescription. The spermicidal jelly used for both methods can be obtained—without a prescription—from pharmacies, grocers, megastores, and online vendors.

Pros and Cons, Risks and Benefits

Wearing a diaphragm for more than twenty-four hours or a cervical cap for more than forty-eight hours is not recommended because of the risk, though low, of toxic shock syndrome (TSS). With prolonged use, the cap or diaphragm may cause an unpleasant vaginal odor or discharge in some people. For those prone to urinary tract, yeast, or bacterial infections, diaphragms may not be a good choice. Cervical caps don't present the same potential issues with UTIs.

Some people also may not like using diaphragms or cervical caps because they find them difficult or awkward to put in or because they don't like the accompanying spermicides. As with condoms, the biggest reason diaphragms and cervical caps fail is that they aren't applied properly, used all the time, or used for all genital contact, from start to finish—so if you feel like they're a drag to put in, then they're probably not a good choice.

But there are also a lot of pros. Both methods can be put in well before sexual activity, so they don't interrupt sexual activity. Diaphragms can be used for sex during menstruation (cervical caps cannot). Both can be used without replacement for a couple of years, making them one of the least expensive methods there is. Like other barrier methods, these do not pose the health risks that hormonal methods may pose, and they may be used by people who cannot use those other methods due to health conditions. Both are comfortable once inserted, and neither partner is likely to feel them during intercourse or other sexual activities.

Spermicides

Spermicides come in many forms: foams, suppositories, tablets, films, creams, and jellies. Used alone, rather than with a barrier method, spermicides are one of the least effective methods of contraception, even with perfect use. Spermicides may also increase STI risks in some users as a result of genital irritation due to the spermicide, which can inflame the genitals and make them thus more prone to infection.

"Homegrown" agents sometimes thought to be spermicides, like lemon juice, vinegar, or castile soap, have not been proven to be very effective.

Contraceptive Sponge

Effectiveness with perfect use:

91% effective (80% for those who have given birth vaginally)

Effectiveness with typical use: 84% effective (68% for those who have given birth vaginally)

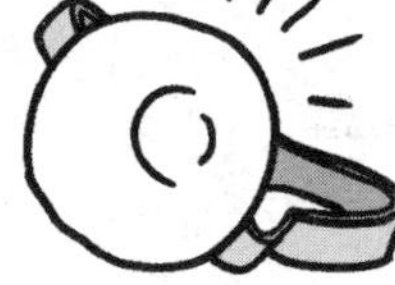

Cost: $

What is it, and how does it work?

The vaginal contraceptive sponge is a device made of polyurethane that looks like a little white bagel: you place it inside your vagina, in front of the cervix. The device works in two ways: it contains spermicide (nonoxynol-9; find out more about it on page 291) that foams from the sponge when it is used (you add water to it before inserting it to produce the foam), and it forms a barrier to the cervix. It has a loop on one side for removal. Like a diaphragm, it should be left in place for at least six hours after intercourse and removed no later than twenty-four hours after insertion to prevent TSS and vaginal irritation from the spermicide. When you're finished using it, you just pull it out and throw it away.

Where and how can you get it?

Contraceptive sponges can be bought over the counter at pharmacies or megastores. No prescription or exam is required.

Pros and Cons, Risks and Benefits

One sponge offers protection for up to twenty-four hours, even with multiple acts of intercourse. Sponges are also inexpensive.

Because of the foaming that comes from the vagina with the sponge, it can be messy and feel socially awkward for some, and it is not a good choice for anyone sensitive to spermicides or prone to yeast infections. It may also carry risks of TSS if left in longer than advised.

Hormonal Methods

Hormonal methods all work by intentionally putting hormones into the bloodstream—via pills, patches, rings, injections, or subdermal (under the skin) implants—that basically hack the fertility cycle, making conception very unlikely when it would otherwise be likely. Whether methods are called combined hormonal contraceptives—which have both synthetic estrogens and progestins—or progestin-only, progestin is the hormone that does the heavy lifting when it comes to how and why these methods work. These methods suppress ovulation—they keep eggs from being released each month by blocking the luteinizing hormone (LH) surge responsible for ovulation, as explained in Chapter 12—and thicken the cervical mucus, making it difficult for sperm to reach the cervix and fertilize an egg. They also make the uterine lining thinner so in the event the two proven ways these methods prevent pregnancy were to fail, a fertilized egg would be unlikely to implant. However, this last way they could work is more theoretical than actual: how these methods are known and proven to work is really about those first two things.

Hormonal methods are very effective when used properly. Skipped or late pills or injections, or patches or rings used incorrectly or sporadically, decrease the effectiveness of hormonal methods. Some hormonal methods are more reversible (easier to use without lasting effects or to stop taking, allowing the hormones to gradually leave your system) than others.

One big downside of hormonal contraceptive use may be a false sense of security in terms of sexually transmitted infections: when people start using a hormonal method, they often stop using safer sex barriers. Hormonal birth control methods provide *no* STI protection, so safer sex is still needed and important when using a hormonal method.

How to use a specific hormonal method and manage problems—like late or missed pills, patches that slide off, or troubles inserting the ring—varies based on the method, so always be sure to ask your healthcare provider about your type and brand, and read the patient information for your medication carefully.

Many people are concerned that certain medications or even what they eat or drink can interact with hormonal methods and make them ineffective. No one has to worry about foods or beverages creating a problem, and the majority of medications, both prescription and over the counter, including antibiotics, have not been found to present issues with contraceptive effectiveness. Some medications, however, can interact in ways that make the hormonal method or that medication less likely to work or to work well, but so long as you make sure your healthcare provider knows which medications you use, rest assured they will make sure you're not using anything that can interact poorly.

Combined Oral Contraceptives, aka the Pill or BCP

Effectiveness with perfect use:
99%+ effective
Effectiveness with typical use:
91% effective
Usual cost: $$,
including cost of GYN exam

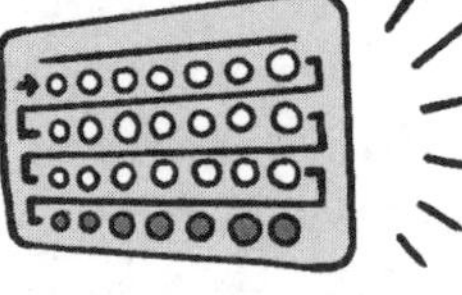

What is it, and how does it work?

The combined birth control pill—meaning it contains a combination of two different synthetic hormones, estrogen and progesterone—is currently the most popular method of birth control in the United States (though IUDs are starting to give pills a run for their money). As long as someone is taking their pill as directed and on time every day of a cycle, the pill provides equally effective protection on every day of that cycle, including during the placebo week. When starting the pill, a backup method of birth control is advisable through the first cycle—one month—of use. A person then takes one "active" pill—a pill with hormones in it—every day for twenty-one days, and then for the last week of the cycle, takes one "inactive" pill—with only inert ingredients—during which time a withdrawal bleed (it's not really a period, but some people still think of theirs that way and call it that) will usually begin.

The pill works by suppressing ovulation and thickening cervical mucus and theoretically by impeding implantation.

TECH TIP

A few great online tools can help you figure out which method or methods of contraception are likely to be your own best fit. Scarleteen has a thorough walkthrough on our website, Planned Parenthood has some quick widgets on theirs, and many other reproductive and general health sites have easy tools for picking a method. So, if you need a little more help after you read through this section, go online and go to our website or Planned Parenthood's or use a search engine to search for "choosing a method of contraception." That'll pull up a range of good tools from reputable sources to help you out.

Where and how do you get it?

In most areas the pill currently requires a prescription from a healthcare provider. Some providers require a sexual health or general exam before they will provide a prescription, others do not. You pick up pills at your pharmacy or health center each month or in whatever number of cycles your pharmacist is willing to dispense them. Part or all of the cost of hormonal methods are sometimes included in health insurance plans or public health care, so costs may be lower than stated above.

Pros and Cons, Risks and Benefits

Beyond a high level of effectiveness when used properly, some benefits of hormonal contraceptives can include reducing some kinds of PMS and menstrual pain, lightening monthly flow, aiding with acne, and reducing risks of many reproductive cancers, PID, and anemia.

The pill can also help with irregular menstrual bleeding, though it does not permanently "regulate" periods—in fact,

"I'm on birth control"

When many people say that, they mean the pill, and many people only know of the pill as a method of effective birth control. But the pill is only one *kind*; there are other kinds, too. The pill is a great method for some people and a totally crap one for others. So, if you're asking a healthcare provider about birth control, and all they're suggesting is the pill, be sure to ask them to consider all your birth control options with you, not just pick this one.

because someone taking the combination pill correctly isn't ovulating, the flow at the end of a cycle of pills isn't a menstrual period. Instead, it is a *withdrawal bleed* because the body is withdrawing from the hormones in the previous active pills. Some people assume it does regulate menstrual cycles because, after they have been on the pill and then have come off, periods have become more regular. But because it usually takes a few years of menstruating for cycles to become regular, what's more likely to be happening, especially if the pill was started in adolescence as it often is, is that periods have become more regular on their own simply as a result of the passage of time.

It's normal, while on the pill, for monthly flow to be lighter than usual and even for someone to miss a period occasionally or only to spot.

The combined pill isn't right for everyone. Some conditions that may make the pill a poor birth control choice or prevent a doctor from prescribing it to young people are high blood pressure, liver disease, hepatitis infection, reproductive cancers or a history of blood clots, unexplained vaginal bleeding, migraine headaches, or depression. Some studies have also suggested that combined hormonal contraceptives, including the pill, may inhibit the normal growth of bone mass that occurs during puberty and that is important for healthy adult development, so if you're under twenty, just ask your doctor about bone mass.

All hormonal contraceptives carry similar possible side effects, to greater or lesser degrees, which often include loss of or changes in libido/decreased sexual desire, vaginal dryness, nausea, headaches, mood changes or depression, tender breasts, weight changes, missed periods or prolonged absence of menstruation, and/or spotting. Serious risks, which generally are rare in patients prescribed the

TECH TIP

With hormonal contraceptives, timing truly is everything. For these methods to work and be highly effective, pills have to be taken every day, and rings, patches, and injections swapped or redone on schedule. If you have a mobile device of any kind, you can use the alarm or calendar functions to easily help you remember. And because they'll only beep just like for anything else—it's not like those alarms will yell out, "Time for birth control!"—no one but you has to know what they're for.

Menstrual suppression

BCPs can be used to suppress menstruation by skipping placebo periods and taking active pill packs back to back. Some brands of the pill are designed expressly for this purpose. Doing so may suppress bleeding for a cycle . . . or it may not. Sometimes bleeding still occurs, and sometimes someone may experience spotting during the weeks afterward.

Medical organizations currently advise that a person should not have fewer than four periods each year, and at this time, no data are available about any long-term effects of menstrual suppression, nor have specific studies been done on suppression in younger people. Given that (1) we don't have those data yet, (2) we do know of certain positive health benefits of menstruation, like helping to rid the vagina of bacteria, and (3) hormonal methods already pose extra risks to younger people in terms of bone mass (and those risks may logically increase when more active pills each month are taken), just check in with a healthcare provider first, before you suppress your period.

pill wisely (taking into account factors that may increase risks), include liver and gallbladder disease, bone density changes, blood clots, heart attack, and stroke. Risks and side effects are more likely with combined, rather than singular, hormonal methods.

Sometimes, the pill isn't the best choice for young people, because remembering to take any kind of medication every day can be difficult—especially if a medication is something someone has to hide and only take in secret. (For those who want or need, for whatever reason, a method they can hide, an IUD, the implant, or a Depo-Provera injection works better for that, and these methods also happen to be the most goofproof and effective reversible methods available.)

Progestin-Only Oral Contraceptives, or Minipills

Minipills are ever-so-slightly less effective than the combination pill. That's mostly because they have a grace period to take them on time of only three hours rather than one of twelve to twenty-four hours. It's their typical use rate where the difference lies, because it's so easy to take a pill late. Minipills work like combined oral contraceptives do, they just don't have any estrogen, and an active pill is taken every day (there's no placebo week like with combined pills).

Minipills are a good option for people who want to use oral contraceptives but can't take combination pills because of the risks estrogen presents in terms of blood clots, high blood pressure, headaches, or other issues or who want to use a birth control pill without the typical side effects estrogen presents.

The Vaginal Ring

Effectiveness with perfect use: More than 99% effective

Effectiveness with typical use: 92% effective

Cost: **$$**, including cost of exam

What is it, and how does it work?

The vaginal ring is a combination hormonal method that works the same way the pill does, and it is used a lot like a tampon or menstrual cup. It's small and flexible; you insert it into your vagina—into the canal, and it then rights itself at the far back of the vagina, circling the cervix—once every four weeks, and you wear it there for three weeks and remove it for the fourth. A new ring is used at the beginning of the next cycle. The hormones are contained in the ring, which releases them into the bloodstream.

Where and how do you get it?

The ring is available by prescription from your doctor, gynecologist, or sexual health clinic.

Pros and Cons, Risks and Benefits

The ring carries the same possible benefits, risks, and side effects as other combined hormonal contraceptives and may be a good choice for those who want a low-maintenance hormonal contraceptive they do not have to remember to take daily. Some people do experience an increase in vaginal infections or irritation while using the ring.

For someone who wants the kind of protection birth control pills offer but who doesn't want to or can't remember to take a pill every day around the same time, the ring provides an easier option.

The person "wearing" the ring or their partner may be able to feel it, but that isn't associated with pain, discomfort, or reduction of pleasure. Sometimes, the ring can slip out, but as long as it's reinserted right away, slipping won't make it less effective. However, it's okay to remove the ring for up to three hours (and no longer than three hours every twenty-four hours; so, for example, taking it out for two on Tuesday morning and taking it out again for more than an hour on Tuesday night won't allow it to be effective), so if someone prefers to not have it in during sex with partners, they don't have to.

The Patch

Effectiveness with perfect use: More than 99% effective

Effectiveness with typical use: 92% effective

Cost: **$$**, including cost of exam

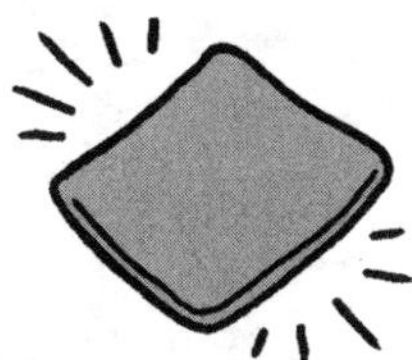

What is it, and how does it work?

The patch contains the same hormones as combined oral contraceptives and works by delivering those hormones into the bloodstream through the skin to suppress ovulation each cycle. The patch is just like a nicotine patch, affixed to the skin on either the upper outer arm or the belly below the waist or the back, where it remains for one week before it is replaced with a new patch in a new place on the body. As with birth control pills, users will have one hormone-free week in the cycle, so for one week they don't wear a patch but are protected from pregnancy during that week, as they are when the patches are worn during the other three weeks.

Where and how do you get it?

The patch is available by prescription from your healthcare provider.

Pros and Cons, Risks and Benefits

The patch is a good choice for people who want to use a hormonal contraceptive but who have trouble remembering pills every day and who don't want to or can't use a longer-acting form of hormonal contraception like an injection or implant (see below and page 365). Patches are generally very resilient and can be worn during bathing, swimming, and showers.

However, if a patch user is late applying a new patch (and the same goes for those using the pill or ring again after the week off), they won't be effectively protected for that week or the next. That is also the case if a patch falls off and stays off for more than a day.

Some people experience skin reactions to the patch. If someone is trying to hide that they're using birth control, the patch may not be ideal (on the other hand, it really does look just like a nicotine patch, so one could always say they were quitting smoking). In addition, the patch *may* be less effective for people who weigh more than 198 pounds. It has also been suggested that the patch presents a risk of stroke higher than that of the birth control pill; fatality from any hormonal contraception method is extremely rare, but it is always something to consider when choosing a method.

The Injection (Depo-Provera)

Effectiveness with perfect use: More than 99% effective
Effectiveness with typical use: 97% effective
Cost: Around **$$**, including cost of exam and office visits

What is it, and how does it work?

Depo-Provera (DMPA) is an injection of progestin that is given to someone by a healthcare professional every three months, four times each year. It works in the same ways that birth control pills do: by preventing ovulation, thickening cervical mucus, and theoretically by thinning the uterine lining.

Where and how do I get it?

Depo-Provera is available through a healthcare provider.

Pros and Cons, Risks and Benefits

The injection is a good choice for someone who wants a really low-maintenance, highly effective method they don't have to worry about remembering about too often. For people who can't take hormonal contraceptives with estrogen, the injection may be a good option. It also affords the user a high level of privacy in use and is pretty goofproof as long as injections are obtained on time every three months.

It's not unusual while on DMPA to have extremely light bleeding or stop monthly flow altogether, which may be a benefit for some people and a downside for others. Some people experience the opposite: persistent or constant bleeding or spotting.

It has been shown in some studies to present some risks of bone density loss, which is a particular concern for people going through a time of life when they need to be developing bone density to get them through the rest of life. If you want the injection, talk with your healthcare provider about this; they may even prescribe you a good calcium supplement to use while using the injection. Studies have shown, however, that bone density returns to normal if and when people stop using the injection.

Frequent spotting is more likely with the injection than it is with combined hormonal methods. Because it's long-acting, that can also mean that, if and when someone stops it, it can take a longer time to leave the body—which can stink if someone stopped because they were having side effects they don't want to deal with. The injection is also the one hormonal method that *is* (the rest aren't) associated with weight gain, whether someone views that possibility as a positive or negative.

The Implant

Effectiveness: More than 99% effective in both perfect and typical use

Cost: **$$$**

What is it, and how does it work?

A birth control implant is a flexible plastic rod inserted by a healthcare professional under the skin of the arm, inside fat that is between the skin and muscle. It works by releasing a progestin (a hormone) slowly and in tiny amounts over time into the bloodstream. That hormone suppresses ovulation and thickens cervical mucus to prevent pregnancy. Hormonal implants are one of the most effective methods of contraception.

How and where do I get it?

Implants are only available through a healthcare provider, who will insert the implant for you. Your healthcare provider will also remove the implant when it's time to swap it out—an implant can be used for up to three or four years—or any time you want to stop using it.

Pros and Cons, Risks and Benefits

Unlike the injection, an implant can be removed immediately if a user just cannot deal with it or no longer wants it. As with ceasing any hormonal method, it usually takes your body at least a few cycles to get back to normal, but removal of the implant should cease many of the most intense side effects pretty quickly. It is very rare for patients to have any complications with insertion or removal.

People using an implant may have very unpredictable vaginal bleeding or spotting. If you know or think you cannot deal with potentially having light spotting as much as all the time, you'll want to consider a different method, because that frequency of spotting is possible with an implant (not very likely, but possible, and it happens this way for some users). The implant also has the same or similar possible side effects as other hormonal methods.

On the other hand, the implant has the capability of making birth control a total no-brainer for a long time. Like the injection, it does not contain estrogen, so it is a hormonal option for people who cannot tolerate estrogens well or use estrogen at all, and it also works immediately, as long as it is inserted between days one and five of the menstrual cycle.

IUDs

Effectiveness: 99%+ effective in both perfect and typical use

Cost: Around **$$$**

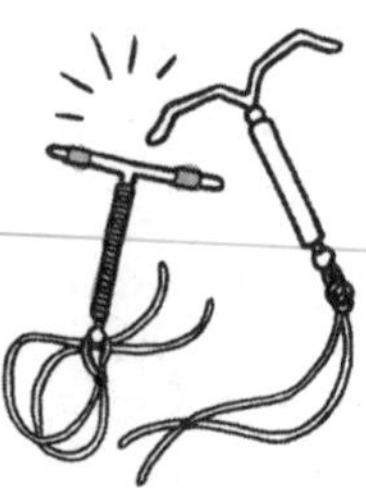

What is it, and how does it work?

An IUD is a T-shaped device that contains either copper or the hormone progesterone and that is placed inside the uterus. IUDs work by getting in the way of and disrupting how sperm cells would otherwise get to and connect with an ovum: think of them as a big-time road block. An IUD is inserted into the uterus through the cervical opening by a healthcare provider. A local anesthetic may be used to manage momentary discomfort or pain with insertion. A soft bit of string is sometimes left outside the cervix so the person with the IUD can then check at least once a month to make sure the IUD is still placed as it should be, but some providers don't recommend string checks: just do whatever your provider recommends, but know that currently string checks aren't considered necessary. Sexual partners cannot feel the IUD itself because it's in the uterus, not the vagina, and most also cannot feel the string. One IUD can net a person anywhere from three to twelve years of highly effective, supereasy contraception, depending on the type of IUD inserted. If someone wants to become pregnant while they have an IUD, they simply have the IUD removed. Someone wanting to keep using an IUD after its time is up just has the previous IUD removed and gets a new one inserted.

Where and how do I get it?

You can get an IUD by seeing your sexual healthcare provider, who will evaluate you as a candidate for the IUD. If they feel you're good to go, they will insert it for you. Like most methods, the cost of an IUD depends on whether someone has any healthcare coverage for the device. The price tag for an IUD without any financial healthcare coverage is usually between $600 and $1,000.

Pros and Cons, Risks and Benefits

Typical side effects of the IUD include cramping during and a little after insertion, increased menstrual flow, and an increased risk of infections for the first three weeks after insertion. Copper IUDs tend to cause longer and heavier bleeding and more cramping during periods. Those with localized hormone do not often have those side effects, and hormonal IUDs can result in less flow, fewer cramps, or more infrequent periods, which some people may like, whereas others may not.

Unlike methods where the user has to do things to make a method work—like putting in a cervical barrier or taking a pill each day—once they're inserted, IUDs just do their thing without any help, which makes them a great choice for people who either find they can't or don't want to administer a method themselves consistently, correctly, and frequently.

Although IUDs are generally considered one of the most highly effective forms of birth control—both in perfect use and typical use, because once they're in, there are no pills to skip or steps to forget—they're not for everyone. They are not advised for anyone who has an active genital or pelvic infection, who has cervical or uterine cancer, who has unexplained vaginal bleeding, or who may be pregnant.

For a long time—including when the first edition of this book was published—IUDs were often not recommended for young people because of concerns about increased risks of infections, greater risk of expulsion, and increased difficulty with insertion of the device and discomfort afterward, particularly if someone hadn't been previously pregnant or given birth. But many studies, including a biggie done in 2013 by the American College of Obstetricians and Gynecologists, gathered and interpreted data from about ninety thousand IUD users, including young people and people who had never been pregnant before. They found that **fewer than 1 percent had any complications.** These findings and others like them—as well as the high effectiveness rate and ease of perfect use—changed the recommendations for IUDs and young people. The ACOG and other reputable major health organizations now recommend IUDs for teens and emerging adults. Until this new research evidence became available, fears about medical complications tended to limit the use of IUDs.

It used to be that IUDs were also recommended only for people in monogamous marriages or other long-term sexually exclusive relationships because increased risks of some health complications due to STIs while someone had an IUD were a concern (which was foolish, because married people and people in long-term relationships can and do get STIs, too). We now know that in the first few weeks—not forever, just in those first few weeks—after insertion of an IUD, people can be more susceptible to developing an STI and possible complications from one, whatever their relationship status. To account for this and play it safe, everyone should be—and usually is—tested for STIs before having an IUD inserted (and, if they have an infection, will need to treat it) and should use condoms and other safer sex barriers for those first few weeks to reduce any STI risks.

Hormones: Without or With?

The ParaGard Copper-T IUD—which contains no synthetic hormones—is a small, T-shaped piece of plastic wrapped with copper. It can remain in the uterus for as long as twelve years but can be removed at any time for any reason, if someone wants to become pregnant or wants to switch to another method. People who have allergies or sensitivities to any part of the other kind of IUD, the kind with the hormone levonorgestrel, people who want a method that can be left in place for as many as twelve years, those who want to avoid any synthetic hormones in their contraception, and people who want to be sure they still get periods every month may find the Copper-T to be their best choice.

The other kind of IUD—the current common brands are Mirena, Skyla, and Liletta—contains a small amount of localized hormone in the device. It is also a small, T-shaped piece of plastic, but it is not wrapped with copper. It contains a very small amount of levonorgestrel, a non-estrogen hormone (so it's okay for those who do not want or cannot use estrogen). That hormone helps prevent a typical and unwanted side effect of the Copper-T: longer, heavier, or more painful periods. The hormone also changes cervical mucus to make it harder for sperm to get to the cervix (the copper is what does that with the Copper-T IUD).

Most using this kind of IUD have shorter, lighter periods, and some people may stop having periods altogether, which some see as a bonus and others are not comfortable with. This kind of IUD can be left in place for a shorter period of time than the other: just three to five years. People who want lighter and shorter periods, who are okay with a possible absence of periods (but accept spotting may still occur erratically), or who have allergies to copper may find a hormonal IUD to be their best choice.

To sort out which would be best for you, talk with your healthcare provider.

WHEN USING ANY KIND OF HORMONAL CONTRACEPTIVE . . .

If at any time, you are experiencing any of the following symptoms, it is very important that you call your doctor:

- Sharp chest pain, coughing blood, or shortness of breath
- Persistent pains in the legs or abdomen
- Severe headaches, dizziness, fainting, weakness, vision problems, numbness in the arms or legs, or vomiting
- Severe depression or mood changes
- Yellowing of the skin, lasting tiredness, loss of appetite
- Breast lumps or heavy vaginal bleeding

Emergency Contraception (EC)

Although it's always best to use a reliable method of birth control, and preferably a backup as well, even reliable birth control sometimes fails. Or sometimes someone just doesn't use a method of birth control at all, even when they don't want to become pregnant. It used to be that a hope and a prayer for no pregnancy was all that was available in these situations. Now we have emergency contraception, which, unlike hopes and prayers, actually works very well to prevent pregnancy.

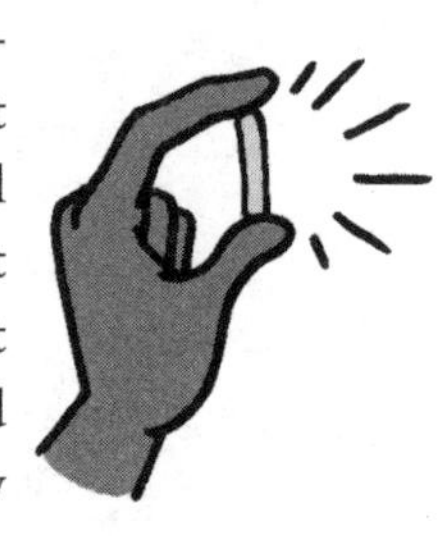

Emergency contraception can decrease the risk of pregnancy by 75 to 95 percent when used within 120 hours (five days) of a risk. When using emergency contraception pills, seven out of every eight people who would have become pregnant will not. EC is relatively inexpensive (usually between $25 and $50, though can be often acquired more cheaply through health clinics), carries very few side effects (far, far, *FAR* fewer than a pregnancy!), and is easy to use.

There are two forms of EC currently available: emergency contraceptive pills (often called the morning-after pill—though it's most effective when used before the next morning—or Plan B)

DID YOU KNOW? . . .

Some people say that ECPs contain a *massive* amount of hormones, which can make EC sound dangerous and scary—but that isn't true. The amount of hormone in most brands of EC is the equivalent of just over four days' worth of minipills: the amount of hormone in one usage of most emergency contraceptive pills is around 1.5 mg of a progestin; one day's worth of a common minipill with the same kind of hormone is usually around 0.35 mg. Plus, unless someone is using combined oral contraceptives as emergency contraception, ECPs usually contain no estrogen, which is the hormone in hormonal contraception that presents more risks and often gives people more trouble when it comes to side effects.

and the IUD. A Copper-T IUD may be inserted for emergency contraception and can reduce the risk of pregnancy by more than 99 percent: only 1 in 1,000 people who use the IUD as EC will become pregnant. The cost of an IUD as a method of emergency contraception is the same as the cost of an IUD inserted at any time. The cost of emergency contraceptive pills, when not covered by healthcare plans, usually ranges between $30 and $60 per use.

Emergency contraceptive pills (ECPs) are the most common form of EC and typically the easiest to access and use. They can be used within 120 hours of a risk, but the sooner the pill or pills are taken, the more likely it is to be effective. The highest effectiveness ratings for ECPs are for use **within 24 hours of a risk.** How to take the kind of EC obtained is always explained in the patient information that comes with it or by your healthcare provider or pharmacist. The pills contain the synthetic hormone progestin, like the minipill, and work the same way: by inhibiting or delaying ovulation and preventing fertilization of the egg.

There are no known serious or long-term side effects of ECPs. Common side effects—which usually last for several days when someone experiences them at all—are nausea or vomiting, headache, dizziness, breast tenderness, spotting, or fatigue. It's also common after taking ECPs for menstrual periods to begin a bit sooner or later than usual in the current or next menstrual cycle.

ECPs can now be obtained over the counter without a prescription for people of all ages in most areas. Sometimes EC is on the shelves of a pharmacy, just like tampons or analgesics; other times it is kept behind the pharmacy counter so that you need to ask for it. If you do not meet the age requirement for over-the-counter purchase where you live, or you live in an area where EC is not available over the counter, period, you will need a prescription to obtain it. You can get that prescription by calling or seeing your regular doctor, gynecologist, general or sexual health clinician or by going into the emergency room or an urgent care center. An office visit may or may not be required to get a prescription. If you ask, some clinics, doctors, or gynecologists may also be willing to give you a prescription for ECPs during your regular annual exam so you can have them on hand in

IS EC ABORTION?

Abortion is the termination of an existing pregnancy. Emergency contraception can only help *prevent* pregnancy. EC is *not* abortion (nor are ECPs mifepristone, RU-486, or the medications used for medical abortion) because it can only work *before* pregnancy has occurred, just as birth control pills do, and it can only work if a pregnancy has not yet happened. It cannot and will not terminate a pregnancy if a person is already pregnant. If that seems confusing, remember that pregnancy is not instant: it often takes several days to a week to occur, which is why EC can be an effective means of preventing pregnancy for a few days after a risk.

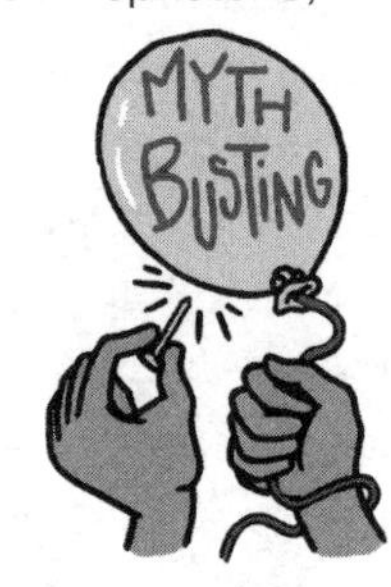

advance in case of emergency. Because EC works best when taken as soon as possible, having either a prescription or a pack of ECPs available, just in case, can make getting it when you need it a whole lot easier.

When you are given a prescription for ECPs, your doctor or clinician should give you clear directions for how to take them. If they do not or if you have additional questions, be sure to ask. You can also ask your pharmacist for additional information.

Some regular birth control pills can also be used as emergency contraception if you cannot access medications designed and prescribed specifically as EC. To find out which pills to take as EC, call the gynecologist, pharmacist, or sexual health clinician who prescribes your birth control pills for instructions or see the Resources section of this book.

ECPs are not advised as regular contraception. There are no known dangers in doing so, but they are not as effective as many other methods of contraception (including combined oral contraceptives or minipills used daily) and would be terribly expensive if used often. ECPs also are not effective preventatively: you can't take them before sex for use as birth control.

Copper-T Intrauterine Device

A copper IUD can also be inserted as emergency contraception up to five days after a pregnancy risk, just like the timing for ECP use. Using an IUD is more effective than ECPs, and if the IUD is right for you, it can then be left in place for as long as twelve years as ongoing birth control. Since IUDs are expensive, it probably won't be a method of EC someone chooses if they don't intend to keep it in afterward. For more information on IUDs, see page 366.

Birth Control Methods Not Generally Recommended for Young People

Withdrawal (aka "Pulling Out")

Withdrawal means that a partner with a penis withdraws from the vagina before ejaculating. It is only about 76 percent effective in typical use, tops, and is known to be less effective for teens and young adults. We don't have clinical trials for withdrawal to say for sure how effective it is in perfect use, but estimates of its "perfect" effectiveness are around 96 percent.

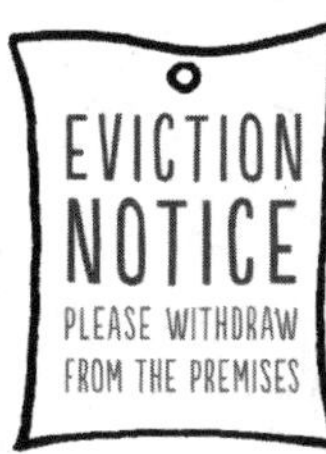

The thing about withdrawal is that for someone to be able to use it effectively they have to be very, very familiar with their own sexual responses with sex with partners. In other words, they need to have the ability to know, *before* it starts to happen at all, when orgasm or ejaculation is around the bend and to withdraw in advance of that happening—not at the time of or just-just before, but in advance. Someone using withdrawal perfectly also needs to be very good at not getting caught up in the moment during parts of sexual response when getting all caught up and lost in it is usually exactly what's happening. When we're at the point when we're about to orgasm, our bodies are actually clouding our minds a little bit, so that's one of the toughest times during sex to think clearly. That person also needs to have the ability to—and be okay with—stopping intercourse right at a time when it often feels best to a lot of people: right around orgasm is usually when more people are feeling and saying, "Please, don't stop." That's something that tends to take a good deal of sexual and life experience, so even for young people who truly intend to use withdrawal correctly, it can be very difficult to do it right, especially consistently.

So, even though withdrawal is more popular with younger people than other age groups—more than anything, that's probably because it's free and no one has to ask anyone for it—as it turns out, it's one of the hardest for young people to use properly.

Withdrawal also puts all the control over reproduction in the hands, per se, of the person who themselves cannot become pregnant. For this person, the potential for pregnancy may be an issue that's less big or immediate for them because it wouldn't be happening inside of and to their own body. And if reproductive coercion is afoot, unfortunately, using only withdrawal as a birth control method makes coercion very easy to accomplish.

Fertility Charting/Natural Family Planning (FAM)

Natural family planning can be done using one of several methods. The least effective methods are counting the days in the cycle to estimate or guess when ovulation might occur on the basis of average fertile times for all people (sometimes called the *rhythm method*) and using online ovulation charts, which only count cycle days to estimate ovulation—these are mostly ineffective methods because there are no specific days during which **everyone** is fertile or infertile. Fertility timing varies: someone may be most fertile on the eleventh day of their cycle; someone else on the sixteenth. Some people even ovulate more than once per cycle. During certain phases of the cycle—namely, the final week of each cycle and during menstruation—conception is generally *less* likely for most people.

So, although a majority of people are unlikely to be fertile just before and during menses, this should never be assumed to be a given, and there is a real risk of pregnancy any time there's been direct vaginal or vulval contact with semen, most commonly during penis-in-vagina intercourse. There are times in the fertility cycle (usually just around and during ovulation, when the mucus of the vagina is most friendly toward sperm and a fertile ovum is available in the fallopian tube) when someone is *more* likely to become pregnant than other times. But, technically, a person can get pregnant at nearly any time in a cycle when live sperm cells enter the cervix, and because cycles differ, there is no one "safe time" for everyone.

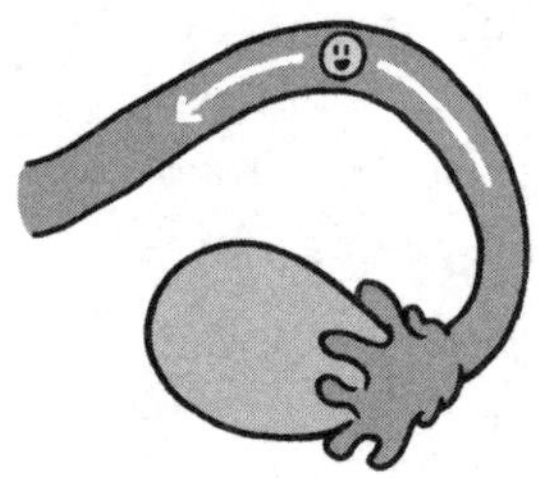

A more effective method of natural family planning is a combination of observing and charting cervical mucus—its texture and consistency are different during different phases of the cycle—and taking basal temperature readings daily; basal body temperature fluctuates as someone's fertility changes over the course of the cycle. Currently, handheld calculators on the market can be used to chart and track fertility, and some fertility websites or software use mucus and basal temperatures to help people chart.

When used properly, FAM can be very effective and is a good choice for people whose health, finances, or religion may prohibit other methods—and/or for couples who *are* prepared for a pregnancy. However, for it to be effective as contraception, not only does charting have to happen daily and consistently but also the results of the charting have to be interpreted correctly and unprotected intercourse can occur *only* on days when someone is least likely to be fertile based on those results. Because FAM can only give a person information on when ovulation probably occurred after a cycle is finished, estimates are based on previous

TECH TIP

Is a Mobile App Telling You When You're Ovulating?

If so, it's probably guessing and will often be wrong. Only one or two current apps ask for the right kind of information needed to accurately predict fertility and sort out whether that's something someone can do accurately in the first place. To find out whether you even could track, chart, and predict these things, an app would need to ask some screening questions, like if you're using a method of contraception that suppresses ovulation (in which case ovulation can't be tracked because it isn't happening) and if your menstrual cycles are regular (if not, you just can't make accurate predictions about fertility). If your fertility could be predicted, for the prediction to be as accurate as it can be, the app needs to know more than just when you had a period. It also needs you to be able to interpret and input daily cervical mucus changes, basal body temperatures, or, ideally, both. If you're going to use FAM, make sure, if you don't do it by hand yourself, any tool you're using really can do accurate planning instead of just claiming it can.

cycles. For teens or emerging adults whose cycles have not become regular yet (which is very common in the first five years of menstrual periods), this isn't doable.

FAM *can* be used well as backup birth control if it is used in this way: on the basis of the charting results, condoms are used for times thought to be the least fertile, and then a person *abstains from intercourse completely* during their most likely fertile times. And, of course, young people can chart their fertility, even if they are not trying to use those results to prevent pregnancy. Charting can enable someone to become familiar enough with their cycles and their stages that, when they're nervous about a possible pregnancy due to birth control failure, they may be able to recognize irregularities. Anyone using hormonal contraceptive methods simply cannot chart fertility because if those methods are being used correctly the person is not ovulating—and thus, fertile—in the first place.

Permanent Birth Control (Sterilization)

"Permanent" methods of contraception—like tubal ligation or vasectomy—are some of the most effective methods there are (IUDs and implants, though, are actually more effective, believe it or not!) and are forever for most people. Most permanent methods are done via surgeries; the current fallopian tube insert is a nonsurgical procedure. These surgeries are safe; tubal ligation, however, is more invasive and irreversible than vasectomy. These procedures make it so that someone's body just is not going to be capable of or able to co-create a pregnancy **for good,** either because that's how someone wants it—some sterilizations can be reversed—or because their permanent method simply is just that: permanent.

For that reason, permanent birth control is rarely offered to young people because of issues with informed consent and because the decision whether to ever reproduce is generally—not always, but often—one people need more time and life experience to make than childhood and adolescence allow them. These options are also more costly than many young people can afford.

What Isn't a Method of Birth Control?

Douching or vaginal washing: You can't rinse or wash sperm cells from or off of the vagina because by the time you get to a wash area they're already well out of reach of water or soap.

Chance: (See also: fate.) Using no birth control at all—or "letting fate decide"—puts people at an incredibly high risk of pregnancy. Within just one year of unprotected intercourse, pregnancy will occur for around 85 out of every 100 people, according to the World Health Organization. Fate isn't a person: it can't decide this for you. If a person chooses not to use a birth control method, fate isn't making that decision, the person is—they're making the decision to take big risks of pregnancy and also to most likely become pregnant or be part of a pregnancy within the year.

IT DOESN'T TAKE A VILLAGE . . . BUT IT'S AWFULLY NICE TO HAVE ONE: BIRTH CONTROL DISCUSSION WITH PARTNERS AND PARENTS

Anyone who needs birth control has at least one other person intimately involved in that need, so which method to use is a decision made solely by one person. When responsibility for contraception is shared, birth control is always more effective.

Ultimately, because the vast majority of birth control methods can be used only by the person who's got the uterus and because that person bears the greatest risk regarding reproductive choices, I feel very strongly that *the final choice on what to use should always lie with that person.* People who can become pregnant who are not currently in relationships and/or who may have more casual sex partners than partners they're sexual with in an ongoing way often make their birth control choices completely independently of anyone else.

If you're a minor or an emerging adult living with your parents or guardians, financially dependent on them, or wanting to use their health insurance for contraception, some birth control options may also involve your folks. If you're a person who could become pregnant by having sex with a partner, you and that partner may need to agree on a given method if it requires their participation in using it correctly; you may even want to split the cost of birth control. If you're hooking up casually, birth control discussion should still be taking place with partners. If you're someone who can't yourself become pregnant but your partner can, you may want to help by offering to pay for part of the birth control method, by helping them research which methods are best for both of you, and, in some situations, by taking responsibility for the burden of providing and insisting on birth control if you don't want to risk becoming a parent.

With any and every aspect of sex, discussion and communication are key to healthy, smart sexual choices and relationships everyone involved feels good about—and birth control is certainly no exception.

Discussion with Partners

If you're the person who could become pregnant, the responsibility of birth control largely rests with you. Because most methods of birth control go in your body, because you're the one who must deal with taking them as well as with any side effects, and because you are the one who may become pregnant and who'd have the biggest burden to carry, now and lifelong, with any pregnancy, it's really **best** that you are the most responsible and have the most say what is best for you. When it's our lives most involved with something, we always want to be the person most in charge.

If you do currently have a sex partner or partners, whether long term or very casual, then you also have a partner to discuss birth control with.

With a casual partner:

▶ Discussion may be as simple as plainly stating what method you use. If your chosen method is condoms or involves backing up with condoms, make clear that you expect and require condom use with sex. If your partner or partners don't like that, they get to not like that and not use a condom . . . with someone else who feels differently about it than you do. If you set that limit and they don't want to respect it, then they get to opt out but also need to understand they're opting out of sex with you.

- Discussion may also involve stating what choice you would make for yourself in regard to an accidental pregnancy should your method or methods fail. That's a biggie if you feel strongly that whatever choice you will want to make isn't negotiable or up for debate.
- If you're *only* using condoms and a casual partner refuses to, discussion will also involve drawing a line and opting out of sex with a risk of pregnancy with that person. (And it's usually safe to assume that people who refuse to use condoms are the most likely to have STIs to transmit because safer sex practices work so well to prevent most STIs, so you may want to opt out of sexual activity with this person altogether.)

With a partner in an ongoing or more committed partnership:

- Discussions about birth control may be more involved. It's fair and sound to

Reproductive coercion

Reproductive coercion is sexual behavior that aims to obtain or maintain power and control in a relationship related to reproductive health and, often specifically, pregnancy. It's when someone tries to make someone pregnant without their consent or against their will, or when someone makes someone a part of their own attempts to become pregnant deceptively. It can include sexual abuse or assault or sabotage of someone's method or methods of birth control.

This is an abuse, and it is never okay. Any relationship in which reproductive coercion is happening is an abusive relationship. Reproductive coercion is also, unfortunately, common in abusive relationships: a special report on reproductive coercion from the American College of Obstetricians and Gynecologists in 2013 found that 25 percent of young women, specifically, in abusive relationships also report reproductive coercion. Everyone should be afforded the right to choose when they do or do not want to take risks of pregnancy, to become or be pregnant, or to parent. Whether someone perpetrates a sexual assault, throws away a partner's birth control pills, or says they use a contraceptive method to a partner when they don't (with the aim of creating a pregnancy without that person's consent), it is always an abuse, sometimes a punishable crime, and **never** okay.

The same goes double for when you don't agree on using birth control at all. If a partner just plain refuses to use birth control, when neither of you is prepared for or wanting a pregnancy, then the only smart thing to do is flatly refuse to have sex with that person. If the issue is just a simple lack of comfort with discussing birth control, either reevaluate your readiness and take a step back from sex until you *can* discuss it or, if your reticence is due to feeling pressured or controlled by a partner, take a step back from *them.*

share birth control expenses or logistics, for instance. If you can't afford birth control all by yourself or feel those expenses should be shared, this may be a requirement of your sexual partnership. Making it clear that one partner shouldn't always be responsible for reminders about birth control or sexual policing when it comes to contraception is also wise. And if you can't afford it and your partner can't afford to contribute either, it may mean making plans to become sexually active at a later date when you both can afford it.

▶ You may use more than one method over time or tailor what you use more jointly based on discussions about personal preferences, changing safer sex habits, or greater desire for or trust in shared responsibility.

If you're using nothing but condoms for birth control with any sort of partner, a bit more negotiation and discussion is sometimes involved. You may have to step up in terms of insisting on condom use, reminding your partner when to put a condom on, or making sure you have plenty of them, and lubricant, on hand. If a partner complains about discomfort, you may have to experiment with different brands or types until you find a condom that works. Making sure that you—not just your partner—know how to use them properly is also essential: don't leave all of this up to someone else. The same goes for a shared method such as abstinence or natural family planning that requires your partner to abstain from sex completely or periodically to be effective.

Sometimes, partners may tell you that a given method of birth control is what they most want to use, even though it's really a method *you* will be using, taking, and largely responsible for. Let's say your boyfriend feels the pill is the best choice for both of you. You can research it, look into it, and weigh all the issues with it. You may come to an agreement that the pill is a choice you both feel good about. Or you may not. If you feel differently, you can certainly explain why (you don't want to take a pill every day; you don't like the side effects or health risks), but you shouldn't be engaging in huge arguments about it because it's *your* body it would be

Birth Control Issues to Discuss with Partners (the Short List)

- **Effectiveness, ease of use, and availability:** Does what you each want work well? Can one or both of you easily access and use the method? Are both of you open to trying different methods to find the best ones for you, which can take some experimenting sometimes?
- **Birth control backup:** Do you need it or want it? If so, what combined methods will you use?
- **Responsibility:** Whose is it? How will you work it together without unduly burdening one partner? How will you pay for it?
- **Failure:** If birth control fails, what would both of you want to do? Are you in agreement on that? How might you handle it? Who would you ask for help?

going in, not his. If he isn't comfortable with sex using any method but the one he has suggested—or he doesn't want to use birth control at all—then he has the power to opt out of sex with you, and you with him. And that'd be the right way to play this rather than trying to talk someone into or out of any kind of health behavior or choice that's mostly about them and mostly involves them that they don't want to do.

Having to opt out is not a fun situation to be in. But being sexually active with a partner with whom you don't agree on a birth control method or who wants to control you in any way involving contraception choices is a really bad idea. A sound golden rule is this: Whichever partner is at risk for more side effects, permanent body changes, big life upheavals, and other consequences of a possible pregnancy should get the final say when it comes to how all of that is prevented.

Reproductive Choice, Sans Uterus

Even when you're not the one who can become pregnant but can be someone who is part of causing a pregnancy, you still get choices and should ideally participate in birth control use and responsibility just as much as your partner (as much as they want you to, anyway). Understand that many methods, such as hormonal birth control like the pill or Depo-Provera, carry risks and side effects for the person using them (and they don't offer any STI protection).

So, although it may seem to you that a given method you don't have to do anything with yourself is best and easiest for *you,* your partner may not feel the same way because they're the one who needs to live with it, short and long term. For instance, they may have a diminished desire for sex due to the chemical changes a method creates, they may have less natural lubrication because of the pill, and they are the one who must remember to take a pill at the same time every day. If a given method that a partner would use, not you, seems like a good choice from your perspective, by all means, bring it up for discussion, but know that the decision is primarily not yours to make, nor are you the best person to be making that decision.

It might be difficult for you to understand the weight of birth control use for people who are using something much more complex and invasive than a condom, for you to comprehend how much someone who *can* become pregnant has to think about it, and how much real estate it takes up in their head. Although it's become a bit of a convention for couples to say, *"We're pregnant!"* **there is no *we* here** unless both people actually *are* pregnant—and someone without a uterus can't be.

In a way, birth control is not unlike safer sex practices, which you know plenty about. Think about the flip-flopping that sometimes goes on in your head when you're making those decisions:

*Do I **really** need to use a condom for oral sex?*

Can I get away with not using one for intercourse just this once?

Didn't I hear their ex cheated—what if they got a disease from them?

When do I ask them about it? How will they react?

Do I even have condoms with me tonight?

You recognize those conflicted feelings: the strong desire to avoid an STI, and sometimes even how it just feels tiresome or kills your buzz to have to bring worries and practical issues to bed with you. Your partner, who can become pregnant, shoulders all those same issues about safer sex, like you, **and** all of those sorts of issues when it comes to pregnancy and birth control. It may feel superstressful for you to think about contraception, but figure that for however stressful it is for you—however much a big, scary deal it feels like for you, who cannot become pregnant—it's that much more stressful and scary for the person who could actually become and be pregnant.

If you're in a long-term or committed sexual partnership, I think it's a great idea to suggest that you can help to shoulder aspects of birth control you can contribute to, like paying for it, helping with transportation to OB/GYN visits, or playing your part when it comes to using a given method.

It may also happen that you someday have a partner who isn't responsible about their part in birth control or who wishes to become pregnant when you really don't wish to be involved in that. In those situations, the burden of birth control via condoms—or by vetoing sex if you don't agree with them about readiness for parenthood—may lie solely on you, and you have every right to insist that your *own* choices be respected. It's also completely okay for you to insist on backup via condom use, if you need or want it for your own security, even if your partner has told you they already use an additional method. Whereas trying to control someone else and what is mostly about their body and life *isn't* okay, setting limits and boundaries of your own when it comes to what you want and need most certainly *is*. Of course, if you ever have any reason to believe you can't trust your partner to be honest and ethical about contraception, the best tack is not to sexually partner with them at all. Trust is an important and vital part of a healthy sexual partnership, and being trustworthy is part of being ready to be sexual with other people.

Sparing vasectomy, the currently available methods *you* can use that are directed by you or reliant upon you are withdrawal and condom use. Withdrawal is easy to mess up, whereas learning to use condoms like a boss is pretty easy. Beyond safer sex issues—only condoms give you and your partners protection against infections—condom use makes for an excellent birth control backup for any other method, so insisting on it and being in charge of that aspect of birth control can be an important role for you.

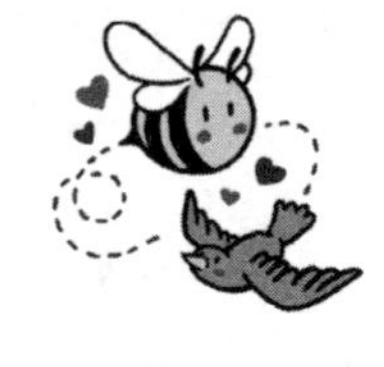

On the other hand, you may feel ready for parenthood when your partner isn't or you may wish not to worry about birth control altogether. In other words, it may be you thinking about the birth control sabotage or about behaving irresponsibly. Thing is . . . well, let's not tiptoe. *That's not okay.* If you're ready for sexual partnership, you need to also be ready to deal with birth control and to respect your partner's

How NOT to Ask Parents o
for Help with Birth Cont

- *"If you don't get it for me/pay for it, I'll get pregnant."* I really hope you're not saying this (especially after all that talk about personal responsibility in choosing to be sexually active). Blackmail of any sort is never very effective, especially when the one who'd pay for it most is the person threatening it. A better way of addressing this issue is to say, *"I am choosing to be sexually active because I feel I'm ready, and I'm asking for your help with birth control because I think I'd benefit from your help so I can do this most responsibly."*

- *"But you didn't use it, and see, you had me!"* Rubbing parents' faces in their own mistakes (when they feel they were mistakes) is a fine way to piss them off and make them really upset—not a good way to come to an agreement or get an endorsement. Sexual shaming also is no more okay to do to parents than it is for them or anyone else to do to you. A better bet may be: *"I know that you had an accidental pregnancy, and I understand, but I don't want the same for myself, and I know I can avoid that by using reliable birth control."*

- *"Then I'll just get it myself and you'll never know."* The only thing this is good for is to pretty much guarantee your parents will henceforth not trust you, and your social and sexual life will suffer fo
be a better approach: *"I really*
able to be honest with you about
being tempted to lie or hide things fr
you, because that's just not the kind of r
tionship I want us to have." Plus, if you do want to just get birth control yourself and not have parents know—which is certainly your right—then telling them about it would be pretty silly.

- *"But [insert friend's name here]'s mother got it for them."* Y'all know the drill on this one, and probably even know what your parent is likely to say about cliffs and friends jumping off them or about *life* not being fair. Like it or not, for the most part, every parent gets to make the parenting choices on the basis of what *they* feel is best for them, their family, and you, if you're their child. If you want your parent to help get you birth control (and so, feel envious of your friend), you can perhaps ask your friend's parent if they would be willing to, even in just casual conversation, mention to your parent that they help your friend with birth control access. But mostly, what you want is your parent's or guardian's help accessing birth control. So, what you want to say, instead, is just this: *"I'd really like your help with getting birth control. Would you be willing to help me?"*

... with both of you. That's not just an ethical issue, it's a practical one: if you don't, and a pregnancy does occur, your partner can hold you legally responsible should they choose to see a pregnancy through to term. So, even though it may feel like it's not your issue, and you do have limited choices in the matter, a good deal of responsibility does still lie with you, and to be a good partner, you need to step up and take charge of the aspects you can control.

Discussions with Parents

If you're a minor, are living at home, or are dependent on your parents financially (even just for health care), they may be people you've got to discuss all or some aspects of birth control with, too.

Although some parents may not be especially jazzed that their children—whatever their age—are sexually active, many *are* going to be supportive of their growing-into-adult children having sex responsibly, which certainly includes using birth control for those kinds of sex that carry pregnancy risks. Some parents are even willing to help pay for contraceptive methods or to make sure you're able to obtain them by doing things like helping you get to and from doctor appointments or to the pharmacy.

Some parents will not be willing to pay for birth control methods and will insist that you're on your own with that. That's fair enough; after all, if you're ready for partnered sex, some of that readiness is about the ability to be responsible for sex, including getting the essentials for yourself. Or your parents may be willing to help but with certain conditions attached, so you may have to do some negotiating with them about with whom, where, when, or in what situations you're sexually active, about what methods you use, or about who will shoulder responsibility, financial and otherwise, should your birth control fail.

As in any other negotiations with parents or guardians about sex, it's smart to not be in a huge hurry or bring a lot of entitlement to the table. It isn't on parents or guardians to manage your sex life for you, especially with things you often could take care of by and for yourself. So, be prepared to be cool and calm and for loaded issues like birth control to take a few discussions, with plenty of time for both you and your folks to think things over and process in between. Be prepared to offer up and make some compromises—understand that it's possible you may have to agree to disagree or may be allowed to use a given method but without their financial or emotional support.

There's a theme here you might have picked up on, whether you're discussing this issue with partners or parents, and that's honest, patient, and compassionate communication. It's certainly not always easy, especially with stuff as loaded as this is, but being able to talk about sexual choices is an important part of sexual readiness overall and it's going to make your sexual life a whole lot easier and a whole lot better, now *and* later. Birth control isn't the only issue where good communication skills come in handy, but it's a biggie.

We tend to only think about reproductive choice in terms of what we do when a pregnancy occurs. But birth control, choosing when and if we will become pregnant, is also part of reproductive choice—the most important part—that benefits from the support of everyone involved.

13

Oh, Baby (or Not)! Reproduction and Reproductive Options

When a pregnancy has occurred, there are two initial, basic choices to make: staying pregnant—with the aim of either parenthood or arranging an adoption—or terminating the pregnancy with an abortion procedure. These are equally viable and valid choices, and any of them may be the best choice for someone. Sometimes any of these choices can be tremendously difficult to make, sometimes very easy, and, most often, somewhere in between. None of these choices is universally right or universally wrong: just like sexual choices, reproductive choices are highly individual, based on our unique wants and circumstances.

Teen pregnancies account for about 25 percent of all accidental or unplanned pregnancies, and *the other 75 percent*—the great majority—*occur among adults of all ages.* So, no matter your age, it's safe to say that if you are or are thinking about becoming sexually active in ways that present risks of pregnancy, you'll want to inform yourself about reproduction, pregnancy, and parenting and become familiar with how reproduction happens, all of the reproductive options, and their practical realities.

[HOW CAN YOU TELL IF YOU'RE PREGNANT?]

By taking a pregnancy test. There is no other accurate way to know for sure early enough in the game to adequately consider the options.

Early physical responses to pregnancy aren't reliable ways to determine preg-

HOW LONG HAVE YOU GOT TO DECIDE?

For such a big decision, once a pregnancy has occurred there isn't much time to make it:

- In most areas, a person who wants to choose abortion has around **five or six months** after pregnancy occurs before they are outside the window for a safe, legal abortion. The later that decision is made, the fewer the options available, the greater the cost, and the greater the health risks (which always increase the longer a pregnancy goes on, abortion or not). So, it's ideal to make this choice sooner rather than later.
- A person who wants to choose to remain pregnant should get to their first prenatal visit at around **8 to 12 weeks of pregnancy.** This is especially vital for pregnant teens. The main reason pregnancy in younger people presents higher physical risks is not so much physiological as behavioral and situational: lack of prenatal care, inadequate nutrition, lack of needed weight gain, and failure to make needed changes to lifestyle factors (quitting drinking or recreational drug use, for example) are the big players in those increased risks. If someone wants or needs financial help from their country, state, or county—for pregnancy health care or assistance when parenting after a birth—they should ask about or file for that help when they go for a first prenatal visit, or before if they need assistance to get that initial health care.
- A person who wants to choose to remain pregnant and arrange an adoption can make that decision and adoption arrangements any time during pregnancy or after birth. But to best secure a home for a child, make open adoption arrangements, or have any or all prenatal care, childbirth costs, or living expenses during pregnancy paid for, it's best to start contacting adoption agencies and pursuing avenues to adoption **as soon as possible after pregnancy occurs.** (Making adoption arrangements early does not change or remove the right of the pregnant person to rescind their decision to give up the child for adoption: someone choosing adoption can always change their mind at any time before they surrender a child.)

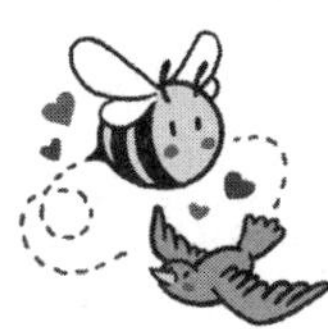

nancy. They usually only occur after at least a few weeks have passed and, most typically, after the first month of pregnancy. Some early things that can happen because of pregnancy can include sore or tingly breasts, a missed period, general nausea, a feeling of tiredness, increased appetite, or having to urinate more often. But these symptoms can also be and often commonly are caused by stress, PMS, puberty, infections, or other illness, or they can even occur psychosomatically (in your head, caused mentally). That's the biggest reason why physical symptoms just are not a good way to try to determine pregnancy.

Some tests are more sensitive than others. You can tell which are more sensitive by looking at the box: those that say they are sensitive to a level of 20 mIU/ml (that is, twenty milli-international units of hCG per milliliter) are more sensitive or

HPTs

Home pregnancy tests (HPTs) work by measuring a hormone called hCG (human chorionic gonadotropin), which is secreted as soon as ten days after conception is complete and which, with only very, very rare exceptions, is a hormone that isn't in the body if there isn't a pregnancy. The most accurate results are found at least two weeks after a pregnancy risk or at the first late or skipped period. A late or missed period is a period that hasn't shown up five or more days later than the very *latest* you'd expect it. So, if you were expecting a period on Tuesday, but you don't have it that same day or a day later, the period is probably not actually late yet because even regular cycles standardly deviate by around two to three days. If, on the other hand, you were expecting it Tuesday, but by Friday at the latest, if it still hasn't shown up by the following Wednesday, it's late.

To know how and when to take an HPT, follow the directions on the box. All tests aren't exactly the same, so the right way to take a test is always the way the directions for a specific test say. When used according to the package directions, home pregnancy tests are just as reliable as clinical tests are.

reliable than those that say they are sensitive to a level of 50 mIU/ml.

False positives are incredibly rare. They may occur in instances in which fertilization or conception has occurred but will not continue to a full pregnancy—bear in mind that as many as half of all fertilizations do not complete to conception. They may also occur with people who take any drugs that contain hCG, such as fertility drugs. (Hormonal birth control methods do *not* contain hCG and do not interfere with pregnancy tests.) False negatives are much more common, but that's often because a test was taken too early or wasn't taken according to the directions.

Blood tests can't usually detect hCG earlier than home urine tests, and they're no more effective. Most healthcare providers will just do the same kind of urine test you can do by yourself at home to test for pregnancy.

A home test should be repeated one week later if it shows a negative result and a period still hasn't arrived. If a test shows a positive result, a visit to a doctor or a clinic should be scheduled to verify the results and to get you directed to whatever kind of health care you will need, whether that's prenatal care or termination preparation.

[PREGNANCY AND DELIVERY BASICS]

Regular prenatal care as well as good nutrition, plenty of rest and activity, reduced stresses, emotional support, and the practical and financial means to obtain all of those things are needed for a healthy pregnancy. Because of increased health risks and social disparities, people who are pregnant as teens or emerging adults need to be *more* dedicated to these issues than older people, not less.

If you or your partner is pregnant and thinking about bringing a pregnancy to term:

- Tobacco, alcohol, and recreational drug use should be stopped, pronto. Fetal health may also be compromised if the person who's pregnant was doing any of those things shortly before pregnancy or when they became pregnant, so someone pregnant with a recent history of smoking, drinking, or doing drugs will need to be honest with their doctor and themselves and ask for whatever help they need to change those habits or address any existing risks. Partners of pregnant people who do any of these things and plan to stick around should also quit because of the way some of those habits can

Within the first few months of pregnancy—the first trimester—a person may experience:

- Feeling more tired than usual
- General nausea or morning sickness
- Frequent urination, gas, constipation, and indigestion
- Physical and emotional symptoms similar to PMS

Often, after the first few months, emotional issues such as feeling irritable or unstable may pass, and into the second trimester, many people begin feeling better about being pregnant than they did in the first trimester, although hormonal changes and new frustrations—like not fitting into clothes, feelings about weight gain, fears and doubts, and other issues—may still cause moods to be erratic. Appetite increases and food cravings as well as food aversions may appear. Weight gain should also have begun by now, and *you will need to make an effort to gain weight* during the rest of the pregnancy.

If someone is choosing to have an abortion procedure, they will usually do so before the end of the first trimester. For information on abortion, see page 398.

Into the second trimester, many of the symptoms from the first few months continue, and a person may also experience:

- Greater fatigue or dizziness
- The pregnancy showing
- Swelling of the ankles and feet
- Changes in vaginal discharge, skin, and hair
- Enlarging breasts
- Headaches or sinus symptoms
- Backaches

In the second trimester, fetal movement a pregnant person can feel also begins and increases throughout the rest of a pregnancy.

In the last few months of pregnancy, the third trimester, many of the symptoms from previous months continue, and, in addition, people usually experience:

- Heavier vaginal discharge
- More intense back and body aches
- Some breast leaking
- Hemorrhoids
- Greater fetal movement
- Trouble sleeping
- Occasional contractions
- Shortness of breath
- Varicose veins
- Clumsiness
- Emotional issues, like feeling seriously sick of being pregnant or big worries about childbirth or parenting

indirectly affect a pregnancy or just to show solidarity and to make changing habits a lot less challenging for the person who's pregnant.

▶ If someone pregnant has an eating disorder or chronically diets, that should be addressed with a healthcare provider. For a healthy pregnancy and child, gaining weight is important.

▶ If someone is sexually active while pregnant, it is vital for them to reduce STI risks because STIs can create health risks for a fetus or pregnant person during pregnancy and at birth.

Labor Day

Labor and childbirth consist of three different stages: (1) labor (subdivided into early or latent labor, active labor, and a transitional phase); (2) childbirth, or delivery; and (3) delivery of the placenta, or afterbirth. The whole process takes around fifteen to twenty-four hours, on average, for first-timers.

Early labor is the longest stage of labor and delivery, lasting many hours or even a couple of days, but it is also the least intense. When short contractions—which feel like very intense menstrual cramps—start to occur within twenty to thirty minutes of one another over a period of a few hours, and the lapse between them gets progressively shorter, early labor has begun. Before that time, usually over a period of days, the cervix has been slowly thinning out (effacement) and sometimes dilating (opening) to up to 3 centimeters.

When contractions are a few minutes apart and become stronger, ***active labor*** has begun, and it generally lasts a few hours. The transitional phase is usually the most difficult and tiring part of labor for most people: contractions are intense, longer, and very close together. The cervix completes dilating during this phase, opening to around 10 centimeters to be ready for delivery. People in the transition phase of labor may feel heavy pressure on the back, rectum, and bladder; body temperature tends to fluctuate erratically; and cramps, nausea, chills, shakes, and an overall feeling of exhaustion and/or serious moodiness or irritability are common and normal. Vomiting or bloody discharge may also occur.

When ***delivery*** begins, many people get a second wind and are glad to be able to start pushing (if you bear down as you might when pushing out a bowel movement, you can get a vague idea of what pushing is like, sans baby). Is it painful? Pretty much always, to varying degrees. But pain during delivery is also often exacerbated by other factors—by being alone, if that isn't desired; by certain hospital environments or birthing approaches; by lack of preparation or knowledge of what's happening; by stress or anxiety, embarrassment, shame, or fear; and, most of all, by the expectation of a lot of pain. So, it is often more painful for plenty of people than it should be, and the environment a person is in, and their state of mind, count for an awful lot.

With a vaginal birth, the doctor, midwife, or birthing coach and/or partner can aid with delivery and help the person who's actually in labor to keep pushing and stay as energized but relaxed as possible.

Midwifery

Before we had OB/GYNs, we had midwives. Through most of human history, midwives or doulas have helped deliver babies and have provided prenatal and postnatal care. Most of the practices Western doctors use today for childbirth are based on techniques midwives developed over the centuries through active learning. You can find references to midwives in the Old Testament. Midwives are still around today; you can see a midwife privately if you are pregnant, and some hospitals and healthcare systems even include midwifery among their available services, so ask your doctor or insurance provider about it. Too, if you're young and pregnant or are otherwise struggling to afford or procure prenatal and delivery care—or are dealing with discrimination in your prenatal care as a result of your age—midwives are often generous with their help and services for young pregnant people in need. For a few places to find a midwife, see the Resources section.

Although typical hospital deliveries have had people in delivery lying down, many are starting to catch on and adapt to use more natural positions that are helped by gravity, like partially sitting or squatting. When the baby begins to "crown," or their head first is visible at the vaginal opening, the birthing partner, midwife, or doctor helps ease them out of the vaginal canal as the person in labor continues pushing, until the entire infant is through the birth canal. The umbilical cord may be clamped, cut, or left in place until after the afterbirth has been delivered.

Just so you know, brand-new babies, even when cleaned off, rarely look like newborns in the movies: most retain a slightly wooly body hair called the *lanugo,* and they often look a little blue and pretty oddly shaped, including the head, which sometimes even looks cone-like. They can look more weird than adorable.

The actual vaginal delivery in full lasts an hour or two on average but sometimes as little as fifteen minutes or as long as a few hours, especially if there are complications during birth.

The final stage of labor is the ***delivery of the placenta,*** or afterbirth—the tissue mass that provided nourishment for the infant during pregnancy. After delivery of the infant, the uterus begins to contract again, and a few more pushes are needed to expel the placenta. This generally takes five to ten minutes.

There aren't hard-and-fast rules on what someone feels emotionally during labor and delivery, and there's no one way everyone feels. Most people are very glad when labor and delivery are over, not just because the exhausting process is complete and they can rest but also because, for most, experiencing the whole process and giving birth to a child—and seeing their child—are seriously satisfying. But it's also normal for people who have just given birth to feel depressed, overwhelmed, or just too plain tired to know *what* they're feeling.

It takes a few days to months after delivery for the physical and emotional aftereffects to wear off. At first, someone who went through labor and delivery may experience physical effects like cramps, discharge (including *lochia,* postpartum bleeding that generally lasts for four to six weeks), exhaustion, and overall genital and breast soreness or discomfort. A wide range of fluctuating emotions can occur, including postpartum depression (which can be a major long-term problem for as many as 25 percent of all people who've delivered) and wild elation, and often swings between the two, as well as decreased sexual desire. Within about six weeks, most people return to feeling normal (albeit "normal" in the way that now includes living with a brand-new infant and a completely changed life).

C-sections

A cesarean section—or C-section—is a surgical birth procedure in which an incision is made in the abdomen and uterus to deliver an infant that way rather than vaginally. A person is given regional anesthesia for a C-section, and the doctor removes the infant through the incisions.

Some people schedule C-sections or plan on them in advance; C-sections are typically suggested or done because of multiple births or vaginal birth complications. C-sections are also usually done with those who are HIV-positive or who have active genital herpes sores during labor.

Because it involves surgery, a C-section can carry more risks. Rates of cesareans are at a record high, and although there are good reasons for some people to have a C-section (sometimes doing one is about reducing risks), many obstetric advocates, midwives, pregnancy and natural childbirth activists, and medical organizations such as the Kaiser Foundation have voiced concern about C-sections being done needlessly or without giving accurate information about options and risks.

If you're pregnant and planning to deliver, talk to your doctor or midwife in advance about your birthing options, and get the facts if your healthcare provider suggests a C-section delivery for you.

Miscarriage: What It Is and Why It Happens

By medical definition, a miscarriage, or "spontaneous abortion," is a pregnancy that naturally (all by itself) ends before twenty weeks—the fifth month—of pregnancy. Experts believe that as many as **50 percent of all fertilizations or conceptions do *not* result in a viable pregnancy**. Miscarrying is just as normal and as common as not miscarrying is.

Often, miscarriage occurs so early and so uneventfully that a person won't even know they've had one or that they were even pregnant in the first place. Many of those incredibly early miscarriages aren't even technically considered miscarriages but rather pregnancies that just didn't complete through the implantation stage.

It's estimated that of people who have become "fully" pregnant and know of their pregnancies—so, those who have been pregnant at least a couple weeks—around 15 to 20 percent will miscarry. Most miscarriages are not preventable once pregnancy has taken place, and they occur when the body is simply unable to sustain a healthy pregnancy—they don't happen because anyone did anything wrong. Miscarriage is the body's natural way to safeguard against an embryo or fetus that will be stillborn, deformed, or unhealthy or a pregnancy that will put the pregnant person's health at risk. Some factors that increase the possibility of miscarriage are as follows:

- Lack of full sexual maturity or growth (in other words, becoming pregnant when very young)
- Poor nutrition
- Cigarette, drug, or alcohol use
- Hormonal imbalances
- Sexually transmitted infections or conditions
- Other reproductive or general medical conditions, like PCOS, uterine malformation, fibroids, lupus, congenital heart disease, severe kidney disease, diabetes, thyroid disease, or exposure to environmental hazards or radiation
- Stress or injury from sexual or domestic abuse

No one can rely, for the record, on any of these things to cause a miscarriage. Someone who wants to terminate a pregnancy safely and effectively must seek out a safe abortion procedure.

Symptoms

Early miscarriage is most common and accounts for about 75 percent of all miscarriages. *Very* early miscarriage is rarely even noticed, nor does it have any visible symptoms; although some spotting or mild cramping may occur, those are often easily mistaken for a period. You often can't have a very early miscarriage verified, so it's one of those situations where you simply may never know whether you had a miscarriage or not.

When miscarriage occurs after the first few weeks and is usually noticeable, symptoms often include mild to severe pelvic and abdominal cramps that may persist for more than a day, vaginal bleeding or spotting, sometimes including a passage of tissue from within the vagina, or a clear fluid drainage.

Early miscarriage rarely requires prompt medical attention or hospitalization. For most people, it is *physically* no different than a crampy period. It's smart to see your doctor or gynecologist after a suspected miscarriage, however, to check up on your health and be sure you did fully miscarry. If, however, very heavy bleeding occurs or spotting lasts more than two weeks, if large clots are passed or a foul-smelling discharge is present, or if cramps are severe or a fever develops, seek medical attention.

No matter *how* someone may have felt about a pregnancy, whether it was planned or unintentional, it is normal and common to experience feelings of grief, regret, guilt, and loss after miscarriage (and it's also normal not to feel upset). These feelings can be tricky when you're a young adult: friends, family, or partners may not have been happy you were pregnant in the first place and may not be sympathetic. For people of all ages, grief and upset after miscarriage is usually worse if there's a lack of support or understanding from those around them, so seeking out support and doing plenty of emotional self-care are key.

Please remember, though, if miscarriage happens to you or to someone you know, it is not your or their fault. Most of the time, just as our body often makes us throw up bad food we've eaten because it knows it's not good for us, our body miscarries when it knows that a pregnancy is not sound for the person who's body it is happening to or for a fetus. That fact alone may not make any hard feelings go away, but blaming yourself (or someone else, if you're not the person who's miscarried) is often a big player in the toughest feelings, so on top of not being truthful, it's also

ALWAYS AN ACCIDENT? NOPE.

Teen pregnancy is often presented as something that must have happened by accident. But a good many teen pregnancies—as many as one in five—*are* intended or planned. According to Kristen Luker in *Dubious Conceptions: The Politics of Teenage Pregnancy* and other experts, one big reason that even good sex education hasn't reduced teen pregnancy rates as much as expected is that some young adults know what birth control is and how and when to use it but *choose* not to use it because they *want* to become pregnant or just don't really care that much whether they do or don't become pregnant.

In many cases, young people who want to become pregnant have the same kinds of motivations older people have: they like and want children, they want to be parents, it feels right for them to do so, and/or they want to parent with the partner they're with now. Sometimes, as with older people, the reasons aren't so great or responsible: to try to cement or force continuation of a relationship, to prove adulthood or sexual development, to try to fill emotional voids or quell loneliness, and/or to get attention they want but aren't receiving.

Maybe one of your goals in life is to be a parent, and there isn't a thing in the world that's wrong with that, as long as you understand that it isn't your only option, even if it seems that way. Even if you know that, and parenting is what you want, it'll keep. You have the right to become pregnant and parent if and when you want to, including when you're young, but it is almost always a whole lot harder—harder to be pregnant, harder to parent—than it will be even just a few years down the road.

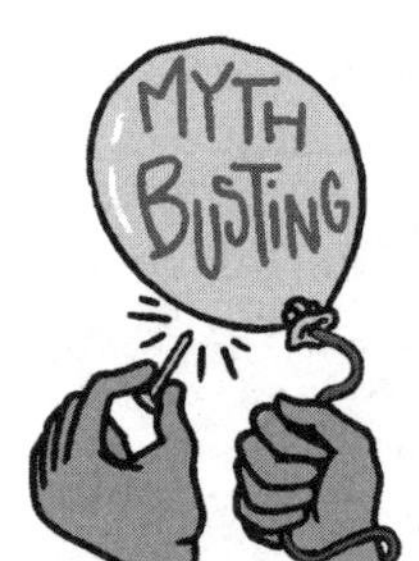

Although few people will ever reasonably suggest that pregnancy and parenting are easy, both are eas*ier* when the people involved are as prepared as they can be, physically, emotionally, financially, and practically. Because a *big* part of parenting is patience, if you just don't feel that you have the patience to wait to become pregnant and be a parent, chances are pretty good you also don't have the patience required to *be* a parent.

There's no rule that young parents can't be good parents. Plenty of teen parents *are* good parents, just like plenty of older parents are. But plenty of people who are or have been young parents will tell you that it would have been a lot easier for them to be better parents, and happier people overall, if they'd waited until they were at least out of high school.

something that's going to make you feel a lot worse.

REPRODUCTIVE OPTIONS: PARENTING, ADOPTION, AND ABORTION

Parenthood

Young Adult Parenting: Perils, Pitfalls, and Perks

Many people have the idea that they'll find a way to cope and can handle pregnancy and raising a child like a pro—sure that, for some reason, it'll be easier for them than it ever was for anyone before, even if they're totally unprepared. But more times than not, it ends up being more difficult than they imagine, especially for the youngest parents. That doesn't mean it's impossible to enjoy or do well. Lots of young parents find parenting fulfilling despite the challenges it brings. But wanting a child or loving a child isn't often enough preparation to ensure a healthy pregnancy—physically or emotionally—or readiness to parent well.

Teens and emerging adults *can* be good parents—**as good as anyone else**. There have always been young parents who have also been excellent parents, who have *enjoyed* being parents, and who have felt very good about the choice they made to parent. (There are also plenty of older people who are terrible parents.) If it's really what you want to do—and you're prepared to manage the realities of parenting—chances are good that you *can* do it and do it *well.*

So, if you're thinking about it, here's a basic reality check to run by yourself, on the house.

You're 100 Percent Responsible for Your Child and Its Upbringing

Sure, that means that the good stuff that happens and all of your kid's accomplishments are things you'll feel really proud to have had a hand in. But with responsibility comes accountability, something many young people haven't yet had to deal with in any major way. If you're late to pick your kid up from day care, you're going to have to pay the late fees and deal with a bummed-out kid, and if you do it repeatedly, you may be asked to find another day care center. The folks in charge aren't going to be real interested in whose fault it is because it's your responsibility. If you have a partner who harms your child, you'll have to deal with both being and feeling responsible. If you make poor parenting choices, you and your kid have to live with them as well as any long-term effects. You're also likely to be very emotionally invested in your child. So, when they're sick or unhappy, you're going to be scared and distracted. When you screw something up, you're likely to feel horrible about it. In many, many ways, your kid becomes your whole life. You're responsible and accountable for most of what your kid does, even through their teen years—legally, practically, and emotionally. Imagine the possibilities. All of them, the good, the bad, and the ugly.

Those possibilities include one parent *not* sticking around or actively parenting. And that potentially leaves you not only dealing with child rearing as a single parent but also dealing with feelings of abandonment, betrayal, and heartbreak—at the same time you're trying to get through a pregnancy or take care of your kid.

One reason choosing to be a parent is such a big deal is that you're not just making a choice for you, you're making choices for a person who can't make their own choices and who has no choice but to live with yours.

Parenting at a Young Age Can Be Lonely

Young parents often feel incredibly isolated. You may (or may not) get plenty of attention, care, and company while you're pregnant and in the first six months or so of your kid's life. But when all the showers and parties have passed, when the novelty of a cute baby has passed, a whole lot of young parents start to feel like they moved to Mars. Many feel far more alone than they felt before they were parents.

Somebody to Love?

For a lot of people, one of the appeals of parenthood is the notion that someone—their child—will love them unconditionally. But, very often, especially once they are out of very early childhood, children don't behave *at all* as if they love their parents unconditionally. So, many people get this one twisted: the unconditional love in a parent-child relationship is supposed to come from the *parent*, not the child.

Parenting Is Hard Work

Just during your kid's first year of life, you'll have bags under your eyes the size of the Grand Canyon, you'll be pretty crabby, and your kid isn't going to say thank you for a couple more years. Postpartum depression—deep and sometimes debilitating depression after childbirth that can sometimes last for many months, during one of the most challenging stages of parenting, no less—is common. Lactating and breastfeeding can hurt like the dickens. Babies often cry more than they gurgle cutely. Having to tend to someone's basic needs and functions literally 24/7—feeding, changing diapers, putting to sleep, entertaining—is exhausting, even with help, and always putting your own needs after theirs can make a parent feel like a walking bottle rather than a person.

They're Awesome, but, Man, Can Kids Cramp Your Style

You may be used to going out for a night with your friends, maybe needing only to okay it with your folks and come up with transportation and spending money. Now you'll need to find a reliable babysitter you feel safe with; try to afford extras when you often already can't pay for the basics; and reschedule things constantly because babies and kids tend to have schedules of their own that don't neatly coincide with yours. You may find that the things that are important to your friends aren't that important to you anymore—and that they're not very interested in what *is* important to you, like your struggle to find good day care, the nightmare dating has turned into, or how many nights in a row you've spent with a colicky, screaming infant. Your friends also may not be very patient with you having to reschedule or cancel a lot because of your kid, as anyone parenting has to do often.

Dating when you have a kid is always more difficult and often frustrating, and if you're co-parenting with a partner, you'll find that the two of you end up with very little alone time and more challenges and conflicts in your relationship than you can shake a stick at. This is all the same stuff older people go through with parenting, but it's often more challenging for younger parents.

Juggling school, college, or work with a kid is also tricky, especially if you're single and young. It's hard to study when a baby is crying or a toddler decides to rip up all the notes for that paper that's 50 percent of your grade and due next week. Many high schools and colleges, unfairly and unfortunately, do not make concessions for people who are pregnant or parenting. Many employers aren't very understanding about letting you take time off because your kid is sick or leave early to get to a day care center before closing time. Even basic things you take for granted, like having the time to take a bath or shower, to take in a movie, to do your laundry, to talk on the phone with friends, or to sit down to eat a meal, will be compromised.

Kids Cost the Big Bucks

Delivery alone—not counting prenatal care or all the stuff you have to buy to prepare, like diapers and cribs—will probably cost around $10,000 for a normal, complication-free birth if you've got good healthcare coverage (if not, then we're talking anywhere from around $30,000 to $50,000). In the first four years alone, raising a child often costs more than attending a four-year public college and there are *no* financial assistance, grants, or scholarships whatsoever—something few people can afford.

Children cost a *lot* of money. Add their costs to the cost of taking care of yourself as well, and you can see why parents are often so stressed out about money.

You need a consistent, reliable means to pay these costs. Your parents may be willing and able to help, but don't just assume they will, especially indefinitely. Your partner may be able to help, but remember that, whether you like it or not, they can leave at any time, and constant child support battles are the norm for single parents. Assuming federal or state aid will pay all the costs is also unrealistic. Most people aren't low income enough or they don't meet other criteria to qualify for many programs—even those who are eligible cannot come close to covering all of their costs with welfare.

Kids Aren't a Cure-All

If you have any major challenges in your life—an abusive partnership, depression, self-destructive behavior, an eating disorder, drug dependence, homelessness—they're likely to remain tough issues when you have a kid. Plenty of young parents find that dropping bad habits or patterns actually seems pretty easy when they first become pregnant or at the beginning of their child's life. But it's typical for those issues to pop right back up in time. When they do, they are often even harder to manage and work through than before, and they directly affect someone besides you. How might your child be affected by growing up around an eating disorder, self-injury like cutting, or an abusive relationship? How are you going to manage putting your needs second when you're depressed? If your own parents or family had big challenges, take a look at how you think these struggles influenced you. Even seemingly small issues, such as poor eating habits or having a hard time making

and enforcing limits, can become pretty big problems when you're pregnant or parenting.

Kids also don't solve relationship problems. Having a baby and parenting add loads of extra stresses that make intimate relationships more challenging, not less.

Our Society Stigmatizes the Hell Out of Young Parents

If you're in your teens, parenting is going to be harder for you than it would be for someone just a few years older, and not just because of their often increased financial, health, legal, or emotional status. A whole lot of people really look down on and strongly discriminate against teen parents. Finding resources and assistance will be harder for you, and often you're going to have to fight for your right both to parent and to be treated like a parent. You'll be walking into parenthood with people assuming—even if you planned your pregnancy—that you're irresponsible and incapable. You're going to need to be able to advocate for yourself and for your kid like a boss.

That may involve battling to get schools or workplaces to provide child care or make allowances for your being a parent; it will probably mean working your buns off to obtain financial assistance, housing, school and work opportunities, health care, and emotional support. It may involve facing up to people who feel very confident that you are not a good parent and that you have no *right* to parent, and they may make it harder for you to do so. It may mean losing the support or presence of friends, family, or partners.

Deciding to parent is a big deal for those of any age. People in touch with reality—whether they're seventeen or forty-five—are often scared when they make that choice, because they have at least some inkling of how big a responsibility it is. So it's normal to be scared (if you're not, at all, chances are you're not really seeing the big picture). It's also normal to feel grossly unprepared, even after the birth. Many parents of every age and social stratum feel like hacks as parents, find that parenting is much more challenging than they thought it'd be, and worry about failing their kids. That's called caring.

That's a big list up there of challenges and pitfalls, which isn't to say that there aren't a lot of really great parts of being a parent. Kids are really cool, and they are often a whole lot of fun to be around. Involved, engaged parenting helps *you* grow as a person; you'll find that a child can teach you things no one else could. It's unique and special to be in a relationship with someone who is literally a part of you and for whom you are the sun, moon, and stars—for some of their life, anyway. Later on, they won't be so dependent and will be able to see your flaws (and will likely let you know explicitly what they are, ad nauseam), but even at that point, a strong, intimate, and meaningful relationship develops when you nurture it well, one you will truly have for their whole life and yours.

If you've become a young parent, you may find that at the same time you're having to learn to take care of a baby, you're also having to learn to take care of yourself, and that's vital. *You* need care as well. It's important that you stay physically

What They Won't Teach You in Childbirth Class

From Aria, a Scarleteen volunteer and former teen momma:

1. Maternity clothes are tools of the Devil. A big stretchy panel on the front of your pants. Nightgowns with big slits in the front that do nothing for coverage. And some of the ugliest bras you've ever seen outside your grandma's dresser drawer. Get used to the "grandpa pants," because you'll be wearing them directly under your breasts until your baby comes. These, my friends, are what you should be shown when you're being taught abstinence in Health class.
2. When you're pushing during childbirth, sometimes your baby's head isn't the only thing that comes out. Imagine: downward pressure on your bowels as the baby moves south. Play with a Play-Doh Fun Factory, learn all about extrusion, and you'll understand what I'm talking about.
3. Newborn babies sometimes arrive complete with an impressive blanket of hair on their back and shoulders. Like those guys you sometimes see on the beach who you think are wearing sweaters.
4. Newborn baby heads are more moldable than clay. You may find yourself holding a little miniature Conehead. Or someone with a high ridge running down the center of their head. Don't worry; these go away within the first week or two. It's a great chance to try out all those adorable baby hats you've no doubt gathered in the last few months.
5. Modesty and Childbirth aren't very good friends. Toward the end, Childbirth gets so whiny and annoying that Modesty goes on vacation for a while.
6. You'll be amazed at how high your cervix seems when a doctor with big hands is checking it. Apparently, mine is located somewhere between my sinuses and my tonsils.
7. Remember all that lung capacity you lost in the last forty weeks? It comes back quickly and is one of the strangest sensations you'll encounter.
8. Remember all that bladder capacity you lost in the last forty weeks? It doesn't. And when you're lying in bed, sometimes you aren't aware that the tank is full. Be sure to remind yourself to get up at least once every three hours. You don't want to have to call the mop-and-bucket lady into the bathroom doorway. Believe me, I know.
9. You'll be told that it is not pain you'll feel during childbirth, it's pressure. This is true in the same way a tornado might be called an air current.
10. At all costs, avoid mirrors after you have your baby. That's a surprise best left for the safety and security of your own home.
11. You may not fall in love with your baby at first sight. This can take a while for some people and is perfectly normal and acceptable. Your baby, however, will. Prepare to feel more needed than you ever have in your life.
12. Babies sleep more than you think. Don't always feel pressured to do the same. Not tired? Do something for yourself. Bathing will turn into an immeasurable joy.
13. Remember those periods you missed during your pregnancy? They're back. And they've brought friends. (For more on lochia, see page 388.)

If You're Considering Parenting . . .

- Talk to other young parents at your school or workplace. Seek out parents around your age who currently have infants and toddlers (if you or friends don't know any, ask your school guidance counselor or job supervisor). Not only can you ask them about what it's like for them emotionally but you can also find out very practical things you need to know, like how the school, college, or job you're at handles young parents. Do they provide day care? Is it safe and sound? What special programs and resources exist in your area for teen or young parents? What do you need to do to obtain those resources and aid, like funds and health care for young parents and kids? How are your local hospitals with young parents? What doctors, midwives, hospitals, or clinics would they suggest?
- Talk to your doctor, gynecologist, clinician, and/or nurse. About one-third of pregnant teens receive inadequate prenatal care, so babies born to young people are currently more likely to be low-birth-weight, to have childhood health problems, and to be hospitalized. And you may have other health risks of your own that can complicate pregnancy or delivery, so you'll need to be sure to spend extra time assessing your overall health. Healthcare pros can fill you in on health issues and help hook you up with resources and support; they can also give you their unique perspective on what you'll be dealing with.
- Spend some time visualizing your life with a kid at every stage of the game: not just when they're babies but when they're five, ten, or fifteen years old. Consider the goals you have for your life, and figure out how you might or might not be able to work toward them while also parenting, with or without help or a co-parent. If you still want to move forward with a pregnancy, sit down with those goals and make some solid plans so that you're more likely to be able to be pregnant and parent without having to give up your other dreams.

healthy and emotionally well; that the relationships you choose are beneficial, balanced, and healthy; that you get downtime by yourself or with your friends and partners. It's vital that you still follow your goals and dreams and that besides becoming the parent you want to be you also get to be the *person* you aspire to be.

The Adoption Option

Adoption in the present day is different from how it used to be. For a long time, adoption meant that a birth parent was always required to give up all legal rights and responsibilities to their child, didn't ever know what happened to their child, and could count on never finding out. For much of history until very recently, many birth parents didn't even have a choice in participating in adoption at all but were forced into it, whether it was what they wanted or not. Things have become more flexible, and there are more options within adoption than there used to be.

The two basic types of adoption are the following:

- **"Closed" or confidential adoption:** A "closed" or confidential adoption means you relinquish all your rights, and you do not meet the adoptive family. The family is generally given information about you, but it is largely very basic and health-oriented information.

- **"Open" adoption:** This is the more common kind of adoption now. Open adoptions vary in terms of how much or how little openness is involved. The least open allow a birth parent to choose the parents for their child on the basis of files of waiting families that they can look through. More open agreements may allow the birth parent to speak with potential parents or families on the phone or in meetings to choose a family. The adoptive parents may be present during pregnancy and delivery, and agreements can even be open to the extent that a birth parent is allowed contact throughout a child's life or is included within the adoptive family.

Adoptions can be arranged in many ways:

- Via licensed public or private adoption agencies
- Independently, with a lawyer or doctor making arrangements between you and the adoptive parent or family
- Privately, between yourself and a couple (although having a lawyer, even among friends, is highly advisable)

The birth parent's pregnancy and prenatal and postpartum costs are usually covered by the adoptive family or the agency, as are their legal fees and sometimes their basic living expenses during the course of the pregnancy. Expenses like fees for counseling or therapy may also be paid. In most areas, how a birth parent can be paid is limited as to the actual amount, the time period, and what she can receive compensation for. So when someone considers how to manage a pregnancy, adoption is the one option where cost may not be a primary concern.

In the United States, by law adoption records remain closed by default, and the adoptive family has all full legal rights to the child. So it's very important when considering adoption to really evaluate and discuss how much openness you want and what you want that to mean if you need for it to be open. If you get to the point of making an agreement, get all of the details *on paper* and get a lawyer involved who is experienced with adoption. Just be aware that even when it is on paper, if adoptive families ever change their minds in terms of how much access or contact a birth parent gets, the adoptive parents are favored by the law and adoption agencies. Open adoptions *may* still result in lack of access or contact with a child, sometimes permanently—something that occurs all too often and that a birth parent usually is unable to do anything about.

The Tough Stuff

Adoption is often very difficult for birth parents. Many pregnant people become emotionally attached to their child during pregnancy, and many find giving the child up after birth to be very traumatic, short and long term. That distress can be escalated when adoption is chosen not because it's what the birth parent really wants but because age, poverty, secrecy, or other issues make abortion or parenting seem impossible. This distress can be heightened further if someone changes their mind about adoption after surrendering a child or has agreed to an adoption they were told or thought would be more open than it turns out to be.

In terms of considering what's best for a child, most children who are placed in adoptive homes do well and have happy, healthy lives. Many people in the world want very much to be parents and can only do so through adoption. But a harsh truth is that, in the United States alone, every year hundreds of thousands of children put up for adoption remain without permanent homes and enter the foster care system. This is more common for children who were not placed for adoption as newborns or infants but when they were older, for children of color, and for special needs children.

To explore adoption, you can ask your doctor, guidance counselor, or social services organization or contact adoption agencies on your own. Make sure you look for someone who will truly advocate for *you* rather than for the adoptive parent or parents. It is also a good idea to talk to other birth parents who gave their children up for adoption and find out about their experiences. National matching services, lists, and other resources are also available that provide adoption services or access to private families.

Abortion: Terminating a Pregnancy

Abortion is a medical procedure performed to remove and end a pregnancy, just like tooth extraction is a medical procedure performed to remove a tooth. Safe, legal, medical abortion procedures are performed through or within a clinic, hospital, or doctor's office, usually on an outpatient basis, and almost always within the first trimester of pregnancy. Legal abortion procedures are very safe: statistically, we know that the health risks are much *greater* for carrying a pregnancy to term than they are for abortion. No long-term health problems have been found, through extensive study, to be associated with legal medical or surgical abortion.

The only safe abortions are legal abortions performed and supervised by qualified healthcare providers. A majority of counties in the United States do not currently have a local provider, so you may have to travel out of your own town or city to obtain one.

At this time, there are two main options for legal abortion: medical abortion and surgical abortion.

Medical Abortion

Medical abortion—sometimes called "the abortion pill"—is available from most abortion providers. Medical abortion is effective up to around seventy days after the last menstrual period, or up until around ten weeks of pregnancy. It does not require any kind of surgery, but instead it is a combination of drugs (usually mifepristone and misoprostol, methotrexate and misoprostol or misoprostol all by itself), given and supervised by a clinician, that causes a process much like a miscarriage.

The drugs do several things: stop embryonic cells from multiplying and dividing to continue a pregnancy, block hormones that would support a developing pregnancy, and cause uterine contractions that empty the contents of the uterus.

A dose of one drug is given in the healthcare provider's office, while the other is taken a day or two later at home.

Usually a few hours after the dose of the second drug, the embryo (not a fetus yet, and certainly not a baby) and other products of conception pass out through the vagina. The experience can be very similar to early miscarriage: there is some cramping and bleeding, from light spotting to heavier bleeding, and what is expelled may contain clots and/or the grayish-looking gestational sac created by the blastocyst. Cramps and bleeding are usually stronger than during a menstrual period. Side effects can include nausea, headaches, vomiting, chills, fever, or bowel problems as well as continued spotting for a week or two. For a person having a medical abortion, it is helpful and most safe if they arrange for someone else—their partner, a friend, family member—to be on call for them, for emotional support, for material needs during the process, or for transportation to an emergency room should any side effects become serious.

Medical abortion should be coupled with follow-up visits to the provider to ensure that a full termination did occur and that the person who had one is in sound health afterward.

Medical abortions are slightly less effective than surgical abortions: anywhere between 1 and 5 percent of patients who choose medical abortion have to have an additional surgical procedure to successfully terminate their pregnancy.

ABORTION LAWS AND MINORS

According to the National Abortion Federation, around half of all people who become pregnant unintentionally choose to terminate their pregnancy with an abortion procedure. People who become pregnant between the ages of fifteen and nineteen years account for about 19 percent of all abortions; people ages twenty to twenty-four account for another 33 percent of those who choose to terminate a pregnancy.

However, in many states, certain laws may restrict teen or general access to abortion with policies that require parents to be notified of a minor's intention to have an abortion (parental notification) or that require a parent's or guardian's written permission for an abortion to be performed (parental consent). Almost all of these policies have options for judicial bypass (getting a judge's permission for the abortion instead of permission from a parent), and some states allow physicians to waive parental notification or consent. Too, court orders have prevented some states from enforcing these laws.

If you are or know a young person who isn't yet a legal adult who is seeking an abortion, you can find out what, if any, legal restrictions exist in your area either by calling your local abortion provider or sexual health clinic or by contacting some of the abortion and reproductive health advocacy groups listed in the Resources section of this book.

Surgical Abortion

Surgical abortions—which are nearly always 100 percent effective—can be performed from the time a pregnancy is confirmed until the middle or end of the first trimester, depending on local and national laws. Surgical abortion is most often performed in the first three months of pregnancy; second-trimester abortions account for less than 10 percent of all abortions. The type of surgical abortion performed depends on the length of the pregnancy and the specific situation and provider.

▶ **Aspiration (sometimes called suction or MVA)** can be done as soon as four weeks from the last menstrual period through about fifteen weeks of pregnancy.

During an aspiration, an injection first numbs the cervix with a local anesthetic. A person can sometimes also choose to have sedation, which makes them less aware or unaware during the procedure. The cervix is then dilated—with slim rods designed to slowly stretch the cervical opening—and a flexible tube is inserted. That tube is either attached to an electric aspirating machine with a gentle vacuum or, for very early abortions, to a handheld syringe. The contents of the uterus are removed through the tube with gentle suction. The entire procedure takes between five and ten minutes.

▶ **Dilation and evacuation (D&E)** is the abortion procedure done in the second trimester. As in the first trimester, local anesthetic is used, sometimes along with other painkillers or deeper sedation. The opening of the cervix is stretched with cervical dilators, just as with a vacuum aspiration procedure. Another sort of dilator may also be used, made of soft fibers that absorb moisture from the body and expand overnight to enlarge the opening in the cervix. Sometimes a drug, misoprostol, may be used with the dilators to soften the cervix. Depending on what is used, how far along the pregnancy is, and individual clinic policies and practices, you may be sent home overnight with a dilator or dilators in place and with antibiotics to prevent infection. If so, you need to return the next day for the second part of the procedure.

After the cervical opening is dilated, the pregnancy tissue is removed through a combination of suction and the use of instruments called forceps. This process takes between five and fifteen minutes, not including the time it takes for dilation or the night that may have passed.

Abortion Costs

Both medical and surgical first-trimester abortions cost about the same, but cost varies very widely by area: on the low end, an abortion and related costs can currently be around $500, while on the high end, it can cost thousands (and the further into a pregnancy someone is, the higher the cost will always be). Some insurance policies or state or county medical aid may cover some abortion costs, but generally only when an abortion is medically necessary rather than elective—that is, when a pregnancy puts the life of the pregnant person or child in danger. Some states and counties do provide funds for elective abortions for low-income people. There are also some grassroots sources for financial assistance for abortion for those who want an abortion but cannot come up with all the funds themselves. For information on abortion funds, see the Resources section.

What to Expect During an Abortion

How You Should Expect to Be Treated

▶ Just like with any other kind of health care, you should be treated with care and respect. Your privacy should be respected in every way. Generally, how you are

TECH TIP

If you're looking for abortion information, an abortion provider, or pro-choice options counseling, be careful where you look on the Internet. Anti-abortion and anti-choice publications, organizations, individuals, and in-person places—like Crisis Pregnancy Centers (CPCs), which are fake clinics that exist only to create intentional misinformation, fear, and guilt and to talk people out of abortion—often have a particularly easy time being shady online. Best bet? Use the Resources section at the end of this book, ask a trusted healthcare provider, or just stick to reproductive health sites and sources online that aren't crowdsourced and that display clear statements in support of all reproductive options and health care, including abortion. If you can't find one, use a search engine and enter current choice-respecting common terms like "right to abortion," "reproductive health care," "options counseling," "contraception," and "pro-choice."

treated is not a problem with abortion providers and clinical staff; providers and their staff take both of these issues very seriously.

▶ Throughout the process, you are counseled by clinic staff to inform you of everything that will happen and to answer any questions you may have. You can also ask for any emotional support from staff. Clinical staff should respect whatever pace you need and decisions you're making (within the limits of what the clinic or provider can offer), even if you come in for an abortion and decide you do not want to go through with the procedure that day. By the way, you *always* can opt out of the procedure at any time before it begins, and staff at your clinic or doctor's office should make that clear. (If you know from the onset that you want more involved counseling or education because you are not sure about abortion yet, you can make an appointment for that all by itself—you don't have to schedule an abortion to receive options counseling.)

▶ You should be helped to feel as emotionally and physically safe as possible, and that usually includes security for the clinic. The office or clinic where you have an abortion should look and be clean and sanitary. Your counselor, nurse, and/or doctor should explain the entire procedure to you and be willing to answer any questions you have at any time before, during, and after the procedure. If you want someone with you, you are often allowed to bring them, although because of health, legal, and safety issues, that person may be permitted only in the waiting room.

What an Abortion Feels Like

Medical abortion may cause heavy cramping at home that can be very uncomfortable, and bleeding occurs, but generally not a lot more than during a heavy menstrual period. You are sent home with medications to take for pain and nausea, should you need them. During surgical abortion, a person is likely to also experience cramping, usually stronger than menstrual cramps, and may feel some strong "pinching" inside their pelvis, not unlike the sensation you feel in your mouth when a dentist gives you an anesthetic injection. Someone who's more nervous, uncertain, scared, or conflicted is likely to experience more pain or discomfort than someone who is more relaxed and resolved.

Common side effects that many people experience following abortion procedures include cramping, nausea, sweating, feeling faint, and, like people who have given birth, depression. Less frequent side effects may include heavy or prolonged bleeding, blood clots, infection due to retained pregnancy tissue or dilators, or infection caused by an STD or bacteria being introduced to the uterus, which can cause fever, pain, and abdominal tenderness. If any side effects persist for more than a week or are severe, call your healthcare provider immediately.

Unloading a Loaded Issue

Because abortion is still such a controversial issue among many people and politicians, it can be tough to choose it or even think clearly and objectively about abortion as a choice. If you decide to get an abortion, you may even have to deal with protesters at your clinic, which can mean being called some pretty nasty names.

All sorts of people have and have had abortions, across all racial, economic, age, marital, identity, and other social lines. According to the Guttmacher Institute:

▶ About 80 percent of those who terminate pregnancies are older than eighteen and are unmarried.

▶ By the age of forty-five, about one in every three people who become pregnant will have an abortion.

▶ The majority of people who have abortions—about six in ten—are already parents.

▶ The majority of people who have abortions do intend to bear and rear children in the future, just not now.

▶ The majority of people who have abortions subscribe to religious beliefs, and 70 percent or more of those who have terminated pregnancies are members of Judeo-Christian religions, including Catholicism.

No matter what you believe, your feelings about abortion—especially when the possibility or event is actual and personal rather than an abstract idea—may not be simple or line up predictably or consistently with your beliefs. Some people who generally are not comfortable with abortion as a whole may decide to have one in a given situation because they truly feel it is best for them, and in their particular situation they feel better about it than their other options. Some who are comfortable with abortion for others or who have had abortions before may, in a certain situation, feel it is not the right choice for them or their children. Plenty of people who do want children have an abortion at some point because they just don't feel capable or able to rear their children adequately at that time because of relationship, financial, lifestyle, health, or emotional issues.

Few reproductive choices are easy to make, but it can be more difficult to choose abortion as an option because of all the personal and political bias against or about it. For that reason, it's important that if you *do* choose abortion—just as you would with any other reproductive choice—you do so because you want to and you feel it is the best choice

DOES ABORTION CREATE TRAUMA THAT OTHER REPRODUCTIVE CHOICES DON'T? NOT REALLY.

Many credible scientific journals, such as the *Journal of the American Medical Association,* have consistently published studies that demonstrate there are no data to support the idea or insistence that abortion is more emotionally traumatic than any other reproductive option is. We have no logical reason to assume nor any sound evidence to support the idea that any one reproductive choice is more or less traumatic for people. In fact, studies support that the majority of people who freely choose abortion for themselves have positive rather than negative psychological responses over the long term.

However, some studies, such as "Emotional Response to Abortion: A Critical Review of the Literature" and "The Psychosocial Factors of the Abortion Experience: A Critical Review," *do* list some factors known to increase the possibility of emotional distress and trauma resulting from abortion. These include being of a very young age, lack of support from partners or community (including the world at large), pressure or coercion to abort, anxiety or distress before the procedure, moral or religious conflicts about abortion, preexisting mental illness or depression, a history of sexual abuse or assault, low self-esteem, and habitual avoidance of responsibility.

In other words, the sorts of factors that make *any* reproductive choice more likely to be traumatic. In fact, the factors above are nearly identical to the at-risk indicators commonly listed for people who give birth and are more likely to suffer from postpartum depression. So, remember, if you or someone you know is pregnant and making a reproductive choice, it is vital that a choice be just that: an option that the pregnant person feels is best for them, first and foremost, and that they choose for themselves based on their unique circumstances, wants, and needs. And whatever the choice, emotional support throughout is crucial.

you can make. You want to do whatever you can for yourself, whatever your reproductive choice, to take the best care of you, physically and emotionally, and that includes making the choices you feel are best for *you, your* circumstances, and *your* life.

Where to Find Sound Help

If you're in the process of making a reproductive choice—whether to parent, adopt out, or abort and any of the choices associated with those—at some point you're going to need to go somewhere to get hooked up with the services you need. It's also helpful to talk about options with someone who is objective, who isn't invested in the choice you make because they aren't an immediate part of your life, and who doesn't have an agenda of their own.

TO TELL OR NOT TO TELL

It's up to you who you tell about a pregnancy, and when and if you tell them—you are not under any obligation, legal or otherwise, to tell any family, friends, or partners about a pregnancy. Who you tell is mostly about who you *want* to tell.

Just be sure that, if you're waiting to tell a partner or parent who you plan to involve in any way or who will be involved—like by covering any of your expenses—or you're not telling them at all, you're being fair about it. For instance, if you plan to count on them financially, it's not fair to wait until your showing to tell your parents you're pregnant. Keeping an abortion from a partner so that you can later try to hurt or manipulate them with it isn't good for anyone. If you deliver a pregnancy, the other person involved who made that pregnancy happen may have parental rights they're entitled to, so a partner who is still around and who is staying around is one you're going to need to inform.

If you feel that telling someone you have to tell about a pregnancy puts you in danger, then it is smart not to tell them by yourself. Instead, seek help, intervention, and support from appropriate resources such as local law enforcement or social services.

No matter what, be sure you tell *someone:* if not family or a partner, a friend, doctor, counselor, teacher, or someone else you trust to provide you support. No matter what choices you make, being pregnant, no matter what choice you make with it, is too hard and complicated to go it totally alone.

Research your options to find the help best suited to you. Your best option for support is usually a center or clinic that provides a number of different services and that makes clear that *all* possible choices are acceptable rather than one that pushes any one choice. General sexual healthcare clinics—which provide a number of sexual health services, such as GYN exams, STI screenings, prenatal care, and abortion—are smart places to go. You can also talk to your gynecologist or general physician. School guidance counselors or student services centers may also offer reproductive options counseling. Any center or clinic you go to should conduct pretty extensive interviews and counseling and lay out your choices to help you evaluate them before offering you services. Once you've made your reproductive choice, any center or clinic you go to for counseling should be wholly supportive of that choice. If your gut tells you something isn't right, trust it and find somewhere else to go.

Remember that you get to make this choice yourself, and you get to come to your own conclusions about what's best. That's also the case even if you became pregnant intentionally with an eye toward parenting and then changed your mind: you are allowed to do that.

HOW TO TELL PARTNERS AND PARENTS ABOUT AN UNEXPECTED PREGNANCY

Let's say the pregnancy test just verified what you already suspected: you're pregnant. At some point, you may need to tell some people about this—your parents, your partner, or whoever it was that contributed the other half of the DNA, and possibly at least a friend or other trusted person so you can get some support and help.

▶ Take some time for yourself. Consider your options and get a good feel for what you think you'd like to do.

▶ Talk to a close friend or two. You'll need some support, preferably from people who are good listeners and who aren't judgmental in terms of whatever your ultimate choice may be in regard to your pregnancy.

▶ Process it as thoroughly as you can in the limited time you have available. Call hotlines or visit pregnancy options counselors if you need to talk it out with someone who can be objective.

Telling Partners

There's no one right way to tell a partner pregnancy has happened—no special finesse, no golden phrase that'll make it all easier or guarantee that it goes well. How partners react can be unpredictable. Someone you thought would handle it badly may take it like a pro and leap to your side, prepared to help you manage it all expertly. Someone you felt sure would be caring and involved may blow you off completely. Even a partner you're very close to and have been with for a long while may behave differently from how you expected.

Your partner may end up being a great ally for you in all this and tremendously supportive. But it's also common enough for pregnancy—even a pregnancy scare—to be the beginning of the end of a relationship. It's entirely possible that your partner may greatly disappoint you, that disagreements about pregnancy may facilitate a breakup, or even that you'll find yourself adrift in this all by yourself. Your partner may try to blame you for the pregnancy or may be angry with you, even though both your bodies were responsible.

In abusive relationships, abuse usually increases with a pregnancy—many abusive relationships that weren't physically abusive before become so. It's hard to look at, but according to the US Department

> In the event you do not want there to be any risk of—or legal requirement for—contact or permissions between yourself and the person whose sperm cells were part of this picture, abortion does not require any consent, notification, or other involvement of that person. Both adoption and parenting do or can.

TECH TIP

It's probably obvious, but just in case it isn't: this is an excellent example of the kind of information *not* to use text, other quick messaging, or social media to tell someone like a partner or parent about. As with other very sensitive issues, this is a situation when it really helps for people to dedicate time and space to be together—face to face or by phone call or video chatting if need be—to discuss it when they're not in the middle of anything else. Such a big disclosure and talk just isn't likely to go well if it's treated like a music video share or reminder to pick up concert tickets.

of Justice, the leading cause of death for pregnant people is homicide (murder), most commonly committed by an intimate partner. (So, if you're in an abusive relationship and think a pregnancy might make things better, please think twice.)

More typically, you'll see a range of behavior while your partner is processing all of this information. They may need time to do that, just like you did. And, just like you, their feelings may be all over the place, and they may bounce between being cool, calm, and collected and totally freaking out. Although it's not easy to make allowances for crappy attitudes or bad reactions, especially when it's you who is pregnant, it often is necessary to give a person a little time to absorb and adjust.

When that adjustment happens, you can start talking about options and about what you want to do and listening to their feelings. You can talk it out together as much as you need to, just bear in mind that it is ultimately *your* choice and should be treated that way by anyone you're talking with, including a partner. This is happening in *your* body. How much a part of this decision they are is not just up to them but up to you.

Trying to Understand Each Other

People who are or who can become pregnant and people who lack the body parts necessary for that to even be possible typically have some big disconnects about pregnancy: neither can really understand how the other feels. Someone who hasn't been or can't become pregnant can't understand how it feels, physically or emotionally, to know you have something basically taking over your body and your life; they can't understand what it's like to have people you don't even know so invested in and opinionated about the choices you make about a pregnancy. People who are pregnant might have difficulty understanding how someone who can't be pregnant—but who was part of the pregnancy happening in the first place—can feel like they have so little control over the situation once pregnancy has occurred or what their experience of the pregnancy is even though it is not in their bodies.

Communicating with each other as clearly as possible can be a big help. A pregnancy usually automatically ups the seriousness of any relationship: a partner who wanted a casual relationship may wake up to find that's no longer possible because of a pregnancy—a scenario that's far less tangible for many people until they've actually experienced it.

The reproductive choice you make may not be what your partner wants. That's a toughie, because if the pregnancy is occurring in your body it is *your* choice to make. Listen to each other. Understand that you don't need to defend your choice but just explain it as best you can. Listen to your partner's feelings and acknowledge that you hear them. Recognize their right to have those feelings as well as the fact that those feelings are just not the ones you can go by most to make your decisions (yours are). You may have to agree to disagree, and that may be really hard. It may mean that you have to gather funds for an abortion on your own or go through a pregnancy without the support or commitment of your partner.

Sometimes, it just takes longer for a partner to accept a decision and really deal with it. Whereas you, as the pregnant person, don't really have the luxury of that time in terms of what you have to do immediately, your partner does. So, you might need to make allowances for the fact that it doesn't feel and isn't as immediate a situation for them to deal with as it is for you.

If you're in a solid relationship and are having trouble dealing with a pregnancy, no matter the choice each of you wants to make, you might consider counseling. Abortion and adoption agencies can usually provide counseling for both partners at a low cost or for free. And if you're considering parenting, your healthcare provider can probably suggest resources where you can get help or can even counsel both of you themselves.

Telling Parents

Telling parents can be tricky, especially if telling them you're pregnant also means telling them for the first time that you've been sexually active, which is a pretty typical scenario when you're young and pregnant.

Your best bet is usually to be as straightforward and honest as possible and to prepare yourself for conflict or disappointment on the part of your parent. A parent is likely to be upset about a young pregnancy (even when it was planned). They may also be upset that you were sexually active at all.

Don't lie. If you didn't use birth control, know you misused something, or used something unreliable, say so. If the sex you had with your partner was consensual, don't say that it *wasn't*. And if it wasn't, don't say that it *was*.

Blaming a parent or guardian in any way for your unplanned pregnancy is also a bad idea: if the sex that resulted in pregnancy was consensual, that was your choice, not theirs.

If you want their help, **ask for it,** whether it's financial or emotional, whether it's about working things out with your partner or making the choice to continue or terminate your pregnancy. Understand that a parent can and may say no. Whereas saying no to emotional support would be pretty lousy, saying no to financial help with pregnancy, abortion, or helping to care for your baby is fair and completely within their rights: it may even simply be outside their ability. Paying for a child is rarely easy, and many parents simply won't have the means to support their children's children, too. Expecting a parent or guardian to cover your pregnancy, parenting, or abortion costs or expecting them to help with parenting your child is expecting a lot. So, if you want help in those areas, you need to ask for it and discuss it, not assume you're entitled to it.

If the worst happens when you tell them, there are ways to deal. If you get kicked out of your house, go to your partner or friend, another relative, or a neighbor. If all of those avenues are closed to you, you can go to your local police station, school, or community center to get hooked up with social services for temporary housing.

[**FOR THE "DADS"**]

It's difficult to be involved in a reproductive choice that you had a part in bringing about but that is not happening in *your* body or directly to you. Ultimately, the reproductive choices a person who becomes pregnant makes are—and should be—*their* choices, just like anything that was happening in and to only your body should be yours. You may have input or feelings about certain reproductive options, and the person who's pregnant may even work to make a choice you can both agree on—but they may also find that the best choice for them isn't one you want. Again, although you had a hand in all this, pregnancy doesn't happen in your body, and the hard truth of the matter is that you can bow out at any time a whole lot easier, socially and practically, than the person who is or was pregnant can. In the United States, single mothers outnumber single fathers four to one. As of 2010, the Office of Child Support Enforcement reported 11.3 million child support cases were in arrears.

There are also practical issues for you to bear in mind. You certainly can choose not to opt in to parenting, but if someone pregnant decides to bring a pregnancy to term, in most areas, you *cannot* lawfully opt out of financial support for the child that you helped create. (This is another reason why, if you know you don't want to risk becoming a father, it's a good idea to make your own proactive reproductive choices by always using condoms or opting out of intercourse.) Even if a pregnant person agrees you do not need to provide financial support, they can *always* change their mind at any time. Also, if you opt out of active parenting or child support at any time, and later change your mind, you may discover that being let back in is difficult and, sometimes, it's just not going to happen. When they're old enough, a child may seek you out because they want a relationship with you; or they may not.

Understand that trying to pressure a pregnant partner into a certain reproductive choice just isn't okay. **It's their choice, not yours, however difficult that might be to accept—their body, not yours.** You can certainly let them know what does feel best to you and what you're capable of managing—money and/or support with adoption, abortion, or parenting; the ability and willingness to parent long term or not. You can also let them know what you can't handle or might need help dealing with: this mostly isn't about you, but you're not nonexistent in this situation either. *You matter.*

Support services are often available for a pregnancy and for whichever reproductive choice is made. If you're having a really hard time, seek them out (see the Resources section for some venues for support). In the case of a pregnancy being carried to term, you can ask your partner's doctor or prenatal clinic for a referral; there are often good support groups and free classes for dads-to-be.

We hear a lot about "deadbeat dads" and young men who ditch their partners when their partners become pregnant and carry a child to term. What we don't hear a whole lot about are the teen fathers who not only stick around but also want to actively parent, of which there are also plenty. Some teen fathers find it difficult to be full participants: their partner's parents may be wary or distrustful of them and may not let them parent actively; friends or family may knowingly or unknowingly encourage them to be inactive or may even ridicule them; or they may merely be given the role of paying for things and left out of caretaking. The expectation that guys will leave or blow off responsibilities may be so high that those who *are* trying to do their part may feel pretty defeated.

If you do want to actively parent, you may have to be very proactive and clear about that and work extra hard to get involved and stay involved, even when it's rough or when people are asking you to prove things you really shouldn't have to. Seek help and support where you need to, and don't be afraid to ask for it.

If you need support dealing with abortion or adoption, ask the abortion or adoption provider for help or resources for you or phone your local sexual health clinic and ask for referrals.

Last, don't forget that people who are or can become pregnant aren't the only ones who do or can make initial reproductive choices. *Every single time you have sex that carries a risk of pregnancy, you are making a choice right there and then.* Using reliable birth control properly is almost always a choice *not* to reproduce—and by using condoms, you can make that choice for yourself, by yourself. Opting out of those risks altogether is also a choice you can control. If you know or feel that you just couldn't handle it if a pregnancy occurred—or just don't want to—or that certain reproductive choices a partner might make with a pregnancy wouldn't be okay with you, then the right choice for you to make for now is to opt out of sex with pregnancy risks altogether. Really, choosing to have or not have sex that carries a risk of pregnancy is the major reproductive choice someone who can co-create a pregnancy but who can't themselves become pregnant can make.

Most of this same advice applies if you're the partner of someone pregnant but you don't have a penis (or you do, but yours wasn't involved in their pregnancy). Same-sex couples can deal with these same kinds of struggles or disconnects and with very different feelings and experiences of a pregnancy. You also can connect to many of the same resources suggested and listed for young dads. Just spare yourself a wasted trip by checking in by phone or e-mail first about how queer-friendly a helping resource is.

[BIG IMPACTS, BIG CHOICES]

Sexuality and partnered sex are about far more than reproduction. But for a majority of people, pregnancy—possible and actual—is a big part of the sex they're having, including efforts to prevent it.

The way human reproduction works can make it challenging to balance and equalize responsibility, power, effort, and awareness between each partner when it comes to sex. This is particularly so when there are any big social agency differentials at play—as there often will be, like one person is a woman in the world and one person is a man, or one person is able to become pregnant and the other person is not. There's a pretty profound difference, for instance, in going to bed with someone, thinking, "Oh, God, what if ***I*** get pregnant?" and going to bed thinking, "Oh, God, what if ***they get*** pregnant?" (In case it's not obvious so far, the former is the way bigger deal.)

There's a profound imbalance when one partner is most ultimately responsible for birth control as well as for shouldering the biggest burdens should a pregnancy occur: making tough choices, quickly making big lifestyle and health changes, taking health risks, footing the bills, giving birth or having an abortion, informing everyone about a pregnancy, being the partner who is visibly pregnant to everyone 24/7—and, in case of rape, going through all of that while also fielding emotional and physical trauma. That is not to say that people who are part of a pregnancy, but not pregnant themselves—especially anyone who actively parents, when parenting is what's happening—have no burdens of their own, nor is it to say that having a child or even being pregnant is only a burden and never a boon.

We ALL make choices about whether or not to reproduce, even those of us with same-sex partners and even those of us with no partners at all. If we all always mindfully make those choices, alone and together, and make an effort to share and own that responsibility as best we can, some of the inherent inequities in reproduction—physical, emotional, social, economic, and practical—can become far more balanced.

It's not as tricky as it sounds. As you've discovered, most birth control methods, when used correctly and consistently, are highly effective. Plenty of sexual activities are just as satisfying—often *more* satisfying—than penis-in-vagina intercourse. Although some of those activities still carry STI risks, and safer sex still must be managed, we can easily choose to eradicate pregnancy risks altogether by engaging in those activities instead of activity with a risk of pregnancy—of course, we can opt out of partnered sex or opposite-sex partnered sex altogether.

When that sort of ownership and sharing of responsibility is taken by all partners; when honest and open communication exists; when full, enthusiastic consent and choice of all partners is *always* a given; **and** when both partners make a conscious effort, always, to share all responsibilities in partnered sex, including owning and nurturing their own sexuality separate from a partner's, it's actually incredibly easy to keep things balanced and for the positive, preventative choices we actively—rather than passively—make to net positive, desired results, both small and great.

How to Change the World (Without Even Getting Out of Bed!)

Well, here we are, at the end of this very (very) big book. Phew!

Take a breath. Put your feet up. Have a cup of tea. Watch a silly puppy video. Relax. Revel in the heady afterglow of newly acquired knowledge that's now (hopefully) beaming from the giant light bulb over your head. But before you shuffle off and ably explain to someone that the clitoris is so much bigger than they even knew, pass along the fact that there's no fist in fisting, point out that there are more than two sexes and genders, remark on the fact that, as easy as it feels, our bodies are sure doing a helluva lot of work to have just one little orgasm, or make a song out of the south-to-north trail of anal sexual anatomy to the tune of "Supercalifragilisticexpialidocious" (like so: "Pubococcygeus-rectum-anus-perineum"), I've got just one more thing I want to tell you.

In a better world, a more balanced, humane and healthy place, your sexuality would be one of the *least* of your challenges. It would be something that grounded you and made you feel more at home in the body you inhabit, that sang the praises of your skin with you in an impressively original harmony. It would be a solace, a source of extra energy and comfort, a way to amplify the joy of the good days and to feel better on the bad ones. It would bring you closer to yourself and to others in a unique, intimate manner, in no one's way but your own; it would be a powerful, individual tool of self-expression and personal growth. It would feel like someone honors you and everyone else, including when it's anything but serious. It would make you feel good, and you'd feel good about it.

I don't need to tell you that we don't live in that world yet: you know that already. Your sexuality is probably challenging, including in a lot of ways it just really shouldn't be or doesn't have to be. If you're a young person who wants to own it, full stop—especially if you're marginalized in more ways than by just being young—you will be met with resistance. If you are someone who wants to reinvent your sexual role or identity, especially around things that really scare the crap out of people when they're questioned or reimagined, like gender roles and alternative sexual or relationship frameworks or structures, you will have some areas of nonsupport and intense resistance. If you are in any way marginal in the world at large—like if you're a woman, of color, transgender or otherwise gender nonconforming, poor, pregnant, queer (including asexual), a teen or young parent, of size, or disabled—then it's very likely that managing and owning aspects of your sexuality will often not come easy or receive latitude. Even for people with the most privilege and people who are almost universally seen and accepted as "normal" when it comes to being a person or having a sexuality, the way a lot of the world approaches sexuality can still create challenges. That place where it can all be comfortable, easy, natural, and accepted is just not the world we live in. Not yet, anyway.

Sometimes, when I'm having a bad day or a hard moment in the sex education or support work I do, I stop what I am doing. I take a deep breath. I close my eyes. Then I picture every single person in the world healthy, happy, and feeling whole in themselves and their sexuality: in body, heart, and mind, no matter where they are with it or the whole of their lives. I picture a world without abuse and assault, sexual or otherwise, in which safety, respect, and consent are simply givens for everyone. I picture a world where no one gets called a fag, a slut, a prude, or a pansy, where those jibes have no power. I picture a world in which institutionalized sexual violence and other violence, which is still so prevalent for certain vulnerable groups—young people, women, especially transgender women, queer people, people with disabilities—is no freaking more, for anyone. I picture a world without shame or fear when it comes to bodies, sexualities, or sexual or gender identities, where difference is embraced and celebrated, and where every voice is acknowledged and treated with care and respect. I picture a world where people only become or stay pregnant or parent when they want to, a world where sexually transmitted diseases and the people who have them are treated the same way as any other kind of illness and the people who have them are. I imagine a world where we don't attack those who are different from us because who they are makes us question who *we* are (oh, save us from the horrors of self-awareness and personal exploration!). I picture a world where sexuality is something we can talk about—and a world where no one has a coronary when some sixteen-year-old says they're ready for s.e.x. and they're feeling really happy and excited about it.

It might seem silly to you (sometimes it seems silly to me, too), but it always makes me feel a little better. It makes me feel hopeful, because I strongly feel that we—and you—*can* get to all of that if we just work on making it all happen. If it wasn't possible, if I knew it was nothing but a pipe dream, I don't think I'd do that. It's only because I know those things truly *are* possible—for me, for you, for everybody else—that I immediately feel more hopeful.

See, the world is made up of an awful lot of people. (Yeah, duh, I know.) And it's *people* who make it the way that it is with most of this stuff, who choose to either start thinking about and doing things a new, better way or enable the same tired, uninspired old crap to continue.

I'm going to ask a favor of you. Humor me.

See if you can't make that same kind of picture in your head, and see if you can picture *yourself* being one of the many kickass people who create and support that world. I'm asking you to recognize and claim the incredible power and potential that you have to make not only *your* world but also *the* world different—better—when it comes to sex and sexuality. Just as I encourage anyone to do with their own sex life, I'm asking you to consider being active, not passive; thoughtful, not careless; compassionate, not cruel (to others *or* yourself) in ways both small *and* great.

You can do this. In fact, I feel pretty sure that you, as a person, and you, as a part of the big group that is made of millions and millions of people at or somewhere near your own age, can probably do all of this better than most people have in the past, including a lot of people much older than you right this very minute, including me.

I ask this of you because I *know* you can do this and because I know it's possible. Some people before you have done an amazing job on this front. Others have mucked it up utterly. All of them had the power to do exactly what it is they did, just as you have the power to do whatever it is you're doing or will do.

Here's the beauty of the thing: this really isn't that hard to do. It's mostly just about changing your mind, which you probably already do at least several times a day, if not a lot more often.

You can do it just by claiming your sexuality for yourself, being its author, designer, and manager (and even when you stumble sometimes, as we all do). Just by coming to it mindfully, with real care, love, and respect for yourself and others, you've won at least half the battle and are approaching it in a radically different way from how a lot of people have and do. Apply that same approach to how you regard and treat the sexuality of everyone else and you've made a giant leap in helping us get to that better place. Hey—it's not every day that powerful activist work is so enjoyable or provides so many personal benefits. Seize that opportunity. Don't let it go. Milk it for all it is freaking worth. Then just go be and do you with all that in your head, heart, and hands.

The American poet, essayist, humanist (and queer person) Walt Whitman, in

Leaves of Grass, said, "We convince by our presence." This is what he meant.

At the start of this book, I asked something of you, too. I asked you to boldly **choose to create a healthy, happy, and fulfilling sexual life that is fantastic for you and for everyone else in it.**

You can be bold and do this, and you can do it brilliantly.

You've got this, and I'm so excited about that, for you and for all the rest of us. Because you've got this and if you just think about, care for, explore, and enact your own sexuality and all of sexuality from that kind of place? Then we're all—you, me, your best friend, your sister, and some dude you don't even know who's rocking out at the bus stop across the street right now—going to start to experience a world and sexualities within that world that are truly more humane and whole, far healthier for everyone, and a reflection of the very best of who we are and can be.

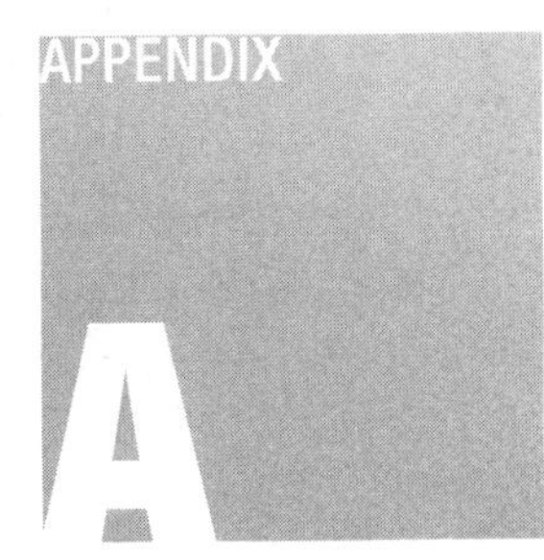

Common Sexually Transmitted Infections: STIs from A to Z

For information on how to safeguard your sexual health, protect yourself and partners from STIs, and deal with life with an STI, see Chapter 10, "Safe and Sound: Safer Sex for Your Body, Heart, and Mind."

[CHLAMYDIA]

Chlamydia is the most common sexually transmitted bacterial infection in the world: it is estimated that there are as many as three million new cases every year in the United States alone. It's the most reported infectious disease of all kinds of infectious diseases (not just STIs) in the United States. In 2014, the Centers for Disease Control and Prevention found 68 percent of all reported chlamydia cases occurred in young people between the ages of fifteen and twenty; the highest incidence rates for chlamydia are in people between the ages of fifteen and twenty-four. Most people who have contracted chlamydia do not know they have it or have had it.

Chlamydia infects the cervix and can spread to the urethra, fallopian tubes, and ovaries. It can cause chronic bladder infections and is strongly associated with pelvic inflammatory disease (PID), ectopic pregnancy, and infertility. For those with a penis, it infects the urethra and can spread to the testicles, which is associated with infertility. Chlamydia can also lead to Reiter's syndrome, which involves eye infections, urethritis, and arthritis and can often cause chronic disability.

How do you get it? Chlamydia is most often spread through unprotected vaginal or anal intercourse, oral sex, shared sex toys, contact during childbirth, and, in rare cases, from hand-to-eye and other nonsexual contact.

How can you tell if you have it? Most people with chlamydia experience no symptoms. When symptoms *are* present, they may include pain or burning while urinating, unexplained vaginal bleeding or spotting, painful intercourse, abdominal pain or nausea, fever, or swelling or pain of the rectum, cervix, or testicles.

Chlamydia is typically diagnosed by a healthcare provider with a urine or genital swab sample (of the vagina, penis, urethra, or anus).

How do you treat it? Chlamydia is usually very easily treatable with antibiotics, and once treated it is no longer present in the body and can't be passed to a partner unless you contract it again. So long as it is diagnosed and treated quickly, long-term impacts are not likely. However, if someone is not treated or has the infection for weeks or longer, long-term impacts, like PID, become increasingly likely. It's very important that any sexual partners someone with chlamydia has been with over a two-month period be tested and treated. Reinfection (repeat infection) rates of chlamydia are very high, usually because all partners aren't treated or, during treatment, partners continue to not practice safer sex, so the infection keeps getting passed back and forth.

How do you avoid it? Chlamydia is nearly always transmitted by unprotected sexual activity, so using latex barriers for vaginal, oral, and anal sex or abstaining from genital sex with partners almost always prevents chlamydia infection.

[GONORRHEA]

Another bacterial infection, gonorrhea is also incredibly common: it's the *second* most reported infectious disease in the United States. About forty million people in the United States have had it. About 75 percent of all reported cases occur in people younger than thirty years.

Gonorrhea appears in warm, moist places such as the cervix, uterus, fallopian tubes, rectum, urethra, mouth, throat, penis, and testicles.

How do you get it? Gonorrhea is usually transmitted by oral, vaginal, or anal contact and can also be passed from an infected person to an infant during childbirth. It is strongly associated with infertility. Those who have gonorrhea and who do not treat it promptly may develop pelvic inflammatory disease (PID). Untreated gonorrhea can also lead to prostatitis or epididymis and narrowing of the urethra, which makes it difficult to urinate.

How can you tell if you have it? If a person has symptoms, they usually appear in the first week after exposure to gonorrhea, but sometimes symptoms appear a month or more after exposure. However, many people do not experience any symptoms.

Someone with a gonorrheal infection may have unusual vaginal or rectal discharge, anal itching, genital soreness, unexplained genital bleeding, or pain when urinating. Gonorrhea of the throat—which is common among people who engage in unprotected oral sex—is usually asymptomatic.

A healthcare provider usually diagnoses gonorrhea with a genital or throat swab test or through a urine sample.

How do you treat it? It is treated with antibiotics. Treatment cures a gonorrheal infection completely, but, like with chlamydia, a person can still contract it again. It's important to treat all current partners when any one partner is diagnosed so that, if the infection is present in more than that one person, it isn't just passed back and forth again and again.

How do you avoid it? Gonorrhea is almost always sexually transmitted, so if you aren't sexually active, your chances of getting it are basically zero. If you are sexually active, you can very effectively prevent gonorrheal infection with basic safer sex practices and screenings.

[HEPATITIS]

Hepatitis A, B, and C are infectious viruses that destroy the liver.

HBV (hepatitis B) is the form of hepatitis spread most commonly via sexual activity (although hepatitis A can be transmitted by oral-anal contact, and hepatitis C is more commonly transmitted by sexual contact than previously thought). Hepatitis A and B have been on the decline in the United States since the 1990s, but the number of hepatitis C infections has been increasing since 2010.

Internationally, one out of three people has been infected with hepatitis B virus, and four hundred million people are carriers of it. In the United States alone, one out of twenty people has been infected with hepatitis B, and there are over one million chronic carriers.

How do you get it? HBV is found in body fluids such as blood, semen, and vaginal fluid, so the most common ways HBV spreads are unprotected sex, sharing drug needles, and tattoos or piercings done with unsanitized tools. It can also be transmitted to an infant during childbirth or breastfeeding.

How can you tell if you have it? Soon after a person is infected, they might get flu-like symptoms such as fever, feeling very tired or easily winded, muscle and joint pain, appetite loss, and nausea or vomiting. Around half of all people infected with hepatitis B don't have any symptoms. A healthcare provider can test for HBV with a blood test.

How do you treat it? Treatments to slow the development of hepatitis B are available, and the vast majority of people fight HBV with natural antibodies and cure themselves over time. Healthcare providers can also help people with hepatitis with a range of medications, supporting health care and lifestyle changes. A diagnosis is very important because some people never develop antibodies to the virus, and thus will always be carriers, and they may develop liver problems or liver cancer later in life. Knowing HBV status is also vital when it comes to knowing if you can infect others.

How do you avoid it? The very best way to prevent infection with hepatitis is to get the vaccine (available for both types A and B). Check in with your healthcare provider to find out whether you've had the vaccine already (chances are good that you have), and if not, ask for it. If you haven't been vaccinated against hepatitis, wear gloves any time you come in contact with body fluids (sexually or in work situations), don't share needles, make sure tattoos and piercings are done with fresh, new equipment, and practice safer sex.

[HERPES]

The herpes virus has been around since at least the ancient Greeks: *herpes* is the Greek word meaning "to creep or crawl."

There are two types of the herpes simplex virus (HSV): type 1 (HSV-1) and type 2 (HSV-2). Type 1 usually infects the mouth (cold sores are always a symptom of HSV-1), and type 2 usually infects the genitals. However, HSV-1 has been more and more commonly reported as the cause of genital herpes in young people, most likely due to the frequency of unprotected oral sex.

Herpes is one of the most common sexually transmitted infections. More than 50 percent of the adult population in the United States has HSV-1, or oral herpes, and about one out of every six people (about 16 percent) ages fourteen to forty-nine years in the United States have HSV-2, the virus that most often causes genital herpes. Many people with either kind of HSV do not have visible symptoms or know what a herpes outbreak, orally or genitally, looks or feels like to know when they are having a symptom. It's most commonly acquired in adolescence, although symptoms may become more prevalent or frequent with age. Since the 1970s, genital herpes infections have increased at least 30 percent, with the largest increase occurring among emerging adults.

How do you get it? Both types can be transmitted sexually (through kissing and oral sex as well as through skin and genital contact). HSV-1 is not limited to the mouth area: if a person with oral herpes performs oral sex, it is possible for the partner to get genital herpes. HSV-1 can also sometimes cause genital-area or anal-area lesions or sores. Most people who contract HSV-1, however, most often contract it in childhood or adolescence from nonsexual contact.

Herpes viruses are spread by contact between an infected area of the body and an uninfected, susceptible area of an uninfected person's body—usually an area with mucous membrane, like the mouth or genitals. This means that herpes can be spread from any affected part of the body—penis, vulva, anus, mouth, eye, lips—with or without fluid sharing.

Sexually, it is most often spread by unprotected vaginal, anal, or oral sex or kissing. Herpes is most contagious when someone has an active sore; however, it may also be spread via asymptomatic shedding, when no sores are visible or perceived to be present.

Safer sex practices and barriers offer protection, but barriers like condoms that do not cover the entire surface of the genitals cannot offer complete protection, even though they do reduce risks. It is believed that barriers provide solid protection—estimates are that they reduce the risk of infection by between 50 and 60 percent—but they do offer less protection than for infections that are transmitted only by fluids, like HIV or chlamydia, not just skin-to-skin contact. Barriers that cover more of the genitals—like dental dams or inside condoms—can provide greater protection.

How can you tell if you have it? *If you experience cold sores or fever blisters, you have oral herpes* and can give it to a partner orally or genitally—something that is often not made clear to people with cold sores. (Those aren't the same as canker sores, by the way. Cold, or herpes, sores appear *on* or *around* the mouth. Canker sores aren't a viral symptom but a mouth injury that occurs *inside* the mouth.)

When symptoms are present with genital herpes, they're usually in the form of a rash or red blisters on the vulva, vagina, or cervix; on the penis, buttocks, or anus; or on the mouth and other areas of the body. Symptoms are generally sore or uncomfortable and tend to recur (happen more than once). When someone first contracts herpes, they might also experience burning while urinating, swollen glands, fever, headache, loss of appetite, and tiredness. When these first symptoms do occur, it's usually within one month of initial transmission, but a rash or sores may not occur for years afterward or may not be visible on the external genitals. However, as many as two out of three people with HSV-1 and almost half of all people with HSV-2 never show or recognize symptoms.

Either form of the herpes virus can be diagnosed by a doctor, usually with a swab of an active sore or via a blood test.

How do you treat it? Herpes isn't curable, in that there isn't treatment to make the virus leave the body. Once it's in there, it's in there for good. However, herpes symptoms and outbreaks—as well as the risk of transmitting it to a partner—can be greatly reduced with oral medications.

How do you avoid it? Most often transmission happens when there *is* an active sore or when a sore is just forming or healing. However, it *can* be transmitted through asymptomatic—as in, without any active sores—shedding, and that is more common in the first few years after someone acquires either type of the herpes virus. People with either form of herpes should avoid unprotected oral or genital contact with others where and when sores are present or when they can feel the tingling sensation that often signals an approaching outbreak. The consistent use of barriers in safer sex substantially reduces the risk of herpes infection.

[HIV]

HIV (human immunodeficiency virus) is a type of virus called a *retrovirus*: it changes a cell's DNA. The HIV retrovirus strongly attacks the immune system and thus massively weakens the body's ability to fight disease and infection, even common infections like flus and colds. AIDS (acquired immunodeficiency syndrome) is an acquired syndrome, or group of symptoms, that can be caused by infection with the HIV virus. **HIV can cause AIDS, but AIDS is *not* an STI: no one can get AIDS from someone else, only HIV.** AIDS is a condition that can develop as a *result* of HIV infection.

HIV is not the most common STI, particularly in developed nations, but it *is* the most lethal. HIV is a very dangerous, potentially deadly infection.

About fifty thousand people in the United States become infected with HIV every year. In 2010, HIV was the seventh leading cause of death for those ages twenty-five to forty-four. Widely (and dangerously) misrepresented as a disease that only or primarily infects gay men, HIV currently infects women, especially women of color, worldwide at higher rates than men. Adolescent and adult women account for about 27 percent of new HIV infections in the United States; HIV has been increasing in those populations for some time.

At least twenty-five million people have died as a result of HIV infection, making it the deadliest epidemic in history. At this time, no one has yet been cured of HIV, but research is still ongoing. Thankfully, however, HIV-related deaths have fallen by around 30 percent since a peak in 2005.

How do you get it? HIV is spread through body fluids (blood, semen, vaginal secretions, and breast milk) via unprotected anal and vaginal intercourse, oral sex (although transmission through oral sex is more rare), shared needles used for injecting IV drugs or body modification, accidental pricks with infected needles, blood transfusions, childbirth, and breastfeeding.

How can you tell if you have it? Initial infection may have symptoms that resemble mononucleosis or the flu within two to four weeks of exposure, but for most people, HIV infection does not show any symptoms for extended periods of time—for some, it is asymptomatic for years. When symptoms are present, they may include sore throat, fever, mouth sores or ulcers, aching or stiff muscles or joints, headaches, diarrhea, swollen glands, rashes or eczema, yeast infections, tiredness, or rapid weight loss.

HIV is diagnosed with a cheek swab or blood test that looks for HIV antibodies. If a cheek swab is done and nets a positive result, a blood test is done to confirm the diagnosis. Because it can take up to three months or more for antibodies to appear, a negative test should always be repeated after a known or suspected risk, and an annual or semiannual HIV screening is strongly advised for sexually active people.

How do you treat it? HIV cannot be cured, but it can be treated and managed, usually through an aggressive combination of antiviral drugs, self-care remedies, nutrition, and consistent health care. Most HIV treatments act to try to protect the immune system from further infection and to fend off or slow the progression of HIV to AIDS. These treatments aren't magic, unfortunately: it is still very hard to live with the physical impact of HIV alone, as well as the impacts of the treatments.

HIV treatment is in a state of constant development and flux, with frequent new treatments and new approaches to treatment. To find and figure out the best course of treatment for you, do your best to choose healthcare providers who stay current, who work expressly in HIV care, and who are always willing to answer all of your questions and concerns. A printed reference book like this can only give the most basic information, and only at the time of writing. With something as potentially serious as HIV and whose management is changing so fast all the time, a healthcare provider who works in HIV care is who you want to get in touch with first and foremost.

How do you avoid it? HIV infection can be very effectively prevented by using condoms for vaginal intercourse, anal intercourse, and oral sex. Prevention methods also include avoiding high-risk sexual practices like anal sex, oral-anal sex, or vaginal sex altogether; avoiding sex with those who use intravenous drugs and not participating in IV drug use yourself; avoiding blood or urine contact with the mouth, anus, eyes, or open cuts or sores; and insisting your partners get annual or semiannual HIV screenings.

Medications called antiretrovirals (PEP or PrEP, post-exposure or pre-exposure prophylaxis) can reduce your risk of acquiring HIV after and before exposure or possible exposure to HIV. If at any time you know or suspect you may have been exposed to HIV very recently, talk to your healthcare provider. You can also talk to them about PrEP, a daily pill that, in recent studies, has been found to be as safe as taking aspirin daily. PrEP can reduce the risk of HIV by as much as 90 percent and is advised for those at very high risk of HIV, like people with HIV-positive partners. It may currently also be prescribed to people who often have sex outside of mutually monogamous relationships, who do not use condoms or only use them inconsistently. The availability of PrEP is currently increasing, so it may soon be available to anyone who wants it and can safely use it. PrEP should not be considered a replacement for safer sex practices like condom use and testing, however, particularly because it does not provide protection for any STIs besides HIV.

[HUMAN PAPILLOMAVIRUS (HPV) AND GENITAL WARTS]

HPV is likely the most common STI in the United States. The Guttmacher Institute reports that nearly three out of every four Americans between the ages of fifteen and forty-nine have been infected with HPV at some point in their lives, and some studies show that at *least* one-third of all sexually active young adults have genital HPV infections. Over five million new cases of HPV infections are reported every year in the United States alone.

There are around thirty different known strains, or types, of HPV that infect the genital tract, some of which are considered high-risk strains because they are associated with some kinds of cancer. HPV is often called genital warts because when some strains are externally symptomatic (not all can be, only some are) the virus appears as tiny cauliflower-like warts on the internal or external genitals. About two-thirds of people who have sexual contact with a partner with a wart-producing strain of HPV will develop warts, usually within three months of contact. Yet, only a teeny sliver of the US population has genital warts; in most cases, HPV shows no external symptoms, although it is still present and highly contagious, and condoms do not offer complete protection against HPV.

HPV infection used to be considered permanent, like herpes infections. However, as the Centers for Disease Control and Prevention reports, more recent study data have found that much of the time HPV resolves itself, leaving the body within a couple of years without creating any health problems. It does not do so in all people, though, and when it doesn't cancers can appear because of it. We don't currently know why it goes away for some people, but not for others, but we do know it's more common for people's bodies to be able to ditch it when they acquire it as a young person than when they are older.

However, no one should ever just assume once they've acquired it that HPV has gone away. Whether the infection is still present in the body is something only a healthcare provider can determine.

How do you get it? It is transmitted through genital contact, usually during vaginal or anal sex, and sometimes through oral or manual sex. Someone who has never had any kind of sexual contact (including sexual abuse or assault) is very unlikely to become infected with HPV. Because barriers like condoms cover only part of the genitals, although using them absolutely does reduce the risk of infection, they are not as helpful at preventing HPV infections as they are at preventing STIs transmitted by fluid sharing. So, it is possible to contract HPV from protected sex, but barriers make it far less likely.

How can you tell if you have it? Again, most HPV cases are asymptomatic: less than 1 percent of people with HPV notice any visible symptoms. When symptoms are present, small, cauliflower-like warts can appear on the vulva, vagina, anus, or penis; inside the urethra; or in the throat, at any time from thirty days to years after infection. People can see some of those body areas and can notice warts; other parts cannot be seen, like the inside of the vagina or urethra. Not all strains of sexually transmitted HPV are wart-causing strains, however.

When warts *are* present, diagnosis by a healthcare provider is pretty simple with a tissue sample, vinegar test, or visual exam of the wart or warts. When no visible symptoms exist, a Pap smear may reveal precancerous conditions likely caused by HPV, and there is also a test for HPV called the digene test that can be run on the same cells swabbed during a Pap smear. A colposcope (a special magnifying instrument used to get a closer look at the vagina and cervix) may also be used to obtain a diagnosis.

Currently, there is no way of testing for HPV for people with a penis if they do not have a wart that can be sampled. If someone's partner is infected, it is generally assumed that he is as well: HPV is very contagious.

How do you treat it? The virus itself is not presently treatable or curable, but in most cases, it resolves itself in time, often within a couple of years.

If warts are present, they can be removed by various methods, namely, cryotherapy (being frozen) or electrocautery, a patient-applied solution, acid solutions, or laser surgery. Those methods are relatively painless and are usually done in a healthcare provider's office on an outpatient basis, not in a hospital, although people with more extensive warts may require surgery. Which method is used depends on the patient, the availability of methods, and the particular warts and strain in question. Even when warts are removed, the virus is still present in the body and can be transmitted to partners.

How do you avoid it? If you're sexually active, to prevent HPV practice safer sex, including getting annual screenings and Pap smears and using barriers, even though latex barriers do not offer as much protection as they do for fluid-borne infections. Avoiding genital contact with partners altogether is also a protection against HPV. Be sure, too, to stay up-to-date with yearly Pap smears, which can diagnose cervical cancer from HPV early enough for effective treatment.

Vaccinations are available for the most high-risk strains of HPV, and vaccination has been found to provide the most effective HPV prevention so far: HPV vaccination is nearly 100 percent effective at protecting patients against four of the most common and risky HPV strains. Vaccination is available for people of any gender, and it's recommended people get the vaccination—which is typically done in a series of three—before becoming sexual with partners, when possible. However, even for people who have already been sexually active (or who have been sexually abused or assaulted), the vaccine can still be used, although it may not be as effective. Ask your healthcare provider about the HPV vaccine.

[MONONUCLEOSIS]

Mononucleosis, or "mono," is a general infection caused by the Epstein-Barr virus and spreads in many of the same ways as a simple flu virus does.

How do you get it? It's often called the "kissing disease" because it's spread mainly by contact with saliva or mucus from someone with mono and because mono is common in adolescents. But it can also be spread by sharing drinking glasses or silverware or by being coughed on by someone who has it.

How can you tell if you have it? Some lucky people with mono experience no symptoms. For most others, though, fever, a sore throat, swollen glands, headaches, reduced appetite, and exhaustion are common.

How do you treat it? Mono isn't treatable. As with a common cold—albeit a really, really bad one, because mono generally feels way more miserable than a cold—you just have to rest and wait it out. That can take a week to over a month, unfortunately. Mono isn't a serious threat to most people's health. If you suspect mono, do see a doctor, however, to make sure it isn't something else with similar symptoms that does need treatment, like strep throat.

How do you avoid it? Because mono is so often transmitted casually, and without sexual contact, the only thing you can really do to avoid it, besides living alone under a rock, is to be sure to avoid intimate contact with someone you know currently has or has been exposed to mono.

[PELVIC INFLAMMATORY DISEASE (PID)]

Pelvic inflammatory disease is a serious bacterial infection of the uterus, uterine lining, fallopian tubes, and/or ovaries. It is dangerous, but not contagious. It's not an STI, but it is most often caused by an STI.

About one million cases of PID are reported in the United States annually, and 20 percent of PID cases are found in teens, who often are unable to get or just don't get reproductive health care, including STI screenings and treatment. When left untreated, PID in one site can progressively infect other reproductive organs. It can, and often does, result in chronic pain and can cause ectopic pregnancy (when an embryo implants in a fallopian tube or somewhere other than the uterus) or permanent sterility (inability to conceive). PID is one of the leading causes of infertility.

How do you get it? PID usually starts in the vagina via an existing sexually transmitted infection. Gonorrhea and chlamydia are the usual causes of PID, especially when they are left untreated or treatment is delayed or incomplete.

How can you tell if you have it? PID symptoms include painful periods that may last longer than in previous cycles, spotting or cramping between periods, unusual vaginal discharge, pain or cramping during urination, blood in the urine, lower back or abdominal pain, fever, nausea or vomiting, and/or pain during vaginal intercourse.

PID is often difficult to diagnose, and it is widely thought that millions of cases each year go undiagnosed or are overlooked. To diagnose PID, a pelvic exam is required that includes a Pap smear and a possible laparoscopy (a diagnostic procedure that can usually be done in an office visit) for your healthcare provider to take a close look at your reproductive system. It is also imperative that you tell your provider if you have been sexually active with a partner and what your sexual history has been, including any known or suspected sexually transmitted infections.

How do you treat it? PID is curable, but a person can become reinfected. A PID infection can result in some permanent health issues even with treatment. It is often treated with a combination of antibiotics, bed rest, and a period of sexual celibacy. In more severe cases, surgery may be required, including the possible removal of reproductive organs.

How do you avoid it? Safer sex practices, especially condoms during vaginal intercourse, offer a high level of protection from PID. Because untreated STIs are often at the root of PID, annual STI screenings greatly reduce the risk of PID.

[PUBIC LICE]

Pubic lice are sometimes known as "crabs." The condition is caused by very tiny parasitic mites that settle in the pubic hair and feed on human blood. About three million new cases of pubic lice are treated in the United States each year, but it is unknown how many people have it at any one time.

How do you get it? Pubic lice are often spread through sexual contact (and latex barrier use doesn't help, because they live in the pubic hair, not on the genitals) but can also be transmitted through bed linens, towels, or clothes because lice can live for twenty-four hours off a human body. Lice are basically people fleas and operate much the same way as fleas do. It is unlikely that pubic lice can be spread by toilet seats, because the feet of lice are not designed to walk on or hold on to smooth surfaces.

How can you tell if you have it? The primary symptom of pubic lice is unmistakable: severe and constant itching in the pubic area within about five days of infection. Some people also get blue spots where they have been bitten. Scratching the itchy areas may spread the lice to other parts of the body with coarse body hair, such as the legs, armpits, mustache or beard, eyebrows, or eyelashes.

Pubic lice can be self-diagnosed, but not easily, because they can be confused with other sorts of mites. A healthcare provider diagnoses pubic lice by looking at a skin sample under a microscope.

How do you treat it? Lotions and shampoos that kill pubic lice are available from a doctor or pharmacy. A person with pubic lice also needs to clean anything that might have lice on it: dirty clothes, bed linens, towels, and the like need to be washed in very hot water. If something can't be washed, it needs to be put in a sealed plastic bag for two weeks to kill the lice and keep them from hopping onto another body in the meantime. It's common to still be itchy for a bit after treatment. Calamine lotion or hydrocortisone creams can relieve itching.

Pubic lice do not cause anything more than discomfort and inconvenience, although people who scratch the bites may get bacterial infections.

How do you avoid it? Latex barriers with sexual partners don't make any difference to pubic lice. So, unfortunately, there's little you can do to avoid pubic lice except avoiding close contact or linen sharing with someone you know has them.

[SYPHILIS]

Syphilis, one of the oldest STIs out there, is a bacterial infection. There are currently fewer that forty thousand reported cases of syphilis in the United States, but there have been considerable increases in the rate of infection over the last ten years in both the United States and Europe. People with untreated syphilis may develop neurosyphilis, a potentially serious disorder of the nervous system. Infants born to mothers with syphilis can be born with very severe mental and physical problems.

In the event you want to get your geek on, syphilis, with gonorrhea, was the target of one of the first abstinence and celibacy campaigns in the United States during World War II. Whereas nearly every other country furnished its soldiers with scads of condoms to protect them, the United States opted for a celibacy campaign. Guess whose country ended up with a syphilis epidemic peaking at over a hundred thousand cases? (The United States.)

How do you get it? Syphilis is spread through skin-to-skin contact when someone touches a sore on a person who has syphilis. The sores are usually on the mouth, penis, vagina, or anus. Syphilis is usually transmitted during oral, vaginal, or anal sexual contact.

How can you tell if you have it? Syphilis has been called "the great imitator" because many of its signs look like those of other diseases. It is also difficult to know whether someone has syphilis because a person might not have any symptoms at all. There are considered to be four stages of syphilis:

1. **Primary: The first symptom of syphilis is an ulcer few people will notice that forms one to six weeks after exposure in the area where the person was exposed.** These ulcers usually disappear in a few weeks on their own, but the person still has the infection and can pass the disease to other people during this stage.
2. **Secondary: A skin rash of large, coin-sized sores.** There are infectious bacteria in the sores, so anyone who touches them can be infected. Mild fever, headache, sore throat, and hair loss are also secondary symptoms. These symptoms usually go away in a few months but recur for up to two years, and again the person is still carrying the bacteria and can infect others.
3. **Latent: During this stage, there are often no symptoms at all, but the infection is still present.** During this time, the infected person likely does not infect others.
4. **Tertiary/Late: People who are infected for a long time may develop many severe problems.** The bacteria can damage the heart, eyes, liver, brain, bones, and joints. People can develop mental illness as a result of the infection, lose their eyesight, develop heart disease, or die.

Syphilis is screened for with microscopic examination of fluid from sores, blood tests, and examination of spinal fluid. It's important that the partners of anyone diagnosed with syphilis also be treated and that anyone treated be retested after treatment to be sure treatment worked.

How do you treat it? Dangerous as it can be, it's easily cured and treated: just a single dose of penicillin can usually cure a person who has had the infection for less than a year. So, annual STI screenings are important as ever. If you're tested once a year, you can rest assured that there's no way you'll be walking around with syphilis for longer than that, even if you've taken sexual risks.

How do you avoid it? Syphilis is generally transmitted only through unprotected sex, so you can prevent syphilis with standard and constant safer sex practices or by abstaining from sexual contact with others.

[TRICHOMONIASIS]

Trichomoniasis ("trich"), infection with the *Trichomonas* parasite, is one of the most common STIs, mainly affecting people younger than thirty-five years. In the

United States, 2.3 million (3.1 percent) cisgender women ages fourteen to forty-nine are estimated to have it.

How do you get it? *Trichomonas* parasites live in warm and damp environments like the vagina, urethra, and bladder. Infection is usually sexually transmitted via direct genital contact but occasionally is spread by sharing damp towels, washcloths, or bathing suits.

How can you tell if you have it? Only about half the people with trich have any symptoms. When symptoms do develop, usually within one to several months, they may include a yellow-green, foul smelling vaginal discharge; vaginal itching or redness; pain during intercourse or urination; and a frequent urge to urinate. Pain during urination and ejaculation, discharge from the urethra of the penis, and a frequent urge to urinate are some symptoms that may be present in infected people with penises.

Healthcare providers diagnose trich by examining genital discharge under a microscope and with a genital exam.

How do you treat it? Antibiotics for an infected person and their sexual partners usually cure the infection, but a second round of antibiotics is sometimes needed. It is also helpful to wear cotton underwear and avoid wearing pantyhose during treatment.

How do you avoid it? It is spread via direct genital fluid contact, so if you aren't sexually active, you aren't likely to acquire trichomoniasis. If you are sexually active, latex barriers during genital sexual activities offer excellent protection against trich.

APPENDIX

B

Bibliography and Recommended Resources

FOREWORD, CHAPTERS 1–4

Chapters covering general sexuality; sex and culture; anatomy; body image and self-esteem; general health; masturbation, arousal, and orgasm; fantasy

Books and Print Sources and Resources

Angier, Natalie. *Woman: An Intimate Geography*. New York: Anchor, 2000.

Arnett, Jeffrey Jansen. *Emerging Adulthood*. 2nd ed. New York: Oxford University Press, 2015.

Bartle, Nathalie, and Susan Lieberman. *Venus in Blue Jeans: Why Mothers and Daughters Need to Talk About Sex*. Boston: Dell, 1999.

Blank, Joani. *Femalia*. San Francisco: Down There Press, 1993.

Bornstein, Kate. *Hello Cruel World: 101 Alternatives to Suicide for Teens, Freaks, and Other Outlaws*. New York: Seven Stories Press, 2006.

Boston Women's Health Book Collective. *Our Bodies, Ourselves for the New Century: A Book by and for Women*. New York: Touchstone, 1998.

Brashich, Audrey D. *All Made Up: A Girl's Guide to Seeing Through Celebrity Hype and Celebrating Real Beauty*. New York: Walker Books for Young Readers, 2006.

Brumberg, Joan Jacobs. *The Body Project: An Intimate History of American Girls*. New York: Vintage Books, 1998.

Cohen, Joseph. *The Penis Book*. New York: Broadway Books, 2004.

Cornog, Martha. *The Big Book of Masturbation: From Angst to Zeal*. San Francisco: Down There Press, 2003.

Costin, Carolyn. *The Eating Disorder Sourcebook: A Comprehensive Guide to the Causes, Treatments, and Prevention of Eating Disorders*. New York: McGraw-Hill, 1999.

Dodson, Betty. *Sex for One: The Joy of Selfloving*. New York: Three Rivers Press, 1996.

Drill, Esther, Heather McDonald, and Rebecca Odes. *Deal With It! A Whole New Approach to Your Body, Brain and Life as a gURL*. New York: Pocket Books, 1999.

Engel, Beverly. *Healing Your Emotional Self: A Powerful Program to Help You Raise Your Self-Esteem, Quiet Your Inner Critic, and*

Overcome Your Shame. Hoboken, NJ: Wiley, 2006.

Espeland, Pamela. *Life Lists for Teens: Tips, Steps, Hints, and How-Tos for Growing Up, Getting Along, Learning, and Having Fun*. Minneapolis, MN: Free Spirit Publishing, 2003.

Gottlieb, Lori. *Stick Figure*. New York: Berkley Trade, 2001.

Hills, Rachel. *The Sex Myth: The Gap Between Our Fantasies and Reality*. New York: Simon and Schuster Paperbacks, 2015.

Hite, Shere. *The Hite Report on the Family: Growing Up Under Patriarchy*. New York: Grove Press, 1996.

Hornbacher, Marya. *Wasted: A Memoir of Anorexia and Bulimia*. New York: Harper Perennial, 1999.

Houppert, Karen. *The Curse: Confronting the Last Unmentionable Taboo: Menstruation*. New York: Farrar, Straus and Giroux, 2000.

Jamison, Paul H. "Penis Size Increase Between Flaccid and Erect States: An Analysis of the Kinsey Data." *Journal of Sex Research* 24, nos. 1–4 (January 1988).

Jukes, Mavis. *The Guy Book: An Owner's Manual*. New York: Crown Publishers, 2002.

Kirberger, Kimberly. *No Body's Perfect: Stories by Teens About Body Image, Self-Acceptance, and the Search for Identity*. New York: Scholastic Paperbacks, 2003.

Komisaruk, Barry R., Carlos Beyer-Flores, and Beverly Whipple. *The Science of Orgasm*. Baltimore: Johns Hopkins University Press, 2006.

Lopez, Ralph I. *The Teen Health Book: A Parent's Guide to Adolescent Health and Well-Being*. New York: W. W. Norton, 2003.

Luciano, Lynn. *Looking Good: Male Body Image in Modern America*. New York: Hill & Wang, 2001.

McKoy, Kathy. *The Teenage Body Book*. Rutherford, NJ: Perigee Trade, 1999.

Moore, Susan, and Doreen Rosenthal. *Sexuality in Adolescence: Current Trends*. New York: Routledge, 2006.

Muscio, Inga. *Cunt: A Declaration of Independence*. Seattle, WA: Seal Press, 1998.

Nagoski, Emily. *Come as You Are: The Surprising New Science that Will Transform Your Sex Life*. New York: Simon & Schuster Paperbacks, 2015.

Neinstein, Lawrence S. *Handbook of Adolescent Health Care*. Philadelphia: Wolters Kluwer, 2009.

Netter, Frank H. *Atlas of Human Anatomy*. Philadelphia: Saunders, 2002.

Paley, Maggie. *The Book of the Penis*. New York: Grove Press, 2000.

Pardes, Bronwen. *Doing It Right: Making Smart, Safe, and Satisfying Choices About Sex*. New York: Simon Pulse, 2013.

Parker, William H., and Rachel L. Parker. *A Gynecologist's Second Opinion*. New York: Plume Books, 2003.

Planned Parenthood Federation of America. *The Planned Parenthood Women's Health Encyclopedia*. New York: Crown Trade Paperbacks, 1996.

Rayne, Karen. *Breaking the Hush Factor: The Ten Rules Every Parent Should Know Before Talking with Their Teen About Sex*. Austin: Impetus Books, 2015.

Reinisch, June M., and Ruth Beasley. *The Kinsey Institute New Report on Sex*. New York: St. Martin's Griffin, 1991.

Robertson, Wrenna, and Katie Huisman. *I'll Show You Mine*. Vancouver, BC: Show Off Books, 2011.

Roffman, Deborah. *Talk to Me First: Everything You Need to Know to Become Your Kids' "Go-To" Person About Sex*. Boston: Da Capo Lifelong Books, 2012.

Salmansohn, Karen. *The Clitourist: A Guide to One of the Hottest Spots on Earth*. New York: Universe Publishing, 2001.

Sandoz, Emily, and Troy DuFrene. *Living with Your Body and Other Things You Hate: How to Let Go of Your Struggle with Body Image Using Acceptance and Commitment Therapy*. Vancouver, BC: Raincoast Books, 2013.

Seidman, Steven, Nancy Fischer, and Chet Meets. *Introducing the New Sexuality Studies, Second Edition*. Routledge, 2011.

Siegel, Daniel J. *Brainstorm: The Power and Purpose of the Teenage Brain*. New York: Jeremy P. Tarcher/Penguin, 2015.

Silverberg, Cory, and Fiona Smyth. *Sex Is a Funny Word*. New York: Seven Stories Press, 2015.

Taylor, Julia V. *The Body Image Workbook for Teens*. Oakland, CA: Instant Help Books, 2014.

Vernacchio, Al. *For Goodness Sex: Changing the Way We Talk to Teens About Sexuality, Values, and Health*. New York: HarperCollins, 2014.

Weschler, Toni. *Cycle Savvy: The Smart Teen's Guide to the Mysteries of Her Body*. New York: HarperCollins, 2006.

Wykes, Maggie, and Barrie Gunter. *The Media and Body Image: If Looks Could Kill*. London: Sage Publications, 2005.

Zaviacic, Miland, and Beverly Whipple. "Update on the Female Prostate and the Phenomenon of Female Ejaculation." *Journal of Sex Research* 30, no. 2 (May 1993).

Online Sources, Websites, and Mobile Apps

About-Face
Combating negative and distorted images of women and girls in the media
http://www.about-face.org

American Academy of Pediatrics Circumcision Policy Statement.
Pediatrics 103, no. 3 (March 1999): 686–693.

ANRED: Anorexia Nervosa and Related Eating Disorders, Inc.
Information about anorexia nervosa, bulimia nervosa, binge eating disorder, and other less well-known food and weight disorders
http://www.anred.com

BioDigital
3D diagrams of human anatomy
https://www.biodigital.com

Centre for Menstrual Cycle and Ovulation Research
Research center with a mandate to distribute information directly to lay people about changes through the life cycle, from adolescence to menopause
http://www.cemcor.ubc.ca

GladRags
Source for alternative menstrual products
http://www.gladrags.com

Health at Every Size
Information and support for Health at Every Size, an approach that acknowledges good health can best be realized independent from considerations of size. It supports people of all sizes in addressing health directly by adopting healthy behaviors.
http://www.haescommunity.org

Intersex Society of North America
Working to end shame, secrecy, and unwanted genital surgeries for intersex people
http://isna.org

KidsHealth
General pediatric and adolescent health information
http://www.kidshealth.org

Kinsey Confidential
An online sexuality information service designed by The Kinsey Institute for Research in Sex, Gender, and Reproduction to meet the sexual health information needs of college-age readers
http://www.kinseyconfidential.org

Lunapads
Source for alternative menstrual products, including Lunapanties
http://www.lunapads.com

Medline Plus: Circumcision
http://www.nlm.nih.gov/medlineplus/circumcision.html

National Eating Disorders Association
Largest not-for-profit organization in the United States working to prevent eating disorders and provide treatment referrals
http://www.nationaleatingdisorders.org

National Youth Rights Association
A youth-led national nonprofit dedicated to fighting for the civil rights and liberties of young people
http://www.youthrights.org

Office of Women's Health, US Department of Health and Human Services: Douching Fact Sheet
http://womenshealth.gov/publications/our-publications/fact-sheet/douching.html

Self-Esteem Support and Information at Mind.UK
http://www.mind.org.uk/information-support/types-of-mental-health-problems/self-esteem

Self-Injury
Self-injury resource founded by a young self-injurer
http://www.self-injury.net

StyleLikeU
Founded by a mother and daughter, a multimedia platform that honors individuals with authentic personal style. Combats fashion's top-down ideology that you need to be "on trend" in order to be "in fashion" and that you need to change yourself physically in order to be beautiful
http://stylelikeu.com

THINX
Washable menstrual underwear (including boxer briefs)
http://www.shethinx.com

US Food and Drug Administration: Breast Implants Home Page
http://www.fda.gov/medicaldevices/productsandmedicalprocedures/implantsandprosthetics/breastimplants/ucm064176.htm

Apps

Binaural: Pure Binaural Beats
A simple sound generator to help with stress reduction, sleep, or focus

Clue
An in-depth menstrual cycle tracking application

Good Blocks
An application to help improve self-esteem by training your mind to stop with bad self-talk and think more positively

Happier
An app designed to help users cultivate more happiness

Journey
A multimedia journaling app

Kindara
A menstrual and fertility cycle tracking application; one of the only apps that claims it can estimate fertility and that asks for the information needed to do so most accurately

Self-Help for Anxiety Management from the University of the West of England
Helpful DIY anxiety management tools

Smiling Mind
A mindfulness and meditation application developed by a team of psychologists with expertise in youth and adolescent therapy, Mindfulness Meditation, and web-based wellness programs

Stop, Breathe, and Think (Tools for Peace)
A meditation app made specifically with young people in mind

Yonder-Outdoor Adventures
It's good for your health and sexuality to get outside! This app can help you find some places near you to get out there.

CHAPTERS 5–7

Chapters covering gender; sexual orientation and identity; media and other outside influences on sexuality, and relationships

Books and Print Sources and Resources

Barker, Meg. *Rewriting the Rules: An Integrative Guide to Love, Sex, and Relationships.* New York: Routledge, 2013.

Bell, Chris, and Kate Brauer-Bell. *The Long-Distance Relationship Survival Guide: Secrets and Strategies from Successful Couples Who Have Gone the Distance.* Berkeley, CA: Ten Speed Press, 2006.

Ben-Ze'ev, Aaron. *Love Online: Emotions on the Internet.* Cambridge: Cambridge University Press, 2004.

Bergman, S. Bear. *The Nearest Exit May Be Behind You.* Vancouver, BC: Arsenal Pulp Press, 2009.

Best, Joel, and Kathleen A. Bogle. *Kids Gone Wild: From Rainbow Parties to Sexting, Understanding the Hype over Teen Sex.* New York: New York University Press, 2014.

Boyd, Danah. *It's Complicated: The Social Lives of Networked Teens.* New Haven, CT: Yale University Press, 2014.

Brill, Stephanie, and Rachel Pepper. *The Transgender Child: A Handbook for Families and Professionals.* San Francisco: Cleis Press, 2008.

Bronson, Howard, and Mike Riley. *How to Heal a Broken Heart in 30 Days: A Day-by-Day Guide to Saying Good-bye and Getting On with Your Life.* New York: Broadway Books, 2002.

Brownsey, Mo. *Is It a Date or Just Coffee?: The Gay Girl's Guide to Dating, Sex, and Romance.* Los Angeles: Alyson Books, 2002.

Canada, Geoffrey. *Reaching Up for Manhood: Transforming the Lives of Boys in America.* Boston: Beacon Press, 1998.

Chomsky, Noam. *Necessary Illusions: Thought Control in Democratic Societies.* Brooklyn, NY: South End Press, 1989.

Colapinto, John. *As Nature Made Him: The Boy Who Was Raised as a Girl.* New York: Harper Perennial, 2001.

Cooper, Barbara, and Nancy Widdows. *The Social Success Workbook for Teens.* Oakland, CA: Instant Help Books, 2008.

Cote, James E., and Anton L. Allahar. *Generation on Hold: Coming of Age in the Late Twentieth Century.* New York: New York University Press, 1996.

Daldry, Jeremy. *The Teenage Guy's Survival Guide: The Real Deal on Girls, Growing Up, and Other Guy Stuff.* Boston: Little, Brown Young Readers, 1999.

Dawson, James, and David Levithan. *This Book Is Gay.* Naperville, IL: Sourcebooks Fire, 2015.

De Rougemont, Denis. *Love in the Western World.* Princeton, NJ: Princeton University Press, 1983.

Easton, Dossie, and Catherine A. Liszt. *The Ethical Slut: A Guide to Infinite Sexual Possibilities.* Oakland, CA: Greenery Press, 1998.

Elkind, David. *All Grown Up and No Place to Go: Teenagers in Crisis.* Cambridge, MA: Perseus Books Group, 1997.

Erickson-Schroth, Laura. *Trans Bodies, Trans Selves: A Resource for the Transgender Community.* New York: Oxford University Press, 2014.

Fausto-Sterling, Anne. *Myths of Gender: Biological Theories About Women and Men.* New York: Basic Books, 1992.

———. *Sexing the Body: Gender Politics and the Construction of Sexuality.* New York: Basic Books, 2000.

Fine, Cordelia. *Delusions of Gender: How Our Minds, Society and Neurosexism Create Difference.* New York: W.W. Norton, 2010.

Ford, Michael Thomas. *The World Out There: Becoming Part of the Lesbian and Gay Community*. New York: New Press, 1996.

Foucault, Michel. *The History of Sexuality: An Introduction*. New York: Vintage Books, 1990.

Fox, Annie, and Elizabeth Verdick. *The Teen Survival Guide to Dating and Relating: Real-World Advice on Guys, Girls, Growing Up, and Getting Along*. Minneapolis, MN: Free Spirit Publishing, 2005.

Gilligan, Carol, and Lyn Mikel Brown. *Meeting at the Crossroads*. New York: Ballantine Books, 1993.

Gordon-Messer, Deborah, Jose Arturo Bauermeister, Alison Grodzinski, and Marc Zimmerman. "Sexting Among Young Adults." *Journal of Adolescent Health* 52, no. 3 (March 2013).

Grant, Linda. *Sexing the Millennium*. New York: Grove Press, 1995.

Gray, Mary L. *In Your Face: Stories from the Lives of Queer Youth*. Haworth Gay and Lesbian Studies. New York: Haworth Press, 1999.

Hanh, Thich Nhat. *True Love: A Practice for Awakening the Heart*. Boston: Shambhala, 2004.

Hatchell, Deborah. *What Smart Teenagers Know . . . About Dating, Relationships, and Sex*. Santa Barbara, CA: Piper Books, 2003.

Hooks, Bell. *All About Love: New Visions*. New York: Harper Paperbacks, 2001.

Huegel, Kelly. *GLBTQ: The Survival Guide for Queer and Questioning Teens*. Minneapolis, MN: Free Spirit Publishing, 2003.

Hutchins, Loraine, and Lani Kaahumanu. *Bi Any Other Name: Bisexual People Speak Out*. Los Angeles: Alyson Books, 1991.

Jacobson, Bonnie, and Sandra J. Gordon. *The Shy Single: A Bold Guide to Dating for the Less-Than-Bold Dater*. Emmaus, PA: Rodale Books, 2004.

Jennings, Kevin, and Pat Shapiro. *Always My Child: A Parent's Guide to Understanding Your Gay, Lesbian, Bisexual, Transgendered, or Questioning Son or Daughter*. New York: Fireside, 2002.

Jones, Jennifer T., and John D. Cunningham. "Attachment Styles and Other Predictors of Relationship Satisfaction in Dating Couples." *Personal Relationships* 3, no. 4 (December 1996).

Katherine, Anne. *Where to Draw the Line: How to Set Healthy Boundaries Every Day.* New York: Fireside, 2000.

Kaufman, Moises. *The Laramie Project*. New York: Vintage Books, 2001.

Kempadoo, Kamala, and Jo Doezema. *Global Sex Workers: Rights, Resistance, and Redefinition*. New York: Routledge, 1998.

Kipnis, Laura. *Bound and Gagged: Pornography and the Politics of Fantasy in America.* Durham, NC: Duke University Press, 1999.

Kulkin, Susan. *Beyond Magenta: Transgender Teens Speak Out.* Somerville, MA: Candlewick Press, 2014.

Lanier, Jaron. *You Are Not a Gadget: A Manifesto.* New York: Vintage Books, 2011.

Lowrey, Sassafras. *Kicked Out*. Ypsilanti, MI: Homofactus Press, 2010.

Mapes, Diane. *How to Date in a Post-Dating World*. Seattle, WA: Sasquatch Books, 2006.

Mukhopadhyay, Samhita. *Outdated: Why Dating Is Ruining Your Love Life.* Berkeley, CA: Seal Press, 2011.

Nagle, Jill. *Whores and Other Feminists*. New York: Routledge, 1997.

Ochs, Robyn. *Bisexual Resource Guide.* Boston: Bisexual Resources Center, 2001.

Orenstein, Peggy. *Schoolgirls: Young Women, Self Esteem, and the Confidence Gap*. New York: Anchor Books, 1995.

Pascoe, C. J. *Dude You're a Fag: Masculinity and Sexuality in High School.* Berkeley: University of California Press, 2007.

Patterson, Charlotte J., and Anthony R. D'Augelli. *Lesbian, Gay, and Bisexual Identities and Youth.* New York: Oxford University Press, 2003.

Pollack, William. *Real Boys: Rescuing Our Sons from the Myths of Boyhood.* New York: Owl Books, 1999.

Queen, Carol, and Lawrence Schimel. *Pomosexuals: Challenging Assumptions About Gender and Sexuality.* San Francisco: Cleis Press, 1997.

Serano, Julia. *Excluded: Making Feminist and Queer Movements More Inclusive.* Berkeley, CA: Seal Press, 2013.

———. *Whipping Girl: A Transsexual Woman on Sexism and the Scapegoating of Femininity.* Berkeley, CA: Seal Press, 2007.

Shandler, Sara. *Ophelia Speaks: Adolescent Girls Write About Their Search for Self.* New York: Harper Paperbacks, 1999.

Smith, Pace, and Kyeli Smith. *The Usual Error: Why We Don't Understand Each Other and 34 Ways to Make It Better.* Austin, TX: Connection Paradigm Press, 2009.

Solot, Dorian, and Marshall Miller. *Unmarried to Each Other: The Essential Guide to Living Together As an Unmarried Couple.* New York: Marlowe & Company, 2002.

Sullivan, Jim. *Boyfriend 101: A Gay Guy's Guide to Dating, Romance, and Finding True Love.* New York: Villard Books, 2003.

Tanenbaum, Leora. *Slut! Growing Up Female with a Bad Reputation.* New York: HarperCollins, 2000.

Van Dijk, Sheri. *Relationship Skills 101 for Teens.* Oakland, CA: Instant Help Books, 2015.

Vaughan, Diane. *Uncoupling: Turning Points in Intimate Relationships.* New York: Vintage Books, 1986.

Zoldbrod, Aline P. *Sex Smart: How Your Childhood Shaped Your Sexual Life and What to Do About It.* Vancouver, BC: Raincoast Books, 1998.

Online Sources, Websites, and Mobile Apps

American Civil Liberties Union (ACLU)
http://www.aclu.org

American Psychological Association: LGBT Section
http://www.apa.org/topics/lgbt/index.aspx

Autostraddle
Friendly and in-depth website for younger, queer-identified women
http://www.autostraddle.com

Bitch Media
Independent feminist media that provides engaged and thoughtful responses to mainstream media and popular culture
http://www.bitchmedia.org

Common Sense Media
A curated library of independent age-based and educational ratings and reviews for movies, games, apps, TV shows, websites, books, and music
http://www.commonsensemedia.org

Executive Summary of The Common Sense Census: Media Use by Tweens and Teens
https://www.commonsensemedia.org/sites/default/files/uploads/research/census_executivesummary.pdf

Everyday Feminism
A popular intersectional feminist digital media website
http://www.everydayfeminism.com

fbomb
A blog/community created by and for teen and college-aged women and men who care about their rights and want to be heard
http://www.thefbomb.org

Families Like Mine
Abigail Garner's site to decrease isolation for people whose parents are lesbian, gay, bisexual, or transgender and to bring voice to the experiences of these families
http://www.familieslikemine.com

Fetto, John, "First Comes Love" (Teen Dating Statistics), *Advertising Age: American Demographics,* June 1, 2003
http://www.adage.com/americandemographics

Gay Teen Resources (GTR)
A site "dedicated to the simple principle that LGBT youth should have a place they could go to online without worrying about being hit on, being outed to family or friends, and where they can find help and links to resources that could offer additional assistance."
http://www.gayteenresources.org

Gender Spectrum
In-depth gender-inclusive and sensitive site, with connected community website, for information and support about gender diversity and identity
https://www.genderspectrum.org

Genderfork
A supportive online community for the expression of identities across the gender spectrum
http://www.genderfork.com

GLAAD
The Gay and Lesbian Alliance Against Defamation
http://www.glaad.org

GLBT Historical Society
Collects, preserves, and interprets the history of GLBT people and the communities that support them
http://www.glbthistory.org

Lambda Legal Defense and Education Fund
National organization committed to achieving full recognition of the civil rights of lesbians, gay men, bisexuals, transgender people, and those with HIV through impact litigation, education, and public policy work
http://www.lambdalegal.org

Beg, Sami A., and P. Anne Loveless. "Media and the Adolescent Mind: From Studies to Action." Medscape.
http://www.medscape.org/viewarticle/569353

NSTeens.org
Help and information for teens about Internet safety, including animated videos, short films, games, and interactive comics as well as teaching materials for educators
http://www.nsteens.org

Parents, Families, Friends, and Allies of Lesbians and Gays
Provides opportunity for dialogue about sexual orientation and gender identity, and acts to create a society that is healthy and respectful of human diversity
http://www.pflag.org

Tolerance.org
The Teaching Tolerance blog: education about diversity, equity, and justice; can find news, suggestions, conversation, and support
http://www.tolerance.org

Too Damn Young
An online resource and community for grieving teens and young adults to let them know they're not alone. The site features expert articles, personal accounts, fiction, poems, and more.
http://www.toodamnyoung.com

The YMCA (Young Men's Christian Association)
http://www.ymca.net

The YWCA (Young Women's Christian Association)
http://www.ywca.org

Apps

Expressing Needs (The Gottman Institute)
A mobile application to help partners improve at expressing their needs to each other

Gratitude Journal (Happy Tapper)
Can be used to share socially or as a self-journal, to help cultivate gratitude and kindness

Voices: Social Justice Articles
A mobile application that pools pieces from a handful of excellent sites: great for intersectional cultural, media, and sexual literacy

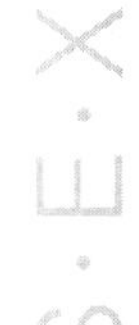

CHAPTERS 8–10, 12–14

Chapters covering sexual readiness; choices and sexual activities; sexual health and safer sex; contraception, reproductive options, and pregnancy

Books and Print Sources and Resources

Bainbridge, David. *Making Babies: The Science of Pregnancy.* Cambridge, MA: Harvard University Press, 2000.

Basso, Michael J. *The Underground Guide to Teenage Sexuality*. 2nd ed. Minneapolis, MN: Fairview Press, 2003.

Beckmann, Charles R. B. *Obstetrics and Gynecology*. Philadelphia: Lippincott Williams & Wilkins, 2002.

Blank, Hanne. *Big, Big Love: A Sourcebook on Sex for People of Size and Those Who Love Them*. Oakland, CA: Greenery Press, 2000.

———. *Virgin: The Untouched History*. New York: Bloomsbury USA, 2007.

Bolles, Edmund Blair. *The Penguin Adoption Handbook*. New York: Penguin Books, 1993.

Boston Women's Health Collective. *Our Bodies, Ourselves*. New York: Simon & Schuster, 2011.

———. *Our Bodies, Ourselves: Pregnancy and Birth*. New York: Simon & Schuster, 2008.

Bright, Susie. *Full Exposure: Opening Up to Sexual Creativity and Erotic Expression*. New York: HarperCollins, Harper San Francisco, 2000.

———. *The Sexual State of the Union*. New York: Touchstone, 1998.

Carmody, Moira. "Ethical Erotics: Reconceptualizing Anti-Rape Education." *Sexualities* 8, no. 4 (2005).

Coles, Robert. *The Youngest Parents: Teenage Pregnancy As It Shapes Lives*. New York: W. W. Norton, 2000.

Davis, Deborah. *You Look Too Young to Be a Mom: Teen Mothers Speak Out on Love, Learning, and Success*. New York: Perigee, 2004.

DePuy, Candace, and Dana Dovitch. *The Healing Choice: Your Guide to Emotional Recovery After an Abortion*. Minneapolis, MN: Fireside, 1997.

Dodson, Betty. *Orgasms for Two: The Joy of Partnersex*. New York: Harmony Books, 2002.

Eisler, Riane. *Sacred Pleasure: Sex, Myth, and the Politics of the Body—New Paths to Power and Love*. New York: HarperCollins, Harper San Francisco, 1996.

Ellison, Peter T. *On Fertile Ground: A Natural History of Human Reproduction*. Cambridge, MA: Harvard University Press, 2001.

Friedman, Jaclyn. *What You Really Really Want: The Smart Girl's Shame-Free Guide to Sex and Safety.* Berkeley, CA: Seal Press, 2011.

Hatcher, Robert A., James Trussel, Felicia Stewart, Anita L. Nelson, Willard Cates Jr., Felicia Guest, and Deborah Kowal. *Contraceptive Technology.* 20th ed. New York: Ardent Media, 2011.

Hite, Shere. *The Hite Report: A National Study of Female Sexuality*. New York: Seven Stories Press, 2003.

———. *The Hite Report on Male Sexuality*. New York: Ballantine Books, 1987.

Jacobs, Thomas A., and Jay E. Johnson. *What Are My Rights?: 95 Questions and Answers About Teens and the Law*. Minneapolis, MN: Free Spirit Publishing, 1997.

Lancaster, Roger N., and Micaela DiLeonardo. *The Gender/Sexuality Reader.* New York: Routledge, 1997.

Langdridge, Darren, and Trevor Butt. "The Erotic Construction of Power Exchange." *Journal of Constructivist Psychology* 18, no. 1 (2005).

Levine, Stephen B. *Handbook of Clinical Sexuality for Mental Health Professionals.* 2nd ed. New York: Routledge, 2010.

Lindsay, Jeanne Warren. *Teen Dads*. Buena Park, CA: Morning Glory Press, 2000.

Lindsay, Jeanne Warren, and Jean Brunelli. *Your Pregnancy and Newborn Journey: A Guide for Pregnant Teens*. Teen Pregnancy and Parenting Series. Buena Park, CA: Morning Glory Press, 2004.

Lorde, Audre. *The Uses of the Erotic: The Erotic As Power*. Tucson, AZ: Kore Press, 2000.

Luker, Kristin. *Abortion and the Politics of Motherhood*. California Series on Social Choice and Political Economy. Berkeley: University of California Press, 1985.

———. *Dubious Conceptions: The Politics of Teenage Pregnancy*. Cambridge, MA: Harvard University Press, 1997.

Marr, Lisa. *Sexually Transmitted Diseases: A Physician Tells You What You Need to Know*. Baltimore: Johns Hopkins University Press, 1998.

Matcher, Robert A., et al. *Contraceptive Technology*, 18th rev. ed. New York: Ardent Media, 2004.

Moen, Erika, and Matthew Nolan. *Oh Joy Sex Toy*. Vols. 1–2. Portland, OR: Periscope Studio, 2014, 2015.

Morin, Jack. *Anal Pleasure and Health: A Guide for Men and Women*. San Francisco: Down There Press, 1998.

———. *The Erotic Mind*. New York: Harper Paperbacks, 1996.

Murkoff, Heidi E., Arlene Eisenberg, and Sandee E. Hathaway. *What to Expect When You're Expecting*. 3rd ed. New York: Workman, 2002.

Newman, Felice. *The Whole Lesbian Sex Book: A Passionate Guide for All of Us*. San Francisco: Cleis Press, 2004.

Oumano, Elena. *Natural Sex*. New York: Plume Books, 1999.

Ponton, Lynn. *The Sex Lives of Teenagers: Revealing the Secret World of Adolescent Boys and Girls*. New York: Plume Books, 2001.

Ryden, Janice, and Paul D. Blumenthal. *Practical Gynecology: A Guide for the Primary Care Physician*. Philadelphia: American College of Physicians/American Society of Internal Medicine, 2002.

Shorto, Russell. "Contra-Contraception." *New York Times*, May 7, 2006.

Shusterman, Lisa Roseman. "The Psychosocial Factors of the Abortion Experience: A Critical Review." *Psychology of Women Quarterly* 1, no. 1 (September 1976).

Silverberg, Cory, Miriam Kaufman, and Fran Odette. *The Ultimate Guide to Sex and Disability: For All of Us Who Live with Disabilities, Chronic Pain, and Illness*. San Francisco: Cleis Press, 2003.

Silverstein, Charles. *The Joy of Gay Sex*. 3rd ed. New York: HarperCollins, 2004.

Soll, Joseph M., and Karen Wilson Buterbaugh. *Adoption Healing . . . A Path to Recovery for Mothers Who Lost Children to Adoption*. Baltimore: Gateway Press, 2003.

Sundahl, Deborah. *Female Ejaculation and the G-Spot*. Alameda, CA: Hunter House Publishers, 2003.

Tone, Andrea. *Devices and Desires: A History of Contraceptives in America*. New York: Hill and Wang, 2001.

Turrell, S. C., et al. "Emotional Response to Abortion: A Critical Review of the Literature." *Women & Therapy* 9, no. 4 (1990).

Venning, Rachel, and Claire Cavannah. *Sex Toys 101: A Playfully Uninhibited Guide*. New York: Fireside, 2003.

Weschler, Toni. *Taking Charge of Your Fertility*. 20th Anniversary ed. New York: Collins, 2015.

Williams-Wheeler, Dorrie. *The Unplanned Pregnancy Book for Teens and College Students*. Virginia Beach, VA: Sparkledoll Productions, 2004.

Winks, Cathy, and Anne Semans. *The Good Vibrations Guide to Sex: The Most Complete Sex Manual Ever Written.* San Francisco: Cleis Press, 2002.

Wiseman, Jay. *SM 101: A Realistic Introduction.* Oakland, CA: Greenery Press, 1998.

Zenilman, Jonathan M., and Mohsen Shamanesh. *Sexually Transmitted Infections: Diagnosis, Management, and Treatment.* Sudbury, MA: Jones & Bartlett Learning, 2012.

Zilbergeld, Bernie. *The New Male Sexuality.* New York: Bantam Books, 1999.

Online Sources, Websites, and Mobile Apps

Abortion Clinics Online (ACOL)
Extensive directory of abortion providers and clinics in the United States
http://www.gynpages.com

American College of Obstetricians and Gynecologists (ACOG) Patient Page
Broad information on sexual and reproductive health from the leading experts in women's health care
http://www.acog.org/Patients

American College of Obstetricians and Gynecologists, Committee on Adolescent Health Care: Adolescents and Long-Acting Reversible Contraception: Implants and Intrauterine Devices
http://www.acog.org/Resources-And-Publications/Committee-Opinions/Committee-on-Adolescent-Health-Care/Adolescents-and-Long-Acting-Reversible-Contraception

Ann Rose's Ultimate Birth Control Links
Extensive information on birth control methods
http://www.ultimatebirthcontrol.com

Babeland
Sexuality information, safer sex supplies, books, and toys
http://www.babeland.com

The Body
A comprehensive multimedia AIDS and HIV resource
http://www.thebody.com

Boonstra, Heather, "Teen Pregnancy: Trends and Lessons Learned." *Guttmacher Report on Public Policy* 5, no. 1 (February 2002)
http://www.guttmacher.org/pubs/tgr/05/1/gr050107.html

The Bump: Breastfeeding
Information, support, and attitude
http://www.breastfeeding.com

Center for Reproductive Rights
Legal advocacy organization to protect reproductive rights
http://www.reproductiverights.org

Center for Sexual Pleasure and Health
A sexuality education and training organization that works to reduce sexual shame, challenge misinformation, and advance the field of sexuality
http://www.thecsph.org/

Centers for Disease Control and Prevention
Sexually transmitted infection data and information
http://www.cdc.gov/std/stats

Childbirth Connection
A *core program of the National Partnership for Women & Families, aiming to improve the quality and value of maternity care through consumer engagement and health system transformation*
http://www.childbirthconnection.org

Dailard, Cynthia, "Legislating Against Arousal: The Growing Divide Between Federal Policy and Teenage Sexual Behavior." *Guttmacher Policy Review* 9, no. 3 (Summer 2006)
http://www.guttmacher.org/pubs/gpr/09/3/gpr090312.html

Early2Bed
An independent Chicago sex supply and toy shop whose website also has extensive sex and sex toy information and education
http://www.early2bed.com

Family Planning Perspectives
A journal of results concerning all aspects of family planning
http://www.jstor.org/journals/00147354.html

Feminist Women's Health Center
Comprehensive and accessible information on birth control methods, abortion and pregnancy, sexual health, and other topics regarding women's health
http://www.fwhc.org

Gay and Lesbian Medical Association (GLMA)
Resources to help LGBTQ people find nondiscriminatory health care
http://www.glma.org

Guttmacher Institute, Fact Sheet: "American Teens' Sexual and Reproductive Health" (May 2014)
http://www.guttmacher.org/pubs/fb_ATSRH.html

HipMama
Political commentary, community, and ribald tales from the front lines of motherhood
http://www.hipmama.com

Journal of the American Medical Association
http://jama.ama-assn.org

The Kinsey Institute
Data from Alfred Kinsey's studies
http://www.indiana.edu/~kinsey/research/ak-data.html

National Network of Abortion Funds (NNAF)
Providing financial aid for abortion services to those in need
http://www.nnaf.org

Not-2-late.com: The Emergency Contraception Website
Constantly updated, comprehensive information on emergency contraception, including a location finder for EC
http://ec.princeton.edu

Oh Joy Sex Toy
A weekly web comic with reviews and education related to sex, sexuality, and the sex industry (Does include 18+ and NSFW content)
http://www.ohjoysextoy.com

Ott, Mary, Susan G. Millstein, Susan Ofner, and Bonnie L. Halpern-Felsher. "Greater Expectations: Adolescents' Positive Motivations for Sex." *Perspectives on Sexual and Reproductive Health* 38, no. 2 (June 2006)
http://www.guttmacher.org/pubs/journals/3808406.html

Our Bodies Ourselves
The blog of the Boston Women's Health Collective
http://www.ourbodiesourblog.org

Planned Parenthood
Current, comprehensive information on sexual health, sexuality, and contraception; includes a locator to find Planned Parenthood clinics
http://www.plannedparenthood.org

Population Council. "Emergency Contraception's Mode of Action Clarified." *Population Briefs* 11, no. 2 (May 2005)
http://www.popcouncil.org/uploads/pdfs/pbmay05.pdf

Pregnant Help: Mom, Dad—I'm Pregnant
Helpful site to guide young people through disclosing a pregnancy to family
http://www.pregnanthelp.com/about_us/blog_detail/mom-dad-im-pregnant

Provide
Seeks to ensure access to abortion for all women, especially those living in low-resource rural and Southern communities, by increasing abortion services, training new abortion providers, and raising awareness about the critical importance of abortion access to women's lives
http://provideaccess.org

San Francisco Sex Information
Information and referral switchboard providing anonymous, accurate, nonjudgmental information about sex via phone or e-mail
http://www.sfsi.org

World Professional Association for Transgender Health (WPATH)
Promotes the highest standards of health care for individuals through the articulation of Standards of Care (SOC) for the Health of Transsexual, Transgender, and Gender Nonconforming People, based on the best available science and expert professional consensus
http://www.wpath.org

Apps

iCondom
MTV Staying Alive's mobile condom locator

Kinsey Reporter (Indiana University)
A global mobile platform for the reporting, visualization, and analysis of anonymous data about sexual and other intimate behaviors

MyPill
Birth control reminder for the birth control pill, patch, or ring

My Sex Doctor
Offers information about sex and sexuality, including puberty and body changes, flirting and relationships, sexual activities, and their associated STI or pregnancy risks

CHAPTER 11

Chapter covering abuse, assault, prevention, and intervention

Books and Print Sources and Resources

Bancroft, Lundy. *Why Does He Do That? Inside the Minds of Angry and Controlling Men.* New York: Penguin, 2002.

Bass, Ellen, and Laura Davis. *The Courage to Heal: A Guide for Women Survivors of Child Sexual Abuse.* 3rd ed. New York: HarperCollins, 1994.

Bean, Barbara, and Shari Bennett. *The Me Nobody Knows: A Guide for Teen Survivors.* San Francisco: Jossey-Bass, 1997.

Cook, Philip W. *Abused Men: The Hidden Side of Domestic Violence.* Westport, CT: Praeger Trade, 1997.

Davis, Laura. *The Courage to Heal Workbook: A Guide for Women and Men Survivors of Child Sexual Abuse.* 1st ed. New York: HarperCollins, 1990.

DeBecker, Gavin. *The Gift of Fear.* New York: Dell Books, 1998.

Feuereisen, Patti, and Caroline Pincus. *Invisible Girls: The Truth About Sexual Abuse—a Book for Teen Girls, Young Women, and Everyone Who Cares About Them.* Emeryville, CA: Seal Press, 2005.

Haines, Staci. *The Survivor's Guide to Sex: How to Have an Empowered Sex Life After Child Sexual Abuse.* San Francisco: Cleis Press, 1999.

Hanna, Cheryl. "The Paradox of Hope: The Crime and Punishment of Domestic Violence." *William and Mary Law Review* 39 (1998).

Harding, Kate. *Asking for It: The Alarming Rise of Rape Culture—and What We Can Do About It.* Boston: Da Capo Lifelong Books, 2015.

Katz, Jackson. *The Macho Paradox: Why Some Men Hurt Women and How All Men Can Help.* Naperville, IL: Sourcebooks, 2006.

Levy, Barrie. *In Love and in Danger: A Teen's Guide to Breaking Free of Abusive Relationships.* Emeryville, CA: Seal Press, 1998.

Maltz, Wendy. *The Sexual Healing Journey: A Guide for Survivors of Sexual Abuse.* New York: HarperCollins, 2001.

Morgan, Robin. *The Demon Lover: The Roots of Terrorism.* New York: Washington Square Press, 2001.

Murray, Jill. *But I Love Him: Protecting Your Teen Daughter from Controlling, Abusive*

Dating Relationships. New York: Regan Books, 2001.

NiCarthy, Ginny, and Sue Davidson. *You Can Be Free: An Easy-to-Read Handbook for Abused Women*. Berkeley, CA: Seal Press, 2006.

O'Hanlon, Bill, and Bob Bertolino. *Even from a Broken Web: Brief, Respectful, and Solution-Oriented Therapy for Sexual Abuse and Trauma*. New York: W.W. Norton, 1998.

Palmer, Libbi. *The PTSD Workbook for Teens*. Oakland, CA: Instant Help Books, 2012.

Raphael, Jody. *Rape Is Rape: How Denial, Distortion, and Victim Blaming Are Fueling a Hidden Acquaintance Rape Crisis*. Chicago: Chicago Review Press, 2013.

Ristock, Janice. *No More Secrets: Violence in Lesbian Relationships*. New York: Routledge, 2002.

Rotman, Isabella. *Not on My Watch: A Bystander's Handbook for the Prevention of Sexual Violence*. 2015. http://www.isabellarotman.com/store/preorder-not-on-my-watch-the-bystanders-handbook-for-the-prevention-of-sexual-violence

Simmons, Rachel. *Odd Girl Out: The Hidden Culture of Aggression in Girls*. Orlando, FL: Harvest Books, 2003.

Snortland, Ellen B. *Beauty Bites Beast: Awakening the Warrior Within Women and Girls*. Pasadena, CA: Trilogy Books, 1998.

Warshaw, Robin. *I Never Called It Rape: The Ms. Report on Recognizing, Fighting, and Surviving Date and Acquaintance Rape*. New York: Harper Paperbacks, 1994.

Online Sources, Websites, and Mobile Apps

Abuse of People with Disabilities: Victims and Their Families Speak Out
http://www.disabilityandabuse.org/survey/survey-report.pdf

Break the Cycle
"Empowers youth to build lives and communities free from dating and domestic violence"
http://www.breakthecycle.org

Centers for Disease Control and Prevention: Intimate Partner Violence
http://www.cdc.gov/violenceprevention/intimatepartnerviolence/index.html

Hatch Youth: Thrown Out/Kicked Out
A basic guide from Hatch Youth to what to know and do if you're kicked out of your home
http://www.hatchyouth.org/index.php?content&view=article&id=37&Itemid=59

Joyful Heart Foundation
Aims to help heal, educate, and empower survivors of sexual assault, domestic violence, and child abuse
http://www.joyfulheartfoundation.org

Leaving Abuse: Family Abuse (and the Effect on Teenagers)
http://leavingabuse.com/family-abuse-and-the-effect-on-teenagers

Love Is Respect
A website that seeks to engage, educate, and empower young people to prevent and end abusive relationships. Includes an online crisis chat, and phone and mobile hotlines
http://www.loveisrespect.org

Miller, Daniel, and Ronald Mincy. "Falling Further Behind? Child Support Arrears and Fathers' Labor Force Participation." *Social Service Review* 86, no. 4 (December 2012). http://www.ncbi.nlm.nih.gov/pmc/articles/PMC3737002

National Center for Victims of Crime: Crime Information and Statistics
https://www.victimsofcrime.org/library/crime-information-and-statistics

National Institute on Alcohol Abuse and Alcoholism: Alcohol and Sexual Assault
http://pubs.niaaa.nih.gov/publications/arh25-1/43-51.htm

Pandora's Project
Dedicated to providing information, support, and resources to survivors of rape and sexual abuse and their friends and family. Pandora's Project offers peer support to anyone who has been a victim of rape, sexual assault, or sexual abuse through a message board, chat room, and blogs.
http://www.pandys.org

ReachOut
A nonprofit organization that meets youth where they are to deliver peer support and mental health information in a safe and supportive online space
http://us.reachout.com

Schwartz, Allan: The Bystander Effect, What Would You Do?
https://www.mentalhelp.net/articles/the-bystander-effect-what-would-you-do

Szalavitz, Maia. "Bystander Psychology: Why Some Witnesses to Crime Do Nothing" *Time,* November 11, 2011.
http://healthland.time.com/2011/11/11/bystander-psychology-why-some-witnesses-to-crime-do-nothing

Teens Experiencing Abusive Relationships (TEAR)
Relationship abuse organization and site founded by a teen survivor
http://www.teensagainstabuse.org

To Write Love on Her Arms
A nonprofit movement dedicated to presenting hope and finding help for people struggling with depression, addiction, self-injury, and suicide
https://twloha.com/home

United Nations: Convention on the Rights of the Child
An excellent overview of and proposal for human rights all young people should be entitled to internationally (most nations have signed this, but the United States has not)
http://www.ohchr.org/EN/ProfessionalInterest/Pages/CRC.aspx

Women of Color Network: Domestic Violence in Communities of Color
http://www.doj.state.or.us/victims/pdf/women_of_color_network_facts_domestic_violence_2006.pdf

World Health Organization: Violence and Injury Prevention
http://www.who.int/violence_injury_prevention/violence/en/

Apps

Choose to Stop (Virtual College)
Tools and support for those who have been in some way abusive and want to stop

Circle of 6
A personal safety application that lets a user choose six trusted friends to add to their circle on the app. If in an uncomfortable or risky situation, a click automatically sends the circle a preprogrammed SMS alert message and the sender's exact location. Also connects to 24-hour hotlines for safety and information as well as to scarleteen.com.

RU Safe (Women's Center and Shelter of Greater Pittsburgh)
A relationship assessment tool to check for abuse and other unhealthy, unsafe behaviors or dynamics

SUGGESTED BOOKS FOR PARENTS AND PARENTS-TO-BE

Arnett, Jeffrey Jansen. *Emerging Adulthood.* 2nd ed. New York: Oxford University Press, 2015.

Gore, Ariel. *The Hip Mama Survival Guide.* New York: Hyperion Books, 1998.

———. *Whatever, Mom: Hip Mama's Guide to Raising a Teenager.* Emeryville, CA: Seal Press, 2004.

Kindlon, Dan, and Michael Thompson. *Raising Cain: Protecting the Emotional Life of Boys.* New York: Ballantine Books, 2000.

Leach, Penelope. *Children First*. New York: Vintage Books, 1995.

Levine, Judith. *Harmful to Minors: The Perils of Protecting Children from Sex*. Minneapolis: University of Minneapolis Press, 2002.

Medhus, Elisa. *Raising Children Who Think for Themselves*. Hillsboro, OR: Beyond Words Publishing, 2001.

Pipher, Mary. *Reviving Ophelia: Saving the Selves of Adolescent Girls*. New York: Riverhead Books, 2005.

Rayne, Karen. *Breaking the Hush Factor: The Ten Rules Every Parent Should Know Before Talking with Their Teen About Sex*. Austin, TX: Impetus Books, 2015.

Roffman, Deborah M. *Sex and Sensibility: The Thinking Parent's Guide to Talking Sense About Sex*. Cambridge, MA: Perseus Publishing, 2001.

Siegel, Daniel J. *Brainstorm: The Power and Purpose of the Teenage Brain*. New York: Jeremy P. Tarcher/Penguin, 2015.

Vernacchio, Al. *For Goodness Sex: Changing the Way We Talk to Teens About Sexuality, Values, and Health*. New York: HarperCollins, 2014.

Weil, Zoe. *Above All, Be Kind: Raising a Humane Child in Challenging Times*. Gabriola Island, BC: New Society Publishers, 2003.

BODY AND SEXUALITY BOOKS FOR YOUNGER READERS

Blank, Joani. *A Kid's First Book About Sex*. San Francisco: Down There Press, 1993.

Blank, Joani, and Marcia Quackenbush. *Playbook for Kids About Sex*. San Francisco: Down There Press, 1981.

Bryan, Jennifer. *The Different Dragon*. Ridley Park, PA: Two Lives Publishing, 2006.

Gravelle, Karen. *What's Going on Down There?: Answers to Questions Boys Find Hard to Ask*. New York: Walter & Company, 1998.

Harris, Robbie H. *It's Perfectly Normal: Changing Bodies, Growing Up, Sex, and Sexual Health*. Cambridge, MA: Candlewick Press, 2004.

———. *Who's in My Family?: All About Our Families*. Cambridge, MA: Candlewick Press, 2012.

Herthel, Jessica. *I Am Jazz*. New York: Dial Books, 2014.

Kilodavis, Cheryl. *My Princess Boy*. New York: Aladdin, 2010.

Loulan, JoAnn, and Bonnie Worthen. *Period.: A Girl's Guide to Menstruation*. Minnetonka, MN: Book Peddlers, 2001.

Madaras, Lynda. *The "What's Happening to My Body?" Book for Girls: A Growing Up Guide for Parents and Daughters*. New York: Newmarket Press, 2000.

———. *The "What's Happening to My Body?" Book for Boys: A Growing Up Guide for Parents and Sons*. New York: Newmarket Press, 2000.

Mayle, Peter. *"What's Happening to Me?" A Guide to Puberty*. New York: Lyle Stuart, 2000.

———. *Where Did I Come From?* New York: Lyle Stuart, 2000.

Richardson, Justin. *And Tango Makes Three*. New York: Little Simon, 2015.

Schiffer, Miriam B. *Stella Brings the Family*. San Francisco: Chronicle Books, 2015.

Silverberg, Cory, and Fiona Smyth. *What Makes a Baby?* New York: Seven Stories Press, 2015.

———. *Sex Is a Funny Word*. New York: Seven Stories Press, 2015.

Spelman, Cornelia Maude. *Your Body Belongs to You*. Park Ridge, IL: Albert Whitman & Company, 1997.

TEN STELLAR TEEN, EMERGING ADULT, OR GENERAL SEXUALITY AND SEXUAL HEALTH INFORMATION WEBSITES

Advocates for Youth
http://www.advocatesforyouth.org

American Social Health Association: I Wanna Know
http://www.iwannaknow.org

Guttmacher Institute
http://www.guttmacher.org

Oh Joy Sex Toy (intended for 18+)
http://www.ohjoysextoy.com

Planned Parenthood
http://www.plannedparenthood.org

RH Reality Check
http://www.rhrealitycheck.org

Scarleteen
http://www.scarleteen.com

Sex, Etc.
http://www.sexetc.org

SIECUS: Sexuality Information and Education Council of the United States
http://www.siecus.org

Teen Source
http://www.teensource.org

TOLL-FREE CRISIS HOTLINES OR TEXT LINES (UNITED STATES)

Alcohol & Drug Abuse Crisis Line: 1-800-234-0420

Centers for Disease Control and Prevention AIDS Hotline: 1-800-232-4636

Centers for Disease Control and Prevention National STI Hotline: 1-800-227-8922

Childhelp National Child Abuse Hotline: 1-800-422-4453

Crisis Text Line: Text keyword SUPPORT to 741-741

Eating Disorders Awareness and Prevention: 1-800-931-2237

Emergency Contraception Information: 1-888-NOT-2-LATE

Gay, Lesbian, Bisexual, and Transgender Youth Support Line: 1-800-850-8078

Gay and Transgender Hate Crime Hotline: 1-800-616-HATE

Love Is Respect Abuse Crisis Line: 1-866-331-9474 (phone) or text keyword LOVEIS to 22522

National Abortion Federation Hotline: 1-800-772-9100

National Domestic Violence Hotline: 1-800-799-7233

National Runaway Safeline: 1-800-786-2929

National Safe Place: Text keyword SAFE to 69866

National Suicide Prevention Hotline: 1-800-273-TALK

National Youth Crisis Hotline: 1-800-442-HOPE

Planned Parenthood: 1-800-230-PLAN

Pregnancy Helpline: 1-800-848-5683

Rape, Abuse, Incest National Network (RAINN): 1-800-656-HOPE

Scarleteen Crisis Text Line: 1-206-866-2279

Self-Injury Hotline: 1-800-DONT CUT

Teen Helpline: 1-800-400-0900

Teenline: 1-800-522-TEEN or text keyword TEEN to 839863

Trevor Project LGBTQ Depression and Suicide Hotline: 1-866-488-7386

General healthcare provider(s):

Name: ______________________ Number: ______________________

Name: ______________________ Number: ______________________

Sexual healthcare provider (for STI testing or treatment, birth control, and more):

Name: ______________________ Number: ______________________

Abortion provider:

Name: ______________________ Number: ______________________

LGBTQA support or advocacy resource(s):

Name: ______________________ Number: ______________________

Name: ______________________ Number: ______________________

Homeless or crisis shelter(s):

Name: ______________________ Number: ______________________

Other:

Name: ______________________ Number: ______________________

Name: ______________________ Number: ______________________

Local hotlines:

Name: ______________________ Number: ______________________

Name: ______________________ Number: ______________________

Name: ______________________ Number: ______________________

Name: ______________________ Number: ______________________

Your core support circle:
Family member(s) or friend(s):

Name: ______________________ Number: ______________________

Name: ______________________ Number: ______________________

A trusted healthcare provider, mentor, or other adult:

Name: ______________________ Number: ______________________

Advocacy organizations:

Name: ______________________ Number: ______________________

Name: ______________________ Number: ______________________

Name: ______________________ Number: ______________________

Index

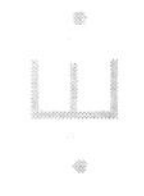